W9-DEK-783

New Arrhythmia Technologies

To our families and the memories of all those
who have inspired us to look toward the future.

New Arrhythmia Technologies

EDITED BY

Paul J. Wang, MD

Director, Cardiac Arrhythmia Service and Cardiac Electrophysiology Laboratory
Professor of Medicine
Stanford University Medical Center

AND CO-EDITORS

Gerald V. Naccarelli, MD

Chief, Division of Cardiology
Professor of Medicine
Penn State University College of Medicine

Michael R. Rosen, MD

Gustavus A. Pfeiffer Professor of Pharmacology
Professor of Pediatrics
Director, Center for Molecular Therapeutics
Columbia University

N.A. Mark Estes III, MD

Director, Cardiac Arrhythmia Service
Professor of Medicine
Tufts New England Medical Center

David L. Hayes, MD

Chair, Division of Cardiovascular Diseases
Professor of Medicine
Mayo Clinic

David E. Haines, MD

Director, Heart Rhythm Center
William Beaumont Hospital

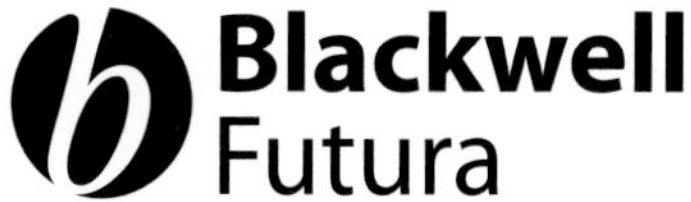

Blackwell Futura is an imprint of Blackwell Publishing

Blackwell Publishing, Inc., 350 Main Street, Malden, Massachusetts 02148-5020, USA
Blackwell Publishing Ltd, 9600 Garsington Road, Oxford OX4 2DQ, UK
Blackwell Science Asia Pty Ltd, 550 Swanston Street, Carlton, Victoria 3053, Australia

First published 2005
ISBN-13: 978-1-4051-3293-0
ISBN-10: 1-4051-3293-0

Library of Congress Cataloging-in-Publication Data

New arrhythmia technologies/edited by Paul J. Wang ... [et al.].
p. ; cm.
Includes bibliographical references and index.
ISBN-13: 978-1-4051-3293-0 (alk. paper)
ISBN-10: 1-4051-3293-0 (alk. paper)
1. Arrhythmia–Treatment–Technological innovations.
[DNLM: 1. Arrhythmia–therapy. 2. Anti–Arrhythmia Agents–therapeutic use.
3. Defibrillators. 4. Electric Countershock–methods. WG 330 N532 2005] I. Wang, Paul J.

RC685.A65N49 2005
616.1′28–dc22 2005004581

A catalogue record for this title is available from the British Library
Commissioning Editor: Gina Almond
Development Editor: Vicki Donald
Set in 9.5/12 pt Minion by Newgen Imaging Systems (P) Ltd, Chennai, India
Printed and bound in Harayana, India by Replika Press PVT Ltd.

For further information on Blackwell Publishing, visit our website:
www.blackwellcardiology.com

The publisher's policy is to use permanent paper from mills that operate a sustainable forestry policy, and which has been manufactured from pulp processed using acid-free and elementary chlorine-free practices. Furthermore, the publisher ensures that the text paper and cover board used have met acceptable environmental accreditation standards.

Notice: The indications and dosages of all drugs in this book have been recommended in the medical literature and conform to the practices of the general community. The medications described do not necessarily have specific approval by the Food and Drug Administration for use in the diseases and dosages for which they are recommended. The package insert for each drug should be consulted for use and dosage as approved by the FDA. Because standards for usage change, it is advisable to keep abreast of revised recommendations, particularly those concerning new drugs.

Contents

Contributors

Michael J. Ackerman, MD, PhD
Director, LQTS Clinic and Sudden Death
Genomics Laboratory,
Mayo Clinic, Rochester, MN, USA

Amin Al-Ahmad, MD
Associate Director of Cardiac Arrhythmia Service
Cardiac Arrhythmia Service,
Standford University Medical Center
Stanford, CA, USA

Mark L. Andrews, BBS
Analyst/Programmer
University of Rochester Medical Center
Rochester, NY, USA

Alexander Bauer, MD
Johns Hopkins Unviersity School of Medicine
Baltimore, MD, USA

William Belden, MD
Fellow in Electrophysiology,
Cleveland Clinic Foundation, Cleveland Clinic
Cleveland, OH, USA

Jesaia Benhorin, MD
Professor of Medicine
The Heiden Department of Cardiology,
Bikur Cholim Hospital
Jerusalem, Israel

Heribert Bohlen, PhD
Director of Axiogenesis AG
Axiogenesis AG
Cologne, Germany

Peter R. Brink, PhD
Professor and Chairman,
Department of Physiology and Biophysics
Health Sciences Center,
Stony Brook University
Stony Brook, NY, USA

David J. Callans, MD
Professor of Medicine, University of Pennsylvania
Hospital of the University of Philadelphia, PA,
USA

Agustin Castellanos, MD
Professor of Medicine, Division of Cardiology
Miller School of Medicine,
University of Miami
Miami, FL, USA

Ira S. Cohen, PhD
Leading Professor of Physiology and Biophysics;
Director of the Institute of Molecular Cardiology
Health Sciences Center, Stony Brook University
Stony Brook, NY, USA

Joseph W. Cormier, PhD
Graduate Research Assistant
Department of Pharmacology,
Columbia University
New York, NY, USA

Jennifer Cummings, MD
Associate Staff
Cleveland Clinic Foundation
Cleveland, OH, USA

Ralph J. Damiano, Jr, MD
John M. Shoenberg Professor of Surgery,
Chief of Cardiac Surgery,
Washington University School of
Medicine at Barnes Jewish Hospital
St Louis, MO, USA

Peter Danilo, Jr, PhD
Senior Research Scientist
Department of Pharmacology,
Center for Molecular Therapeutics,
Columbia University
New York, NY, USA

Paul J. DeGroot, MS
Senior Principal Scientist and Bakken Fellow,
Cardiac Rhythm Management Research,
Medtronic Inc.
Minneapolis, MN, USA

Aseem D. Desai, MD
Assistant Professor of Medicine, Cardiac
Electrophysiology, University of Chicago Hospitals;
Director, Implantable Deice Therapy
Cardiac Electrophysiology,
University of Chicago Hospitals
Chicago, IL, USA

J. Kevin Donahue, MD
Associate Professor of Medicine
Johns Hopkins University School of Medicine
Baltimore, MD, USA

Kenneth A. Ellenbogen, MD
Director, Electrophysiology and Pacing
VCU School of Medicine
Richmond, VA, USA

Shauntelle Elliott, RN
Clinical Research Coordinator
Jackson Memorial Medical Center
Cardiac Arrhythmia Service,
Miami, FL, USA

Gregory Engel, MD
Cardiac Electrophysiology Fellow
Cardiac Arrhythmia Service,
Standford University Medical Center
Stanford, CA, USA

N. A. Mark Estes III, MD
Director, Cardiac Arrthythmia Service,
Tufts New England Medical Center;
Professor of Medicine,
New England Medical Center
Boston, MA,
USA

Bernd Fleischmann
Director, Institute of Physiology
University of Bonn
Bonn, Germany

Steven Girouard, PhD
Director, Basic Research
Guidant Corporation
St Paul, MN, USA

Ian W. Glaaser, PhD
Graduate Research Assistant
Department of Pharmacology,
Columbia University
New York, NY, USA

Michael R. Gold, MD
Chief of Cardiology and Director of
Heart and Vascular Center
Medical University of South
Carolina
Charleston, SC, USA

Bruce D. Gunderson, MS
Principal Scientist, Medtronic Inc.
Minneapolis, MN,
USA

David E. Haines, MD
Director, Heart Rhythm Center,
Cardiology Division,
William Beaumont Hospital
Royal Oak, Ml,
USA

M. Halbach, PhD
Institute of Neurophysiology,
University of Cologne
Cologne, Germany

David L. Hayes, MD
Chair, Divison of Cardiovascular
Diseases
Mayo Clinic
Rochester, MN, USA

Jurgen Hescheler, MD, PhD
Director, Institute of Neurophysiology
University of Cologne
Cologne, Germany

Munther K. Homoud, MD
Assistant Professor of Medicine,
Tufts University School of Medicine
Tufts New England Medical Center
Boston, MA, USA

Alberto Interian Jr, MD
Professor of Medicine; Interim Chief,
Division of Cardiology;
Director, Electrophysiology
Miller School of Medicine,
University of Miami
Miami, FL, USA

Robert S. Kass, PhD
David Hossack Professor of Pharmacology
(in the Center of Neurobiology and Behavior)
and Chairman
Department of Pharmacology,
Columbia University
New York, NY, USA

Elizabeth S. Kaufman, MD
Associate Professor of Medicine
MHMC Arrhythmia Service
Cleveland, OH, USA

Edmund Keung, MD
Director, VA National ICD Surveillance Center and
Western Pacemaker Surveillance Center
Associate Chief, Cardiology Section
San Francisco VA Medical Center
San Francisco, CA, USA

Kan Kikuchi, PhD
Johns Hopkins University School of Medicine
Baltimore, MD,
USA

Bradley P. Knight, MD
Director of Cardiac Electrophysiology
Cardiac Electrophysiology,
University of Chicago Hospitals
Chicago, IL, USA

Peter R. Kowey, MD
Chief of Cardiology, Main Line Health System
Professor of Medicine, Jefferson Medical College
Wynnewood, PA, USA

Dhanunjaya R. Lakkireddy, MD
Fellow in Electrophysiology
Cleveland Clinic Foundation
Cleveland, OH, USA

Anson M. Lee, BS
Medical Student
Washington University School of
Medicine at Barnes Jewish Hospital
St Louis, MO, USA

Mark S. Link, MD
Assistant Professor of Medicine
Tufts University School of Medicine
Tufts New England Medical Center
Boston, MA, USA

Charles J. Love, MD
Professor of Clinical Medicine
Director, Arrythmia Device Services
Director, Electrophysiology
Section and Laboratory
OSU Division of Cardiovascular Medicine
Columbus, OH, USA

Amy D. McDonald, BS
Johns Hopkins University School of Medicine
Baltimore, MD, USA

Scott A. McNitt, MS
Associate Professor
University of Rochester Medical Center
Rochester, NY, USA

Spencer J. Melby, MD
Washington University School of Medicine
St Louis, MO, USA

Arthur J. Moss, MD
Professor of Medicine
University of Rochester Medical Center
Rochester, NY, USA

Robert J. Myerburg, MD
Professor of Medicine and Physiology; American Heart
Association Chair in Cardiovascular Research
Miller School of Medicine,
University of Miami
Miami, FL, USA

Gerald V. Naccarelli, MD
Bernard Trabin Chair in Cardiology
Professor of Medicine
Chief, Division of Cardiology
Director, Cardiovascular Center
Penn State University College of Medicine
Hershey, PA, USA

Girish Narayan, MD
Falk Cardiovascular Center,
Stanford University Hospital
Stanford, CA, USA

Andrea Natale, MD
Co-Section Head, Electrophysiology and Pacing
Director, Center for Artial Fibrillation and
EP Laboratories
Cleveland Clinic Foundation
Cleveland, OH, USA

Derick R. Peterson, PhD
Associate Professor, Biostatistics and
Computational Biology
University of Rochester Medical Center
Rochester, NY, USA

Ming Qi, PhD
Research Assistant Professor, Pathology and Lab Medicine
University of Rochester Medical Center
Rochester, NY, USA

Robert F. Rea, MD
Associate Professor of Medicine,
Mayo Clinic
Rochester, MN, USA

James A. Reiffel, MD
Professor of Clinical Medicine
Columbia University
New York, NY, USA

M. Reppel, PhD
Group Leader
Institute of Neurophysiology,
University of Cologne
Cologne, Germany

Kelly Richardson, MD & Jennifer L. Robinson, MS
Electrophysiology Fellow
Stanford Hospital
Stanford, CA, USA

Richard B. Robinson, PhD
Professor of Pharmacology
Department of Pharmacology,
Center for Molecular Therapeutics,
Columbia University
New York, NY, USA

Jennifer Robinson
Research Associate
University of Rochester Medical Center
Rochester, NY, USA

Dan M. Roden, MD
Professor of Medicine and Pharmacology;
Director, Oates Institute for Experimental
Therapeutics
Vanderbilt University School of Medicine
Nashville, TN, USA

Michael R. Rosen, MD, PhD
Gustavus A Pfeiffer Professor of Pharmacology;
Professor of Pediatrics; Director, Center for
Molecular Therapeutics
Columbia University
New York, NY, USA

Donald G. Rosenberg, MD
Professor of Clinical Medicine,
Division of Cardiology
Miller School of Medicine,
University of Miami
Miami, FL, USA

Heather M. Ross, MS, APRN
Nurse Practitioner
Center for Adult Congenital Heart Disease,
St Joseph's Hospital and Medical Center
Phoenix, AZ, USA

Tetsuo Sasano, MD
Johns Hopkins University School of Medicine
Baltimore, MD, USA

Robert A. Schweikert, MD
Staff Physician
Department of Cardiovascular Medicine,
Cleveland Clinic
Cleveland, OH, USA

Rahul Seth, BS
University of Rochester Medical Center
Rochester, NY, USA

Erik Sirulnick, MD
Electrophysiology Fellow
Falk Cardiovascular Center,
Stanford University Hospital
Stanford, CA, USA

Jeffrey A. Towbin, MD
Professor of Pediatrics
Texas Children's Hospital
Houston, TX, USA

Atul Verma, MD
Fellow in Electrophysiology
Cleveland Clinic Foundation
Cleveland, OH, USA

G. Michael Vincent, MD
Professor of Medicine
Department of Medicine, LDS Hospital
Salt Lake City, UT, USA

Paul J. Wang, MD
Professor of Medicine,
Stanford University School of Medicine;
Director, Cardiac Arrhythmia Service and
Cardiac Electrophysiology Laboratory,
Stanford Hospital and Clinics
Stanford University Medical Center
Stanford, CA, USA

Jonathan Weinstock, MD
Assistant Professor of Medicine,
Tufts University School of Medicine
Tufts New England Medical Center
Boston, MA, USA

Bruce L. Wilkoff, MD
Director of Cardiac Pacing and
Tachyarrhythmia Devices,
Department of Cardiovascular Medicine,
Cleveland Clinic Foundation
Cleveland
OH, USA

Mark A. Wood, MD
Professor of Medicine
Virginia Commonwealth
University Medical Center
Richmond, VA, USA

Yang Xue, BS
University of Michigan Medical School
Fremont, CA, USA

Wojciech Zareba, MD, PhD
Associate Professor of Medicine
University of Rochester Medical Center
Rochester, NY, USA

Li Zhang, MD
Assistant Professor of Medicine
Department of Medicine, LDS Hospital
Salt Lake City, UT, USA

Preface

New Arrhythmia Technologies is designed to serve as an up-to-date text on the rapidly advancing field of arrhythmia innovations. The breadth of the topics covered mirrors the expansive nature of the growing field of arrhythmia evaluation and therapy. The text begins with a comprehensive discussion of new pharmacologic agents for arrhythmia management and new antithrombotic agents, particularly for atrial fibrillation, and proceeds to include chapters on future arrhythmia therapies utilizing pharmacogenomics, structural approaches to novel antiarrhythmic drug therapy, embryonic stem cell-derived cardiomyocytes, and gene and cell therapy for sinus node and A-V nodal dysfunction and cardiac tachyarrhythmias. The numerous advances in noninvasive rhythm monitoring, implantable hemodynamic monitoring, functional status monitoring, and non-invasive mapping are discussed. There have been important advances in risk stratification for sudden death and the identification of relationships between the gene defect and the response to therapy. Because of the central role that out-of-hospital cardiac defibrillation has played in improving survival of sudden cardiac death, a chapter has been devoted to this topic.

In the exploding field of new arrhythmia devices, the text covers sensors and sensor algorithms, new electrode and lead designs for both pacing and defibrillation, advances in lead extraction, new resynchronization devices and left ventricular lead delivery systems for cardiac venous and epicardial placement, and new pacing indications. In the field of defibrillation, chapters are devoted to important advances in arrhythmia prevention and termination algorithms, sensing and discrimination algorithms, new ICD lead design and lead-less systems, optimization of defibrillator waveforms, new ICD indications, and web-based monitoring.

There have been remarkable advances in the development of techniques and devices for the surgical and catheter ablation of arrhythmias. A series of chapters are devoted to the explosion in surgical devices and techniques for atrial fibrillation, novel epicardial access techniques, innovative catheter control devices, new energy sources for catheter ablation, and new ablation paradigms.

We believe that *New Arrhythmia Technologies* provides a unique view into the latest in arrhythmia innovations through the eyes of the experts in the field.

PW

Acknowledgements

We wish to thank the contributors who have generously provided their expertise and time to this project. We would like to thank the efforts of Vicki Donald and Gina Almond of Blackwell Publishing for making this dream a reality. We wish to thank Michael Homer, BS for his administrative assistance. We also wish to thank all of the many unacknowledged assistants and colleagues who have been critical to the editing of each manuscript. Finally, we wish to thank the families of all the editors and contributors who tolerated us as we completed these chapters and this project.

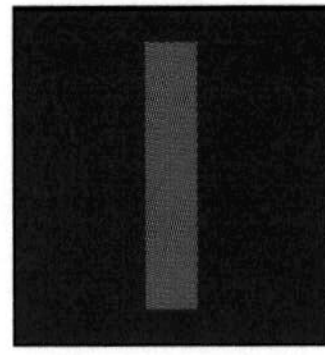

PART I

Advances in antiarrhythmic pharmacologic therapy

CHAPTER 1

New antiarrhythmic pharmacologic therapies and regulatory issues in antiarrhythmic drug development

Heather M. Ross, MS, APRN, *Peter R. Kowey*, MD, & *Gerald V. Naccarelli*, MD

Introduction

Until the 1980s, the majority of approved antiarrhythmic drugs were developed for use in the treatment of ventricular arrhythmias. Since that time, antiarrhythmic drug development has concentrated on the management of atrial fibrillation. Antiarrhythmic drugs that have proven useful in cardioversion and maintenance of sinus rhythm include Class IA sodium channel blockers: quinidine, procainamide, and disopyramide; Class IC sodium channel blockers: flecainide and propafenone; and the Class III agents: sotalol, dofetilide, and amiodarone. In addition, intravenous ibutilide is effective in the termination of atrial fibrillation. Quinidine, flecainide, propafenone-IR and -SR, sotalol, dofetilide, and ibutilide have FDA approval in the United States for the treatment of atrial fibrillation. Due to subjective adverse symptoms, end-organ toxicity, proarrhythmic potential, and lack of safety data in structural heart disease, Class IA agents are being used less frequently than in the past. Class IC drugs have been limited to use in patients with minimal or no structural heart disease. Sotalol and dofetilide can provoke torsade de pointes, and amiodarone use is often limited due to potential end-organ toxicity. In response to these limitations, the pharmaceutical industry has pursued the development of more effective and safer antiarrhythmic drugs for the treatment of atrial fibrillation. Drug development to treat ventricular arrhythmias continues as well, though to a lesser extent than for atrial fibrillation.

Theoretically, an ideal antiarrhythmic drug for the treatment of atrial fibrillation would have the following characteristics: (1) suppress phase 4 automaticity and thus atrial triggers; (2) prolong atrial refractory periods in a use-dependent fashion; (3) slow intraatrial conduction; (4) atrial selectivity to minimize ventricular proarrhythmic effects; (5) prolong AV nodal refractoriness and slow AV nodal conduction for the purpose of rate control; (6) a half-life long enough for once a day usage; (7) low potential for subjective, end-organ and proarrhythmic side effects; (8) safety for use in patients with structural heart disease, incorporating no significant negative inotropic effects or drug interactions.

Antiarrhythmic pharmaceutical development is currently moving in two general directions. First, efforts are being made to modify existing agents in an attempt to ameliorate safety and efficacy concerns. Second, pharmaceutical companies are working to develop agents with novel therapeutic mechanisms in an effort to achieve more effective drug therapy than is offered by existing compounds. Dofetilide and propafenone-SR are the most recently approved antiarrhythmic agents for the treatment of atrial fibrillation. In addition, new data suggest that carvedilol may have a role in treating atrial fibrillation. Investigational antiarrhythmic drugs abound. Non-antiarrhythmic drugs, such as ACE inhibitors, angiotensin receptor blockers, and HMG CoA enzyme inhibitors, also appear to have a role in suppressing atrial fibrillation in certain patient subtypes. This chapter will review the efficacy of the newly approved and currently investigational antiarrhythmic drugs that hold promise in the treatment of atrial fibrillation and other arrhythmias.

Newly approved agents

Termination of atrial fibrillation

In patients with more persistent atrial fibrillation, only oral dofetilide has a Class I indication for the termination of atrial fibrillation, based on the results of SAFIRE-D (Symptomatic Atrial Fibrillation Investigative REsearch on Dofetilide) and EMERALD (European and Australian Multicenter Evaluative Research on Atrial fibriLlation Dofetilide) clinical trials. Dofetilide prolongs action potential duration nearly twofold more in the atria than in the ventricles. This may explain the drug's effectiveness in converting atrial fibrillation to sinus rhythm. Both studies tested doses of 125, 250, and 500 μg of dofetilide twice daily compared with placebo. In EMERALD, sotalol 80 mg twice daily was also tested [1–6]. SAFIRE-D included 325 patients with persistent atrial fibrillation. The majority of patients had structural heart disease and 40% had a depressed ejection fraction. In SAFIRE-D, a 32% conversion rate by day three was noted, superior to the 1% placebo conversion rate ($p < .001$) [1]. EMERALD included 535 patients with persistent atrial fibrillation or atrial flutter. In EMERALD, 500 μg of dofetilide twice daily achieved a 29% rate of converting atrial fibrillation to sinus rhythm, proving more efficacious than sotalol (6%; $p < .05$) [2].

Further data regarding the efficacy of dofetilide in terminating atrial fibrillation come from the DIAMOND-CHF (Danish Investigations of Arrhythmia and Mortality ON Dofetilide) trial in which 391 patients who had atrial fibrillation at baseline had more frequent spontaneous conversion to sinus rhythm with dofetilide (12% at 1 month and 44% at 12 months) compared with placebo (1% at 1 month and 13% at 12 months; $p < .001$) [4, 5].

Suppression of atrial fibrillation

Oral procainamide, disopyramide, flecainide, propafenone, and sotalol are as effective as quinidine for the prevention of atrial fibrillation with efficacy rates averaging about 50%. Comparative trials have demonstrated that Class IC drugs and sotalol are better tolerated than Class IA agents. Recent data suggest that amiodarone is the most effective agent for maintaining sinus rhythm [7]. The Canadian Trial of Atrial Fibrillation (CTAF) demonstrated that patients treated with amiodarone had a lower recurrence rate (35%) versus sotalol or propafenone (63%) ($p < .001$). However, side effects requiring drug withdrawal was higher ($p = .06$) in the amiodarone-treated group [7, 8].

Dofetilide blocks the rapid potassium delayed rectifier current (I_{Kr}). Reverse use-dependent effects may minimize its electrophysiologic effects at rapid rates, such as those occurring with supraventricular tachyarrhythmias. By prolonging action potential duration, dofetilide has no negative inotropic effects and may even be a positive inotropic agent [3]. In addition to being an effective agent for medical conversion of atrial fibrillation to sinus rhythm, dofetilide (500 μg twice daily) had a 58% efficacy in maintaining sinus rhythm at 1 year post-cardioversion compared with only 25% in a placebo group in the SAFIRE-D trial ($p < .001$) [1]. Results of maintaining sinus rhythm in the EMERALD trial were similar [2]. In both studies, efficacy appeared to be dose related. In DIAMOND-AF, 1 year efficacy rates for maintaining sinus rhythm was superior in the dofetilide treated patients at 79%, compared with 42% in placebo patients ($p < .001$) [6]. DIAMOND-CHF found that dofetilide was superior to placebo in maintaining sinus rhythm after conversion from atrial fibrillation (HR 0.35; CI = 0.22–0.57; $p < .001$) [5].

Prospective trials of dofetilide did not demonstrate efficacy high enough to attain FDA approval in the suppression for paroxysmal atrial fibrillation; however, clinical experience suggests efficacy rates similar to other Class III, IA and IC drugs. Dose adjustment based on creatinine clearance and in-hospital initiation under telemetry conditions has been shown to decrease the incidence of drug-induced torsade de pointes [6].

For the suppression of recurrent paroxysmal atrial fibrillation, comparative trials have demonstrated that Class IC drugs and sotalol are equally effective and better tolerated than Class IA drugs [7]. Although these drugs have reported efficacy rates of about 50% at 1 year, up to 70% of patients who have remained on Class IC drugs after a year of treatment experience rare recurrences and minimal side effects that do not require drug discontinuation [7, 9].

In early 2004, a twice-daily formulation of propafenone became available in the United States. In the RAFT and ERAFT trials, propafenone-SR demonstrated statistical dose-related efficacy that was at least as effective as the immediate release form of the drug [10, 11]. In RAFT, propafenone-SR significantly lengthened the time to the first symptomatic atrial arrhythmic recurrence at all doses tested, compared with placebo [10]. These studies yielded a very favorable dose–response curve. The findings from ERAFT were consistent with RAFT, although the 225 mg twice-daily dose was not tested [11]. Plasma levels of propafenone were more likely to maintain therapeutic levels with the sustained formulation of the drug. The sustained release formulation is available in 225, 325, and 425 mg tablets, dosed twice daily rather than three times daily as with the immediate release formulation. The 325 mg twice-daily dose of sustained release of propafenone appears to be roughly equivalent to the 150 mg three times a day dose of the immediate release formulation [10].

Carvedilol possesses complex electrophysiologic properties, related to its Vaughan Williams Class II dose-related antiadrenergic (β_1, β_2, and α) effects. In addition, carvedilol has direct membrane-stabilizing activity (Class IA), prolongs repolarization by blocking potassium channels (Class III), and inhibits L-type calcium channels (Class IV). Carvedilol carries no known proarrhythmic activity. Carvedilol inhibits several native potassium channels responsible for repolarization in cardiomyocytes, including the rapidly and slowly activating components of the delayed rectifier current (I_{Kr} and I_{Ks}) and the transient outward current (I_{to}). Carvedilol does not affect the inward rectifier current (I_{KI}) which prolongs the action potential duration and effective refractory period to repeat excitability [12–14].

In a post-cardioversion trial comparing carvedilol to bisoprolol, carvedilol had a 14% lower rate of atrial fibrillation relapse during the 1 year period following cardioversion [15]. Carvedilol was also compared with two other β_1 selective blockers, metoprolol and atenolol, in a study of postoperative atrial fibrillation as a complication of cardiac surgery. Postoperative atrial fibrillation occurred in 8% of carvedilol-treated patients, versus 32% of patients receiving metoprolol or atenolol, for a 75% risk reduction. This occurred despite significantly poorer baseline left ventricular function in the carvedilol group [16].

Carvedilol was compared with amiodarone in a placebo-controlled trial of patients with chronic atrial fibrillation undergoing electrical cardioversion. Patients were randomized to receive carvedilol, amiodarone, or no antiarrhythmic drug for 6 weeks before and after external transthoracic cardioversion. Successful cardioversion was achieved with carvedilol and amiodarone pretreatment (87% and 94%), versus no antiarrhythmic prophylaxis (69%). Patients in both drug-treated groups immediately had longer fibrillatory cycle length intervals preconversion and longer atrial effective refractory periods 5 min post-conversion than unprotected patients. More patients who experienced a relapse of atrial fibrillation within 7 days were untreated (44%), compared with those receiving either carvedilol (29%) or amiodarone (19%) treatment [17].

Approaches to new antiarrhythmic drugs

Modifications: targeted improvements with new antiarrhythmic drugs

The pharmaceutical industry is currently devoting notable attention to the development of improved Class III antiarrhythmic drugs with enhanced efficacy and safety profiles. These agents are among the most effective currently available antiarrhythmic drugs for the suppression or cardioversion of atrial fibrillation and ventricular tachycardia [7]. Unfortunately, many patients and healthcare providers find the adverse effects associated with these agents, particularly the risks of end-organ toxicity and proarrhythmia, to be untenable.

There are currently more than a dozen new Class III compounds in development [18–23]. These are targeted to various potassium channels, with varying degrees of specificity or breadth. Some agents additionally block calcium channels, and others have beta blockade or sodium channel-blocking capacity (Table 1.1).

Within this category of new antiarrhythmic drugs as improved versions of existing potassium channel-blocking compounds, there are two particularly novel developments to note. Scientists have been able to target blockade of the ultrarapid potassium rectifier current (I_{Kur}), which exists only in atrial tissue, thereby affording atrial specificity and theoretically eliminating the risk of torsade de pointes as a result of ventricular action potential delay. Second, the ability to block the acetylcholine-dependent potassium current ($I_{K,Ach}$) offers another new specificity in targeting antiarrhythmic drug effects to the atria [18].

Cardioversion of atrial fibrillation

Tedisamil is currently in Phase III trials in the United States to evaluate for an indication for cardioversion of atrial fibrillation. Tedisamil is a Class III agent with blockade of I_{Kr}, I_{to}, I_{Ks}, I_{Kur}, and I_{KATP}, as well as sodium-channel-blocking properties. This new compound will theoretically offer an alternative to intravenous ibutilide, without risk of torsade de pointes [19, 20, 27].

Table 1.1 Investigational antiarrhythmic drugs, with mechanism of action [18, 20, 22, 24–26].

Modifications of existing compounds	*Novel mechanisms of action*
Azimilide (I_{Kr}, I_{Ks})	Piboserod (5-HT4)
Dronedarone (I_{Kr}, I_{Ks}, β_1, I_{Ca}, I_{to}, I_{Na})	ZP-123 (GAP 486)
RSD-1235 (I_{Kur}, I_{to}, I_{Na}, I_{KAch})	AAP10 (connexin modulator)
GYKI-16638 (I_{Kr}, I_{K1}, I_{Na})	GsMtx4 (stretch receptor antagonist)
AZD7009 (atrial repolarization delay)	
AVE1231 (atrial repolarization delay)	
ATI-2042 (I_{Kr}, I_{Ks}, β_1, I_{Ca}, I_{to}, I_{Na})	
Tedisamil (I_{Kr}, I_{to}, I_{KATP}, I_{Na}, I_{Kur})	
AVE-0118 (I_{Kur})	
Ersentilide (I_{Kr}, β)	
Trecetilide (I_{Kr}, I_{Na})	
Almokalant (I_{Kr})	
Terikalant (I_{Kr})	
SB237376 (I_{Kr})	
HMR1402 (I_{Ks})	
HMR1556 (I_{Ks})	
L768673 (I_{Ks})	
Ambasilide (I_{to}, I_{K1}, I_{KAch}, I_{Kur}, I_{Na})	
NIP142 (I_{Kur}, I_{KAch})	
CP060S (I_{Na}, I_{Ca})	
KB-R7943 (I_{Na}, I_{Ca})	
Cariporide (I_{Na}, I_H)	
DTI0009 (adenosine A1 blocker)	
Tecadenoson (CVT-510) (long-acting adenosine A1 blocker)	
Abanoquil (α_{1A} blocker)	
E3174 (angiotensin II blocker)	
KB130015 (thyroid antagonist)	

Suppression of atrial fibrillation

Azimilide is an I_{Kr} and I_{Ks} blocker that does not appear to have any reverse use dependence. Thus, azimilide maintains its electrophysiologic effects over both slow and fast heart rates. Azimilide, similar to amiodarone, blocks both I_{Kr} and I_{Ks}, which is thought to minimize the risk of torsade de pointes compared with only I_{Kr} blockade. Azimilide has demonstrated efficacy in treating atrial fibrillation based on clinical trials in the Azimilide Supraventricular Arrhythmia Program (ASAP). The most effective dose appears to be 125 mg daily, averaging about 50% suppression of paroxysmal atrial fibrillation. Lower doses have produced inconsistent effects in suppressing atrial fibrillation compared with placebo. One pivotal study of 125 mg daily did not show statistical benefit in suppressing paroxysms of atrial fibrillation [28].

Because of this, ongoing trials include A-STAR (Azimilide Supraventricular Tachy-Arrhythmia Reduction) to further assess the efficacy of azimilide in suppressing paroxysmal atrial fibrillation and A-COMET (Azimilide CardiOversion MaintEnance Trial) to assess its role in maintaining sinus rhythm in persistent atrial fibrillation post-cardioversion [29]. In A-COMET II, azimilide will be compared with placebo and sotalol.

ALIVE (AzimiLide post-Infarction surVival Evaluation) found azimilide to have neutral effects in a placebo-controlled trial of post-myocardial infarction patients with a hazard ratio of 1.0 with a mortality rate of 11.6% in both the placebo and azimilide-treated groups. In addition, the time to the development of atrial fibrillation was longer ($p = .04$) in the azimilide group [30]. Safety data from trials thus far show that azimilide appears to have a low incidence of drug provoked torsade de pointes. Subjective toxicity is minimal, but a low incidence of drug-induced neutropenia has been reported [30, 31].

Dronedarone is an amiodarone-like compound without the iodine moiety. To date, end-organ toxicity has not been reported. Electrophysiologically, dronedarone blocks I_{Kr}, I_{Ks}, I_{to}, fast sodium, and calcium channels. Dronedarone prolongs the action potential duration in the atria and ventricles with no significant reverse use dependence. Other electrophysiologic effects similar to amiodarone include α, β, and muscarinic blocking effects. Dronedarone appears to slow sinus rates less than amiodarone. However, its AV nodal refractory period prolonging effect should confer some rate control benefits [32].

In the DAFNE (Dose Adjustment For Normal Eating) trial, dronedarone 400 mg twice daily was superior to placebo in preventing recurrent atrial fibrillation. The median time to recurrence was 59.9 days in the dronedarone group compared with 5.3 days in the placebo group ($p < .05$; RR = 0.45; CI = 0.28–0.72). Higher doses of dronedarone were ineffective and associated with a higher incidence of gastrointestinal subjective adverse effects [33]. Ongoing studies at the 400 mg twice-daily dose include ADONIS (American African trial with DrONnedarone In atrial fibrillation or flutter for the maintenance of Sinus rhythm) and EURIDIS (EURropean trial In atrial fibrillation or atrial flutter patients receiving Dronedarone for the maIntenance of Sinus rhythm). Both of these studies have demonstrated that dronedarone suppresses recurrent atrial fibrillation at a dose of 400 mg twice daily [24].

Another novel compound group is the atrial repolarization delaying action agents, which will theoretically allow for adequate dosing to suppress atrial arrhythmias effectively, without risk of torsade de pointes due to concomitant repolarization delay in ventricular tissues. Drugs featuring I_{Kur} blockade offer particular hope in this category [18].

RSD-1235 is an atrial selective potassium channel blocker with little effect on ventricular repolarization. In the CRAFT trial RSD-1235 was shown to have a dose-related ability to terminate atrial fibrillation [34].

AVE-0118 is a biphenyl derivative that blocks the atrial delayed rectifier current and I_{ACH} with little effect on ventricular tissue. Early basic studies demonstrate that it prolongs the atrial effective refractory period, even after atrial remodeling has occurred from persistent atrial fibrillation [35].

Rate control of atrial tachyarrhythmias

Tecadenoson is an adenosine analog with selective A_1 receptor agonist activity. This avoids hypotension that is associated with stimulation of the A_2 receptor, and is commonly experienced with intravenous administration of adenosine. Tecadenoson has completed enrollment of phase III trials for ventricular rate control in paroxysmal supraventricular tachycardia. Enrollment continues in trials to examine tecadenoson as an agent for ventricular rate control in atrial fibrillation. This drug will be indicated only for rate control and not suppression of atrial fibrillation [25].

Treatment of ventricular arrhythmias

Advances in cardiac care have significantly improved survival after myocardial infarction. Compared to the past, early revascularization and thrombolytic agents have minimized the size of myocardial scar compared to 20 years ago. However, a significant number of patients still carry myocardial scar, and thus border zone areas, prone to development of anisotropy and reentrant ventricular arrhythmia circuits. While catheter ablation for ischemic monomorphic ventricular tachycardia is relatively successful, it is a highly specialized procedure not accessible by all patients. As with atrial fibrillation, significant numbers of patients with ventricular tachycardia rely on pharmacologic therapies for arrhythmia suppression. Similar problems regarding safety and efficacy exist with preparations used to suppress ventricular arrhythmias in this growing population.

As there is more enthusiasm for developing antiarrhythmic drugs for the treatment of atrial fibrillation, very few drugs are being developed for the treatment of ventricular arrhythmias. Gap junction modulators may have use in treating ventricular tachyarrhythmias. Multiple new drugs, such as azimilide and dronedarone, are being studied in patients with ICDs to determine if they are effective in suppressing recurrent ICD shocks.

Early animal studies are examining new compounds with combined Class IB and Class III antiarrhythmic properties for the suppression of ventricular tachycardia. *In vivo* studies with dog and rabbit models have been encouraging, suggesting further development of the compound GYKI-16638. To date, however, human studies have not commenced [21].

Innovations: compounds with novel antiarrhythmic mechanisms

As our understanding of the wide range of etiologies for atrial fibrillation onset improves, scientists have begun to develop antiarrhythmic agents with entirely new mechanisms of action. Gap junction (connexin) modulators, such as AAP10 and ZP123, offer promise for the treatment of atrial fibrillation in the setting of dilated cardiomyopathies. Stretch receptor antagonists, including GsMtx4, may gain significant efficacy in the treatment of individuals with hypertrophic hearts, diastolic dysfunction, and valvular regurgitation [18].

There has been some indirect association that 5-hydoxytryptamine (5-HT) can cause atrial fibrillation. Piboserod (an atrial-selective 5-HT receptor antagonist) was developed as a result of this theory. Clinical results to date, however, have been disappointing [20].

Data exist from multiple studies that angiotensin converting enzyme inhibitors and angiotensin receptor blockers are useful for the suppression of atrial fibrillation, by mechanisms not previously thought to have any significant antiarrhythmic effects [23, 35, 36–38]. More recent data from AFFIRM suggest that these drugs may be particularly useful in as antiarrhythmic agents in patients with significant heart failure [39, 40].

Antiarrhythmic therapy choice based on survival data from clinical trials

DIAMOND-MI studied the effects of dofetilide compared with placebo in patients with post-myocardial infarction with ejection fraction of $\leq 35\%$. A total of 1510 patients were recruited (749 dofetilide; 761 placebo) with a minimum follow-up of 1 year. Dofetilide was titrated under telemetry conditions for the first 3 days of dosing. Dofetilide had neutral mortality effects when compared with placebo in the post-myocardial infarction setting (230 dofetilide versus 243 placebo deaths, HR = 0.94, $p = .23$). Dofetilide had no adverse or beneficial effect on cardiac mortality or arrhythmic death. Pharmacologic conversion of atrial fibrillation was more frequent in the dofetilide group ($p = .002$) [41].

The DIAMOND-CHF trial randomized 1518 patients admitted to the hospital with heart failure and an ejection fraction of $\leq 35\%$ to dofetilide ($n = 762$) or placebo ($n = 756$). During follow-up, 311 (41%) died in the dofetilide arm, versus 317 (42%) deaths in the placebo arm ($p =$ NS;

HR = 0.95; CI = 0.81–1.11). These results are remarkable for 25 (3.3%) cases of torsade de pointes in the dofetilide group versus 0% in the placebo treated patients. Hospitalizations for heart failure were statistically lower ($p = .001$) in the dofetilide group (30%) than the placebo group (38%) [5, 6].

In DIAMOND-AF, total mortality was 44.6% in the dofetilide group, no different than the 45.1% mortality rate in the placebo group. DIAMOND-AF also demonstrated that heart failure hospitalizations were nonsignificantly lower ($p = .14$, HR = 0.69; CI = 0.51–0.93) in the dofetilide group (29.3%) versus the placebo group (39.7%) and in all cases hospitalizations were also lower in the dofetilide group ($p = .003$) [5, 6].

The ALIVE trial randomized patients to placebo versus 75–100 mg/day of azimilide. Key inclusion criteria included acute myocardial infarction within 6–21 days; ejection fraction 15–35%; and abnormal heart rate variability of ≤ 20 U. Azimilide also appears to be safe to use in the post-myocardial infarction population since the demonstrated hazard ratio of mortality was 1.0 compared with placebo. In ALIVE, time to the development of atrial fibrillation was longer ($p = .04$) in the azimilide group [31].

The role of dronedarone in treating patients with left ventricular dysfunction will depend on the final results of the ANDROMEDA trial, which will have a combined primary endpoint of mortality and hospital admissions secondary to heart failure. The ANDROMEDA trial, studying the safety of dronedarone in patients with left ventricular dysfunction, was prematurely terminated due to statistically nonsignificant higher mortality in the antiarrhythmic treated arm of the study [27]. Further analyses of these data will determine if dronedarone will be safe to use in this patient population.

Genetics and genomics

With the mapping of the human genome, genetics and genomics are becoming increasingly well understood for their role in affecting drug metabolism. Humans are endowed with polymorphisms, relatively common expressions of specific patterns in genetic code [42]. For example, some individuals carry a genetically coded inability to metabolize compounds via the cytochrome P450 system. This genomic variation, or polymorphism, is significant in considering medications, such as amiodarone, that require this system for adequate metabolism and avoidance of lethal toxicities. As a poignant example, erythromycin, the commonly used antibiotic, may cause prolongation of the QT interval with resultant development of torsade de pointes when ingested by an individual who is also taking amiodarone [43].

In addition to effecting toxic drug responses, genomic variations may also affect therapeutic efficacy. This phenomenon is becoming understood with respect to several analgesic preparations, and is extended to other classes of drugs including antiarrhythmic agents. The pharmaceutical industry is on the cusp of understanding how to modify various preparations in an effort to tailor the effect to an individual's specific genetic needs [26, 42].

Regulatory issues

The development of drugs for arrhythmia indications is tricky business. Evidence of efficacy constitutes a significant hurdle, but demonstration of safety is even more daunting. Multiple studies, which prove that the drug can be utilized safely in the appropriate patient population with an acceptable risk, are required for registration. In addition, studies must be designed and executed in such a way so as to extract relevant and useful information about how to dose the drug and how to monitor patients. There must be a safety experience that is at least large enough to identify adverse effects that will occur with moderate frequency when the drug is available for general use, recognizing that rare side effects may not be recognized even within a robust dataset.

The first step in antiarrhythmic drug development is a careful characterization of the drug's electrophysiologic effects. This includes a full description of its activity at specific ion channels and other cell targets, followed by *in vivo* experiments to demonstrate a composite electropharmacologic profile. One would prefer to see how the drug performs in well-validated arrhythmia models as an index of its potential clinical utility, though the predictive value of animal models of this kind may be low.

It may at least be possible in this early phase to define an electrical effect as a function of blood or tissue concentration to begin to approximate a target dose in humans. It is important to understand that an excellent understanding of the drug's actions in this early phase will facilitate development in later phases, both with regard to issues of efficacy and safety.

Most antiarrhythmic drugs have complex pharmacology. This fact places a significant burden on early phase clinical development to understand basic pharmacological principles, such as distribution, metabolism, and elimination. Such factors are especially important in this realm. Because most antiarrhythmic drugs have a relatively narrow toxic/therapeutic ratio, factors that increase or decrease drug exposure are very important to the drug's safe use. The electrocardiogram provides a crude tool to delineate electrophysiologic effects in some, but not all, cases. For example, it is not possible to observe changes in atrial refractoriness on the surface electrocardiogram, greatly complicating the evaluation of atrial specific agents. It may be necessary to conduct invasive electrophysiologic studies to define the drug's activity in these cases, or utilize previously implanted pacemakers for this purpose. With opportunities to develop and study parenteral as well as oral formulations, decisions about the best methods of drug delivery should be made in early stages so as to properly focus the overall development program.

The next phases of development are considered the critical path, for it is here that so-called "proof of concept" studies are devised and carried out. At this point, patients without significant comorbidities are exposed to the investigational drug at various doses with the goal of demonstrating activity in the target arrhythmia. Investigators face a fine line between recruiting too few patients in the interest of economy, and spending too much on what might not necessarily be a pivotal trial. Nevertheless, this phase of study must clearly demonstrate efficacy and safety at achievable drug concentrations to permit the program to go forward, and to generate the correct hypotheses for late-phase clinical development.

It is in this intermediary phase of development that many other things must be learned about the new agent. In addition to defining a useful dose range, drug and device interactions must be defined. Particular attention must focus on those agents, such as anticoagulants, that are used frequently in patients with cardiac arrhythmia. Safety issues must be more carefully defined to allow for proper focusing of later clinical development. Although longitudinal studies will follow, adequate exposures to define intermediate term tolerability are necessary to set the stage for those very important longer-term safety trials. It is in this stage of development that special populations, such as those with organ impairment or the elderly, may be studied to determine entry criteria for the pivotal trial experience.

Pivotal efficacy studies are tailored to study critical issues related to the putative safety and efficacy of the new chemical entity. It is important that these studies are designed creatively to maximize the yield of information and to allow for proper drug labeling if successful. Studies can be conducted for various indications. In the case of atrial fibrillation, the drug can be considered for conversion to, or maintenance of, sinus rhythm or both. Placebo-controlled studies may be used as long as the patient is protected against the complications of inordinately high heart rates and thromboembolic events. Studies of sufficient duration (at least 12 months) are necessary to assess chronic tolerance. The relevant patient population must be studied here, as inclusion and exclusion criteria for the trials will be used for product labeling.

The development of drugs for ventricular arrhythmia indications is much more difficult and challenging. In previous times, suppression of premature ventricular depolarizations or prevention of inducible ventricular tachycardia in the electrophysiology laboratory were accepted as surrogates of efficacy. This is no longer the case; direct suppression and/or prevention of sustained ventricular tachycardia/fibrillation (VT/VF) are now the gold standard. For parenteral compounds, the intravenous amiodarone development program sets the standard [44, 45]. In this program, patients with frequently recurring VT/VF, refractory to conventional agents, were treated in dose ranging and positive comparator studies. Prevention of recurrent sustained arrhythmia was the primary endpoint. Approval for prophylaxis of high-risk patients, such as those after myocardial infarction, is a lofty goal that is unrealistic, short of conducting mega-trials, because of low event rates.

Oral drug development for ventricular arrhythmias may be less complex. Although prevention of inducibility can be used to "prove the concept," a controlled study to assess sustained arrhythmia recurrence is expected for approval. The most expeditious and practical way to accomplish this is with placebo-controlled studies in patients with implantable defibrillators and a minimum baseline shock frequency. This also avoids the need for a positive comparator that greatly increases the complexity of blinding and multiplies the number of patients that need to be enrolled.

Longer-term safety data are desirable in the development of any antiarrhythmic agent, and particularly in patients with structural heart disease whose substrate and organ function can change over time. Although this may not be possible within the context of controlled trials, long-term extension and "compassionate use" experience may help to provide needed information. These experiences may also serve to increase the size of the overall database for regulatory review, expected to be in excess of 2000 patients for most drugs.

Approval of a potent antiarrhythmic drug in the modern era does not necessarily translate into widespread use. Restrictions may be placed on distribution and access based on safety issues. Dofetilide provides the most recent example in which concerns about adjustments for altered renal function and risk of torsade de pointes prompted the FDA to impose requirements for physician registration and central pharmacy distribution. One would expect that such measures would not be necessary for drugs devoid of major safety concerns. Nevertheless, we expect that there will be increasing emphasis on techniques of postmarketing surveillance so that major but unexpected safety issues can be identified and addressed as soon as possible in the drug's real-world experience.

It is reasonable to assume that drugs with novel mechanisms of action and with new indications will be developed in years to come. For example, with the proliferation of ablation techniques and their wider application, drugs can be developed and studied that are intended to suppress the arrhythmias that develop postablation. We have already seen drugs come forward that have targets other than conventional ion channels. As this work progresses, it will be important to remain open to creative protocols and to innovative development programs that will facilitate bringing these new products to clinical use expeditiously. No matter how this is done, it is of paramount importance to emphasize the most fundamental treatment principle, that the benefit of the drug must clearly exceed the risk. Clinical trials preserve the ability to precisely determine the magnitude of both sides of the therapeutic equation.

Conclusion

The search for effective, safe antiarrhythmic drugs continues with constant development activities on the part of pharmaceutical corporations. Efforts to modify existing structures promise enhanced safety with established mechanisms of action. In particular, efforts to modify amiodarone to create a safe and well-tolerated Class III antiarrhythmic drug are driving the development of several new compounds currently in clinical trials and regulatory examination. The investigation and development of drugs with novel mechanisms of action holds the potential reward of enhanced antiarrhythmic efficacy, particularly for the control of atrial fibrillation and, to a lesser extent, ventricular tachycardia.

The continually evolving understanding of the role played by genetics in drug metabolism will yield additional improvements in antiarrhythmic drug efficacy in the future. Hopefully, today's early stages of genomics research will result in the development of drugs that can play a role in an antiarrhythmic regimen specifically designed to fit a patient's genetic structure, enhancing not only efficacy, but significantly, safety as well.

References

1 Singh S, Zoble RG, Yellen L *et al.* Efficacy and safety of oral dofetilide in converting to and maintaining sinus rhythm in patients with chronic atrial fibrillation or flutter: the symptomatic atrial fibrillation investigative research on dofetilide (SAFIRE-D) study. *Circulation* 2000; **102**: 2385–2390.

2 Greenbaum R, Campbell TJ, Channer KS *et al.* Conversion of atrial fibrillation and maintenance of sinus rhythm by dofetilide. The EMERALD study (abstract). *Circulation* 1998; I-633.

3 Mounsey JP, DiMarco JP. Dofetilide. *Circulation* 2000; **102**: 2665–2770.

4 Torp-Pedersen C, Moller M, Bloch-Thomsen PF *et al.* Dofetilide in patients with congestive heart failure and left ventricular dysfunction. *N Engl J Med* 1999; **341**: 857–865.

5 Pederson OD, Bagger H, Keller N, Marchant B, Kober L, Torp-Pederson C (For the Danish Investigations of Arrhythmia and Morality ON Dofetilide Study Group). Efficacy of dofetilide in the treatment of atrial fibrillation-flutter in patients with reduced left ventricular function: A Danish Investigations of Arrhythmia and Mortality ON Dofetilide (DIAMOND) substudy. *Circulation* 2001; **104**: 292–296.

6 Prystowsky EN, Freeland S, Branyas NA, Rardon DP, Fogel RI, Padanilam BJ, Rippy JS. Clinical experience with dofetilide in the treatment of patients with atrial fibrillation. *J Cardiovasc Electrophysiol* 2003; **14**: S287–S290.

7 Naccarelli GV, Wolbrette DL, Khan M, Bhatta L, Hynes J, Samii S, Luck J. Old and new antiarrhythmic drugs for converting and maintaining sinus rhythm in atrial fibrillation: Comparative efficacy and results of trials. *Am J Cardiol* 2003; **91**: 15D–26D.

8 Naccarelli GV, Wolbrette DL, Bhatta L, Khan M, Hynes J, Samii S, Luck J. A review of clinical trials assessing the efficacy and safety of newer antiarrhythmic drugs in atrial fibrillation. *J Interv Card Electrophysiol* 2003; **9**: 215–222.

9 Fuster V, Rydén LE, Asinger RW *et al.* ACC/AHA/ESC guidelines for the management of patients with atrial fibrillation:executive summary: a report of the American College of Cardiology/ American Heart Association Task Force on Practice Guidelines and the European Society of Cardiology Committee for Practice Guidelines and Policy Conferences (Committee to Develop Guidelines for the Management of Patients With Atrial Fibrillation). *J Am Coll Cardiol* 2001; **38**: 1231–1265.

10 Pritchett ELC, Page RL, Carlson M, Undesser K, Fava G [For the Rythmol Atrial Fibrillation Trial (RAFT) Investigators.] Efficacy and safety of sustained-release propafenone (propafenone SR) for patients with atrial fibrillation. *Am J Cardiol* 2003; **92**: 941–946.

11 Meinertz T, Lip GYH, Lombardi F *et al.* (On behalf of the ERAFT Investigators.) Efficacy and safety of propafenone sustained release in the prophylaxis of symptomatic paroxysmal atrial fibrillation (The European Rythmol/ Rythmonorm Atrial Fibrillation Trial (ERAFT) Study). *Am J Cardiol* 2002; **90**: 1300–1306.

12 Cheng J, Niwa R, Kamiya K, Toyama J, Kodama I. Carvedilol blocks the repolarizing K^+ currents and the L-type $Ca2^+$ current in rabbit ventricular myocytes. *Eur J Pharmacol* 1999; **376**: 189–201.

13 Karle CA, Kreye VA, Thomas D *et al.* Antiarrhythmic drug carvedilol inhibits HERG potassium channels. *Cardiovasc Res* 2001; **49**: 361–370.

14 Maltsev VA, Sabbab HN, Undrovinas AI. Down-regulation of sodium current in chronic heart failure: effect of long-term therapy with carvedilol. *Cell Mol Life Sci* 2002; **59**: 1561–1568.

15 Katritsis DG, Panagiotakos DB, Karvouni E *et al.* Comparison of effectiveness of carvedilol versus bisoprolol for maintenance of sinus rhythm after cardioversion of persistent atrial fibrillation. *Am J Cardiol* 2003; **92**: 1116–1119.

16 Merritt JC, Niebaur M, Tarakji K, Hammer D, Mills RM. Comparison of effectiveness of carvedilol versus metoprolol or atenolol for atrial fibrillation appearing after coronary artery bypass grafting or cardiac valve operation. *Am J Cardiol* 2003; **92**: 735–736.

17 Kanoupakis EM, Manios EG, Mavkaris HE *et al.* Comparative effects of carvedilol and amiodarone on conversion and recurrence rates of persistent atrial fibrillation. *Am J Cardiol* 2004; **94**: 659–662.

18 Camm AJ, Savelieva I. Advances in antiarrhythmic drug treatment of atrial fibrillation:Where do we stand now? *Heart Rhythm* 2004; **1**: 244–246.

19 Singh S. Trials of new antiarrhythmic drugs for maintenance of sinus rhythm in patients with atrial fibrillation. *J Interv Card Electrophysiol* 2004; 10(S1): 71–76.

20 Choudhury A, Lip GY. Antiarrhythmic drugs in atrial fibrillation: an overview of new agents, their mechanisms of action and potential clinical utility. *Expert Opin Investig Drugs* 2004; **13**: 841–855.

21 Matyus P, Varga I, Rettegi T *et al.* Novel antiarrhythmic compounds with combined class IB and class III mode of action. *Curr Med Chem* 2004; **11**: 61–69.

22 Castro A. Bianconi L, Santini M. New antiarrhythmic drugs for the treatment of atrial fibrillation. *PACE* 2002; **25**: 249–259.

23 Weiss JN, Garfinkel A, Chen PS. Novel approaches to identifying antiarrhythmic drugs. *Trends Cardiovasc Med* 2003; **13**: 326–330.

24 Hohnloser, SH. EURIDIS and ADONIS:maintenance of sinus rhythm with dronedarone in patients with atrial fibrillation or flutter. Paper presented at the European Society for Cardiology Congress 2004, 29 Aug.–1 Sep., Munich, Germany.

25 CV Therapeutics. "Tecadenoson (CVT-510)" http://www.cvt.com/prod_atrial.html. Accessed 19 September 2004.

26 Roden DM. Antiarrhythmic drugs: Past, present, and future. *PACE* 2003; **26**: 2340–2349.

27 Hohnloser SH, Dorian P, Straub M, Beckmann K, Kowey P. Safety and efficacy of intravenously administered tedisamil for rapid conversion of recent-onset atrial

fibrillation or atrial flutter. *J Am Coll Cardiol* 2004; **44**: 99–104.

28 Connolly SJ, Schenell DJ, Page RL, Wilkinson WE, Marcello SR, Pritchett ELC. Dose-response relations of azimilide in the management of symptomatic, recurrent, atrial fibrillation. *Am J Cardiol* 2001; **88**: 974–979.

29 Page RL. A-STAR and A-COMET trials (abstract). *Europace* 2002; **3**: A-2.

30 Pratt CM, Singh SN, Al-Khalidi HR *et al.* The efficacy of azimilide in the treatment of atrial fibrillation in the presence of left ventricular systolic dysfunction: results from the azimilide postinfarct survival evaluation (ALIVE) trial. *J Am Coll Cardiol* 2004; **43**: 1211–1216.

31 Camm AJ, Karam R, Pratt C. The azimilide post-infarct survival evaluation (ALIVE) trial. *Am J Cardiol* 1998; 81(6A): 35D–39D.

32 Sun W, Sarma JSM, Singh BN. Electrophysiological effects of dronedarone (SR33589), a noniodinated benzofuran derivative, in the rabbit heart. Comparison with amiodarone. *Circulation* 1999; **100**: 2276–2281.

33 Touboul P, Brugada J, Capucci A, Crijns H, Edvardsson N, Hohnloser S, Radzik D.(on behalf of the DAFNE Investigators). Dronedarone for the prevention of recurrent atrial fibrillation after cardioversion. Results of a randomized placebo-controlled, double–blind, multicenter study (abstract). *PACE* 2002; **24**: 574.

34 Billman GE. RSD-1235. Cardiome. *Curr Opin Investig Drugs* 2003; **4**: 352–354.

35 Tamargo J, Caballero R, Delpon E. (2003) New mechanistic targets for the treatment of atrial fibrillation. In: Papp JP, Straub M, Ziegler D. eds. Atrial Fibrillation: New Therapeutic Concepts. IOS Press, Ohmsa, Amsterdam, 2003: 133–155.

36 Pederson OD, Bagger H, Kober L, Torp - Pedersen C. Trandolopril reduces the incidence of atrial fibrillation after acute myocardial infarction in patients with left ventricular dysfunction. *Circulation* 1999; **100**: 376–380.

37 Madrid AH, Bueno MG, Rebollo JMG *et al.* Use of irbesartan to maintain sinus rhythm in patients with long-lasting persistent atrial fibrillation. A prospective and randomized study. *Circulation* 2002; **106**: 331–336.

38 Kuhlkamp V, Schirdewan A, Stang K *et al.* Use of metoprolol CR/XL to maintain sinus rhythm after conversion from persistent atrial fibrillation. *J Am Coll Cardiol* 2000; **36**: 139–146.

39 Khand AU, Rankin AC, Martin W *et al.* Carvedilol alone or in combination with digoxin for the management of atrial fibrillation in patients with heart failure? *J Am Coll Cardiol* 2003; **42**: 1944–1951.

40 Van Noord T, Tieleman RG, Bosker HA *et al.* Beta-blockers prevent subacute recurrences of persistent atrial fibrillation only in patients with hypertension. *Europace* 2004; **6**: 343–350.

41 Kober L, Bloch-Thomsen PE, Moller M *et al.* on behalf of the Danish Investigations of Arrhythmia and Mortality ON Dofetilide (DIAMOND) Study Group. Effect of dofetilide in patients with recent myocardial infarction and left ventricular dysfunction:results of the DIAMOND-MI study. *Lancet* 2000; **356**: 2052–2058.

42 Anderson JL, Carlquist JF, Horne BD, Muhlestein JB. Cardiovascular pharmacogenomics: current status, future prospects. *J Cardiovasc Pharmacol Ther* 2003; **8**: 71–83.

43 Liu, BA, Juurlink DN. Drugs and the QT interval – caveat doctor. *New Eng J Med* 2004; **351**: 1053–1056.

44 Kowey PR, Levine JH, Herre JM *et al.* Randomized, double-blind comparison of intravenous amiodarone and bretylium in the treatment of patients with recurrent, hemodynamically destabilizing ventricular tachycardia or fibrillation. The Intravenous Amiodarone Multicenter Investigators Group. *Circulation* 1995; **92**: 3255–3263.

45 Scheinman MM, Levine JH, Cannom DS *et al.* Dose-ranging study of intravenous amiodarone in patients with life-threatening ventricular tachyarrhythmias. The Intravenous Amiodarone Multicenter Investigators Group. *Circulation* 1995; **92**: 3264–3272.

2

CHAPTER 2

New frontiers in antithrombotic therapy for atrial fibrillation

James A. Reiffel, MD

Atrial fibrillation (AF) is associated with alterations in atrial size (enlargement), mechanics (reduced emptying characteristics and flow velocity), and prothrombotic hemochemical changes [1–10]. These modifications can result in stagnant atrial flow (especially in the appendage) and in alterations of several coagulation factors, fibrinolytic balance, nitric oxide secretion in the atria and the consequences of its reduction, and, to a lesser extent, platelet derived factors [1–10]. These effects raise the probability of atrial clot formation. Some of the hemochemical alterations that contribute to thromboembolic risk in AF are aspirin sensitive, such as P-selectin, (β-thromboglobulin, and platelet factor 4. Most, however, are not affected by aspirin, but their procoagulant actions can be reduced by warfarin, including, for example, factor VII, fibrinogen, D-dimer, prothrombin fragment 1.2, thrombin–antithrombin complex, altered fibrinolytic balance, increased superoxides (which degrade NO).

Mobile atrial thrombi may produce systemic embolization, resulting in end-organ dysfunctional events, such as stroke, visual loss, coronary occlusion, and bowel or limb *necrosis*. Risk for embolism in AF is independent of whether or not rate-related, irregularity-related, or other AF-related symptoms are present. Importantly, it has been recently appreciated that risk for embolism in the AF patient at risk may persist, in at least some patients, even if (and after) sinus rhythm has been restored, as was clearly demonstrated in trials, such as RACE and AFFIRM [11, 12]. Possible explanations for persistent risk include (Table 2.1) recurrent episodes of unappreciated asymptomatic AF, incomplete reverse atrial remodeling in NSR with residual flow impairment, and negative atrial inotropic effects of drug or ablative therapy. Atrial size 6 months after cardioversion, for example, is reduced if NSR is maintained as compared with that seen if AF recurs, but atrial size is not necessarily reduced to normal [13]. Moreover, the longer AF persists prior to cardioversion, the slower and less extensive is the reduction in atrial size following cardioversion [14]. Atrial contractility may also be reduced by negative notropic effects of antiarrhythmic agents being used to maintain sinus rhythm [15]. Similarly, there data exists to suggest that following catheter ablative procedures for the cure of AF, significant atrial enlargement and mechanical dysfunction can persist or develop? [16].

Multiple clinical trials have increased our knowledge base about the risk factors for AF-associated thrombus formation and emboli, and about optimal preventative therapies [17–20]. The incidence of embolic risk has been shown to be low (<1–2%/year) in patients with AF who are <65 years of age and have no associated high-risk markers while the incidence is higher in patients with certain identified risk factors, including in most series,

Table 2.1 Possible reasons for persistent thromboembolic risk following restoration of sinus rhythm in patients with AF.

Asymptomatic (undetected) AF recurrences
Persistence of atrial enlargement and/or atrial dysfunction (absence of complete reverse remodeling)
Atrial dysfunction induced by pharmacotherapy
Atrial dysfunction resulting from ablative injury
Concomitant, nonatrial sources of emboli

older age, hypertension, diabetes, heart failure, prior transient ischemic attack (TIA) or emboli, rheumatic valvular disease, and combinations of these factors, among others, to a yearly incidence as high as 10% or more. Patients at low risk may require no antithrombotic therapy, although physicians generally administer aspirin. Guidelines based upon results from large placebo-controlled aspirin and warfarin trials indicate a need for potent anticoagulation (with warfarin, at present) in the presence of highest risk markers and a preference for warfarin over aspirin with an intermediate risk profile, as warfarin has had superior efficacy to aspirin for stroke prevention in each comparative trial performed [17–20]. The benefit has outweighed an increased risk for bleeding. Low-dose aspirin has shown no benefit over placebo. The reader is referred to the October 2001 ACC/AHA/ESC AF management guidelines [17] for the most widely agreed upon current therapy recommendations.

Notwithstanding the benefits of warfarin in substantially reducing embolic events in AF patients, warfarin is commonly underutilized in AF patients. Both patients and physicians generally dislike warfarin therapy.

Patients dislike warfarin for many reasons

Warfarin dosing requirements vary widely, even in the same patient over time. Its anticoagulant efficacy and risk profile has to be determined by prothrombin time (PT) monitoring – frequently at initiation and no less than monthly during follow-up. Obtaining a PT is associated with inconvenience, discomfort, and costs to patients. Warfarin has multiple food interactions, and either rigid dietary consistency has to be maintained or frequent PT checks are required during diet alteration since reduced or elevated levels occur during dietary changes, with resultant recurrent thrombotic risk or hemorrhagic risk, respectively. Additionally, warfarin has many known and as of yet unknown drug interactions. Accordingly, dosing alterations and increased PT surveillance are often required when concomitant drug therapies are changed or if patients begin or change over-the-counter dietary aids or supplements.

Physicians also dislike warfarin for many reasons

Prothrombin time monitoring is one of life's true nuisances. It is extraordinarily time consuming for physicians and their staffs. Many busy offices need to employ an anticoagulation nurse or establish an anticoagulation clinic just to monitor PTs and adjust warfarin doses. Their support is a significant overhead burden to the physician. Physicians must remember to order the increased surveillance if concomitant drug therapy is changed or dietary changes or supplements are learned about. Monitoring must also be increased if conditions exist that alter gut flora (with vitamin K formation), absorption, or hepatic function as these each can affect production of coagulation proteins by the liver and thus the patient's warfarin requirements. Some data exists to indicate that generic warfarin and proprietary Coumadin may not always have equivalent effects [21], raising the potential for concern any time formulation substitution occurs. This may account for excursions out of the therapeutic range when formulation substitution takes place and/or the need to increase PT surveillance if substitution is encountered by the physician. Furthermore, current anticoagulation guidelines leave unsettled many other aspects of warfarin therapy frequently encountered by physicians, such as the optimal anticoagulant coverage to be used during warfarin initiation prior to attaining adequate anticoagulant effects or the optimal approach to be used during periods where warfarin must be withheld and then restarted because of an intercurrent invasive procedure.

Under use of and additional management difficulties with warfarin

Because of the above concerns and issues, many AF patients with embolic risk markers who should be given warfarin often are not. In some reports this has amounted to under use in approximately 40% or more of appropriate patients [22–24]. Warfarin is often not used when physicians perceive a likely or demonstrated problem with patient compliance with medications and/or PT follow-up or when physicians perceive an undue alteration in the risk/benefit ratio such that an enhanced likelihood of bleeding is suspected because of neurological disturbances, occupational or recreational hazards, and the like.

Even when warfarin is used appropriately, it is difficult to manage adequately. Patient noncompliance, food interactions, drug interactions, formulation variability (all noted above), plus the effects of intercurrent illnesses can each contribute to significant PT variability and international normalized ratios (INRs) deviating above and below the target therapeutic range. In light of the above reasons, safer, more consistent, more user-friendly, effective alternatives to warfarin have long been desired by physicians and by patients with AF. Currently, several alternatives to warfarin are being examined (Table 2.2). They include combinations of antiplatelet agents, factor Xa inhibitors, direct thrombin inhibitors (DTIs), catheter-implanted left atrial appendage occluders (which ultimately endothelialize), and left atrial resection or plication. While the physical approaches directed at the left atrial appendage are appealing, unless atrial clot only forms in the appendage, these approaches may merely reduce the risk but not abolish it, and therefore may not eliminate the need for anticoagulant therapy. Large long-term clinical trials to address this issue have not yet been performed. Thus, pharmacologic alternatives to warfarin remain prominent targets of investigation, at least for the near-term future. The ideal such agent would likely have at least the following characteristics:

- Maximal efficacy
- Rapid establishment of anticoagulation and rapid offset of action
- Minimal risk
- Minimal side effects
- Simple administration
- Predictable response within and among patients
- No food interactions
- No drug interactions
- No coagulation test monitoring
- Cost effectiveness.

While no such agent currently exists, the pharmacologic approaches being examined include the combination of aspirin and clopidogrel, in the ACTIVE trial [25]; a once-weekly parenteral factor Xa–specific pentasaccharide [26], idraparinux compared with vitamin K antagonists in patients with AF in the AMADEUS trial [27]; and DTIs [28–45], such as the oral DTI, ximelagatran, in the SPORTIF trials [45–48]. ACTIVE has a two-armed protocol consisting of: ACTIVE W (warfarin indicated) – 6500 patients, studying the antiplatelet combination versus the vitamin K antagonist warfarin – and ACTIVE A (warfarin not indicated) – 7500 patients, studying the combination versus aspirin alone. Enrollment began in 2003. The discussion above concerning platelet factors as being lesser in number that those hemochemical changes in AF which require warfarin to address may suggest that the combination being studied in ACTIVE could ultimately be found to have limited utility. AMADEUS is a multicenter, randomized, open label, noninferior, phase 3 study of 5700 patients undergoing treatment for 6–24 months with idraparinux compared with warfarin in patients with AF, with a primary endpoint of stroke and systemic emboli. However, parenteral injections are likely to have less appeal and compliance than a simple, effective, oral program, which may limit the utility of the results of this trial. Unfortunately, oral factor Xa agents are not yet available for investigation.

Thus, the oral thrombin inhibitors now under development appear most likely to approximate the ideal anticoagulant profile noted above in contrast to the other agents being studied. The latest of the oral thrombin inhibitors in its clinical studies is ximelagatran [28–45]. Ximelagatran has been approved for use in several European countries. Data for this agent was submitted to the FDA for consideration for US approval in 2004. The initial response of the FDA advisory committees

Table 2.2 Alternatives to warafarin currently being explored for patients with AF.

New antiplatelet strategies (combination therapy)
Oral (in clinical trials)
Factor Xa inhibitors
Parenteral (in clinical trials)
Oral (not yet available for study)
Oral thrombin inhibitors
Oral (in clinical trials)
Catheter-implanted left atrial occlusion devices
Surgical (thoracoscopic) left atrial appendage resection or plication

was to request additional information to be acquired and made available concerning ximelagatran, and not to approve it for release at this time. Further trials with it may be needed. Importantly, ximelagatran's clinical data with regard to its anticoagulation profile in both AF and venous thromboembolism treatment and prophylaxis did suggest significant efficacy and importance for AF patients. It was felt that additional long-term safety information and analysis was needed.

Since ximelagatran has proven efficacious for anticoagulation in AF patients, and since it is likely that it, or another DTI, will ultimately become available for use in the United States before another type of oral anticoagulant dose becomes available, the experience to date with ximelagatran will be detailed below. This will not only familiarize the reader with this agent but will also show it as a potential model for DTI in general, with regard to the nature of trials that will be needed for approval and the issues that clinicians will face should this agent reach the American marketplace. Specifically, a discussion of the AF studies with this agent, the SPORTIF trials [45–48], will follow, as will a discussion of the implementation considerations that would have to take place if a warfarin alternative (regardless of whether or not it is ximelagatran) does become available. Please recall that in the sections below the reader must keep in mind that it may be ximelagatran and/or it may be another DTI that eventually receives FDA approval for clinical use in the United States. and that at this point in time ximelagatran in this discussion is only being used as a model to introduce the concepts that will have to be considered in any new era of anticoagulation. If it is another agent, then the material discussed below with regard to pharmacokinetics, uses in renal and hepatic dysfunction, interactions, etc. would have to be modified according to the profile possessed by the alternative agent.

Thrombin plays a central role in thrombogenesis as a final step in the coagulation pathway and may be active in both the circulating and clot-bound form [28–35]. DTIs have been and are continually developed both as oral alternatives to warfarin and as parenteral alternatives to heparin and low molecular weight heparins since the latter remain less than optimally effective being unable to inactivate clot-bound thrombin. Moreover, warfarin and heparinoids act at multiple targets within the coagulation sequence with efficacy rates that are influenced by many patient variables. By targeting a single coagulation factor, the DTIs are expected to provide a more reliable response. By inhibiting thrombin, they inhibit thrombin-mediated activation of factors V, VIII, XIII, fibrinogen, and platelets. They do not induce thrombocytopenia as is sometimes seen with heparin congeners. Three DTIs have already been approved and are available for clinical use: hirudin, bivalrudin, and argatroban. Each of these is administered intravenously and each has been used in unstable coronary syndromes and for the prevention of postoperative venous thromboembolism.

Ximelagatran is the prodrug form of melagatran and has a pharmacokinetic profile as follows [28–35]. Ximelagatran is better absorbed (in the small intestine) than the poorly absorbed melagatran, and is then rapidly converted to melagatran, the active agent, which is a synthetic active site-directed inhibitor of thrombin. There have been no age, race, weight, or gender differences in melagatran's pharmacokinetics. So far, ximelagatran has no known food or drug interactions aside from erythromycin and zithromycin, which increase its absorption. Peak levels are seen within 30 min after taking ximelagatran orally and peak melagatran levels are achieved within 2–3 h, regardless of whether the pill is taken intact, crushed, or dissolved. Of the peak concentration, 20–30% is still apparent at 12 hours, which is still above the minimal therapeutic level required, thus allowing bid dosing. Melagatran is excreted primarily via the kidneys (80%) with a plasma half-life of 3–5 h (up to 9 h with renal impairment) and is not metabolized by the cytochrome P450 system, nor does it affect or is it affected by drugs that are. Melagatran has a linear dose/AUC relationship and has minimal binding to plasma proteins (<15%), unlike warfarin. The pharmacokinetic variables have been studied for reproducibility and have proven stable over time with very low intrapatient variability. These pharmacokinetic characteristics provide for a profile that has rapid onset of action (a few hours), steady-state effects after 1 day dosing, and the ability to washout effective anticoagulation by holding 2–3 doses before a procedure but have adequate reanticoagulation with readministration of 1–2 doses. The drug can be removed by dialysis or charcoal hemofiltration.

Clinical trials with ximelagatran in AF

To date, ximelagatran has been studied in clinical trials for the treatment of venous thromboembolism and for prophylactic prevention of phlebitis and venous thromboembolism after large joint orthopedic surgery in high-risk patients [36–39]. In each of these circumstances it has compared favorably with conventional therapies (enoxaparin, daltaparin, warfarin). Ximelagatran has shown similar to superior rates of efficacy with similar to lower rates of bleeding [36–39]. FDA approval for ximelagatran for these indications is being sought.

Ximelagatran has also been studied for the prevention of systemic thromboembolism in patients with nonvalvular (nonrheumatic) AF (excluding patients with prosthetic heart valves or anticipated elective cardioversion) in the SPORTIF program, consisting of the SPORTIF II, III, IV, and V trials [45–48]:

- SPORTIF II: a dose-guiding trial
- SPORTIF IV: a long-term follow-up trial of patients in SPORTIF II
- SPORTIF III: an open-label trial studying the efficacy of ximelagatran versus warfarin in AF patients with high-risk markers
- SPORTIF V: a double-blind trial studying the efficacy of ximelagatran versus warfarin in AF patients with high-risk markers.

SPORTIF II

SPORTIF II [45] was a 12 week, randomized, parallel-group, dose-guiding study of nonvalvular AF patients with at least one high-risk marker (see above) for stroke and systemic embolism, most commonly hypertension. The primary endpoint was the number of thromboembolic events and bleeding episodes. Three groups (n = 187) received ximelagatran at 20 (n = 59), 40 (n = 62), or 60 (n = 66) mg twice a day, given in double-blind fashion without coagulation test monitoring. The fourth group, given warfarin (n = 67] was managed and monitored to achieve and maintain INR values in the 2.0–3.0 range. A total of 254 patients received the study drug. One nonfatal ischemic stroke and one TIA occurred in the ximelagatran patients. One major bleed occurred in the warfarin patients. The number of total bleeds (major plus minor) was low in both groups, with a slight dose-related trend in the ximelagatran arms. The 60 mg bid group resulted in the same bleeding event rate as warfarin. SPORTIF IV is a long-term [5 years) continuation of SPORTIF II for patients who elected to remain on study drug, at 36 mg bid of ximelagatran (n = 125) versus INR-adjusted warfarin (n = 42). To date, the rate of significant bleeding has been less with ximelagatran than with warfarin. In these trials, ximelagatran has occasionally been associated with elevations of hepatic chemistries. ALT was increased to >3 times the upper limit of normal in eight patients taking ximelagatran in SPORTIF II, but resolved in both those who did and who did not discontinue the drug. Much more data regarding such observations is available from the SPORTIF III and V trials [46–48] and from the venous thrombosis trials.

SPORTIF III and V

The SPORTIF III and V trials [46–48] were designed to compare long-term ximelagatran with warfarin in high-risk AF patients (similar to SPORTIF II) with nonvalvular AF. Total enrollment was 7329 patients. SPORTIF III was carried out in 260 centers in 23 non-North American nations and included a total of 3467 patients. SPORTIF V involved 410 centers in the Unites States and Canada. SPORTIF III compared open-label ximelagatran, 36 mg bid and dose-adjusted warfarin (INR target 2.0–3.0).

SPORTIF V studied double-blind, double-dummy ximelagatran 36 mg bid and dose-adjusted warfarin, where each patient took two agents:either bid ximelagatran and dummy warfarin (with sham PTs) or dummy ximelagatran and active warfarin (with real PTs). In both trials, the primary outcome events were all strokes and systemic emboli. In both studies, secondary endpoints included death, stroke, emboli, myocardial infarction (a composite endpoint), ischemic stroke, TIA, emboli (another composite endpoint), and any bleed or treatment cessation. Tertiary endpoints included disabling stroke, and stroke or emboli in patients who were at least 75 years old. SPORTIF III and V were designed as noninferiority trials.

In SPORTIF III [46, 47], 91% of ximelagatran patients had persistent AF versus 93% with warfarin; about 40% in each arm had cardioversion attempted at some point prior to randomization. The duration of AF was <1 year in 22% and 21% of ximelagatran and warfarin patients respectively, and 1–5 and >5 years in 44/44% and 33/35% respectively. Patients had to have at least two ECGs demonstrating AF in order to enter the trial with at least one within 2 weeks of randomization. Of the patients, 66% had two or more risk markers (see above) with hypertension being the most common. In the warfarin patients, the time in range for the INRs was 66% for INR 2.0–3.0 and 81% for INR 1.8–3.2.The demographics for SPORTIF V patients were virtually identical.

In SPORTIF III [46, 47], by intention to treat analysis, the primary endpoint stroke and systemic emboli was reached in 56 (2.3%/year) warfarin patients and 40 (1.6%/year) ximelagatran patients by 21 months of follow-up ($p < .05$ for noninferiority and .10 for superiority for ximelagatran versus warfarin). By on-therapy analysis the results were 52 (2.2%/year) and 29 (1.3%/year) for warfarin and ximelagatran, respectively ($p = .018$). There was no significant difference for patients over the age of 75 versus those younger than 75 years. For the composite endpoint of stroke, systemic emboli, or death (time to first event) there was a trend favoring ximelagatran (124 warfarin patients, 103 ximelagatran patients ($p = .18$) by intention to treat analysis and 116 warfarin versus 96 ximelagatran patients ($p > .2$). For an analysis of either primary event or major bleed or death, the rates were 4.6%/year for ximelagatran versus 6.1%/year for warfarin ($p = .022$) by on-therapy analysis, a relative risk reduction of approximately 25% favoring ximelagatran. Intracerebral bleeding was 0.2% for ximelagatran and 0.5% for warfarin ($p = ns$). Major bleeding was 1.3 versus 1.8% for ximelagatran versus warfarin ($p = ns$). Any bleeding was 25.5% for ximelagatran versus 29.5% for warfarin ($p = .007$), mainly representing hematuria, epistaxis, and bruising. The incidence of congestive heart failure (2.9% versus 3.9%/year) and myocardial infarction (1.0% versus 0.5%/year) and total mortality (3.2% versus 3.2%/year) were not statistically different for ximelagatran versus warfarin, respectively.

The results in SPORTIF V [48] were very similar, that is, again ximelagatran proved to be noninferior to warfarin. By intention to treat analysis, the primary endpoint (stroke and systemic emboli) was reached in 37 (1.2%/year) warfarin patients and 51 (1.6%/year) ximelagatran patients by 24 months of follow-up ($p = .13$ for ximelagatran versus warfarin). The p-value for on-therapy analysis was .9. Intracerebral bleeding was 0.06% for ximelagatran and 0.06% for warfarin ($p = ns$). Major bleeding was 2.4% versus 3.1% for ximelagatran versus warfarin ($p = ns$). Any bleeding was 37% for ximelagatran versus 47% for warfarin ($p < .0001$), mainly representing hematuria, epistaxis, and bruising.

As with SPORTIF III, elevations in ALT to >3 times normal was seen with ximelagatran (6.0%) (versus 0.8% with warfarin, $p < .001$) in SPORTIF V [48], almost all of which was again in the first 6 months. Elevations in hepatic enzymes were handled in the same way in SPORTIF V as in SPORTIF III, and again the ALT values dropped in patients who either stopped drug or who remained on it.

Because of the identical inclusion and exclusion criteria in SPORTIF III and V and the identical approach to data analysis, the SPORTIF program planned a pooled analysis of both trials a *priori*. When the data for SPORTIF III and V were pooled, the results were consistent with the independent data from each trial [46–48]. For example, ximelagatran and warfarin were essentially identical for the primary endpoint, by intention to treat analysis, with a risk reduction favoring ximelagatran of only 0.03 ($p = .94$). The incidence of major bleeding in the pooled dataset was 2.5% with warfarin and 1.9% with ximelagatran ($p = .054$). The incidence of total bleeding was again less with ximelagatran. In addition, an analysis was done on the combined dataset of what was termed the "net clinical benefit," that is, the total of primary endpoints, major bleeding, and death. The total of these events indicated that ximelagatran was the preferable agent, being 6.2% with warfarin and 5.2% with ximelagatran ($p = .038$).

SPORTIF III, and V [46–48], therefore, would appear to support the following conclusions:

In nonvalvular AF patients with high-risk markers for emboli, ximelagatran is at least as effective as INR-dosed warfarin in preventing stroke and systemic emboli.

Ximelagatran is associated with less bleeding.
Ximelagatran offers fixed dose oral administration without coagulation test monitoring.
Ximelagatran appears to require monitoring of hepatic function during its administration.

However, precise advice to physicians with regard to the handling of hepatic testing and any abnormalities encountered awaits ultimate determination by the FDA following any resubmission of this agent. Certainly, monitoring of liver function for a short period of time, were that to be the outcome (with withdrawal of the agent if hepatic abnormalities are encountgered) would likely be less onerous than life-long monitoring of the INR as is required with warfarin.

What can we expect if ximelagatran (or an alternative DTI) is approved and released for use by the FDA?

If ximelagatran (or an alternative DTI) is approved for use by the FDA, practitioners will require assistance in integrating the drug into their clinical practice. If we assume that such approval is forthcoming, and if we limit our discussion to the use of ximelagatran (as a model for a DTI) in AF patients, the following questions will need to be addressed: (1) Which patients will be candidates for treatment with ximelagatran and which patients will not? (2) What process(es) will be required to transfer a patient from warfarin to ximelagatran? (3) Which patients might possibly require transfer from ximelagatran to warfarin, and how?

Because of ximelagatran's short half-life pharmacokinetic profile, as was reviewed above to some extent we might model the approach to the latter two questions on our experience in shifting between heparin or low molecular weight heparin congeners and warfarin.

Which AF patients will be candidates for ximelagatran?

Patients with AF who will be candidates for ximelagatran (or another DTI) will include: (1) those AF patients with markers of increased risk for thromboembolic events, as were noted above *and* (2) who do not have any of the exclusion criteria that were used in the pivotal SPORTIF III and V trials [46–48]. The former includes those patients with AF who are now considered for treatment with warfarin, while the exclusions used in SPORTIF will somewhat reduce this group. To enrich their population for events, the SPORTIF III and V trials modified the risk identifiers and only enrolled patients with persistent or paroxysmal chronic nonvalvular AF plus one or more of the following: prior stroke, TIA, or SEE; hypertension; LV dysfunction; 75 years or more of age; 65 years or more of age with diabetes or coronary artery disease. The exclusion criteria in SPORTIF III and V, which were for ethical reasons as well as to provide an enriched population for events, included patients under the age of 18 years, pregnant patients, patients who were to undergo elective cardioversion, patients with prosthetic heart valves, and patients with chronic valvular heart disease (primarily rheumatic). It is unlikely that ximelagatran will be approved by the FDA for use in patients who possess the criteria used for exclusion in SPORTIF because ximelagatran's utility has not yet been proven in these populations.

Which AF patients will not be candidates for ximelagatran (or another DTI)?

The above problems notwithstanding, ximelagatran was proven noninferior to warfarin in a wide spectrum of patients, both with AF and with venous thromboembolic disorders [36, 39, 46–55], and it seems highly likely that the same relationship would also hold true in most AF patient groups where the two agents have not yet been tested head to head. Thus, it is likely that ximelagatran (or another DTI) will ultimately be used off-label in clinical practice in some additional patient groups, such as those with valvular heart disease (excluding those with prosthetic heart valves) and in those who are to undergo elective cardioversion but are otherwise identical to the population described above. Currently, prospective phase 4 studies with ximelagatran are being planned – including a cardioversion trial. Nonetheless, for ethical reasons related to uncertain effects on a fetus or uncertain efficacy in the setting of an intracardiac foreign body, some AF groups should be excluded from even off-label treatment with ximelagatran, were it to be released, such as pregnant or lactating patients and patients with prosthetic heart valves. The same restrictions would hold true for any additional new alternative to warfarin unless trials including subjects inclusive of these conditions were part of the clinical development process with that agent and were positive.

Moreover, as for many pharmaceutical agents, pharmacokinetic and safety considerations will also limit the use of ximelagatran (or any other new alternative). More specifically, some patients might best be excluded from treatment with ximelagatran because of expected uncertainties or concerns regarding dosing or safety monitoring. Accordingly, ximelagatran should not be given to patients with an inability to evaluate changes in liver function tests due to hepatic disease or, perhaps, due to use of concomitant agents that could confound interpretation of hepatic function tests, since the clinical trial results with ximelagatran suggest that monitoring of ximelagatran's effects on hepatic function will be a requirement for its use. Ximelagatran would also best be avoided in patients with advanced or unstable renal disease because ximelagatran is a renally excreted agent. Additional exclusions that might be considered by the FDA would be those used in the SPORTIF III and V trials as contraindications to both ximelagatran and warfarin. These included: recent stroke or TIA (where the risk of creating a hemorrhagic infarct is a concern); acute coronary syndrome (where multiple other agents that affect coagulation, in a combined regimen, are standards of care at present); increased risk of bleeding; other contraindication to anticoagulation; recent drug addiction, alcohol abuse, or both; or breast feeding. (With regard to acute coronary syndromes, however, trials with ximelagatran are being performed and to date look promising.)

Which patients might switch from warfarin to ximelagatran?

Patients that are likely to be switched from warfarin to ximelagatran (or an alternative DTI) include: (1) patients noncompliant with PT testing schedules; (2) patients with an inability to achieve and maintain stable INR values; (3) patients with experienced or potential food or drug interactions with warfarin; (4) patients with nonbleeding complications of warfarin; (5) patients with a preference for ximelagatran; and (6) patients of physicians with a preference for ximelagatran.

Because ximelagatran is administered without the need for routine coagulation test monitoring [17, 41–56], it would be the preferred agent in patients currently treated with warfarin who are unreliable with PT monitoring schedules or in whom stable INR values in the target range cannot be achieved and maintained due to genetic resistance [57], bowel disease, dietary factors, concomitant therapeutic drug alterations, or the like. Such patients are likely to be switched from warfarin to ximelagatran. Although some blood test monitoring will be required when ximelagatran is used, such tests will primarily be related to hepatic function testing and are likely to be intensive only during the first 6 months of therapy. Therefore, the burden will be much reduced as compared to testing during warfarin treatment over the chronic course of administration. Additionally, because a multitude of compounds – prescription agents, over-the-counter drug, and dietary supplements – interact with warfarin, whereas ximelagatran has been free of food and drug interactions to date (excluding erythromycin and zithromycin), many patients using "polypharmacy" regimens are likely to be switched from warfarin to ximelagatran. In such subjects, the predictable and stable therapeutic levels with ximelagatran, in contrast to those with warfarin should enhance both ximelagatran's efficacy and safety profile as compared to warfarin's in this specific subgroup of patients. Finally, there are rare patients who have experienced nonbleeding complications from warfarin, including serious dermal reactions [58]. Such patients could be given ximelagatran instead. In light of the above, it is likely that many patients, when made aware of the features of ximelagatran, whether by their healthcare provider or by self-research using the Internet or other resources, will choose to terminate their current therapy with warfarin and be switched to ximelagatran as a preferable alternative. The ability to use a drug with a fixed dosing regimen – no need for coagulation test monitoring, no impact for restrictions on diet, and no interaction with the majority of drugs or supplements commonly encountered – will be incredibly attractive to most patients in contrast to the restrictions on life-style that warfarin therapy imposes.

Similarly, ximelagatran is likely to be more appealing to prescribers as well. An additional benefit for many physicians will be the ability to reduce the size, cost, and burden of running a coagulation monitoring program.

What process will be required to change from warfarin to ximelagatran (or an alternative DTI)?

Transferring a patient from warfarin to ximelagatran (or an alternative DTI) will have to be achieved through a consideration of their relative pharmacokinetic profiles. Elimination of warfarin effect (warfarin washout plus resynthesis of clotting proteins) will take longer than the attainment of steady state with ximelagatran [40, 43, 44, 59–61]. The elimination half-life of warfarin has been reported to be as long as 37–53 h [59–61], being somewhat variable due to different degrees of genetic sensitivity [59, 60].

In most patients in my experience it takes 48 h or more to become significantly subtherapeutic after discontinuing warfarin. In contrast (see above) ximelagatran dosing yields significant melagatran serum concentration and activity in 2–3 h [40, 43, 44]. Accordingly, and as determined by any sense of urgency, one would have to either accelerate the elimination of warfarin effect or delay the administration of ximelagatran until the INR is nearing the lower therapeutic margin. Thus, the options for changing from warfarin to ximelagatran could reasonably include:

- All patients: stop warfarin, give vitamin K, start ximelagatran in 12–24 h.
- Low-risk patients: discontinue warfarin and defer initiating ximelagatran until the risk of bleeding from combined therapeutic actions is presumed low enough, for example, until the INR is <2.0 (using daily INR monitoring), or for an arbitrary period of 3 days (which may depend upon the INR value when warfarin is stopped), or whichever comes first.
- High-risk patients: discontinue warfarin, then start ximelagatran after the INR is <2.5 (using daily INR monitoring).

High-risk patients might include those with a prior embolic stroke or SEE, or with multiple other ACCP or ACC/AHA/ESC risk markers [17–20]. The above suggestions are formulated on considerations of minimizing embolic risk upon warfarin discontinuation while minimizing bleeding potential during the period of overlap of the therapeutic agents' actions. They are similar to the approaches commonly used in my experience when transferring a patient from warfarin to LMWH (which also act rapidly and require no routine coagulation monitoring). Notably, if upon approval of ximelagatran by the FDA, the package insert for ximelagatran offers alternative suggestions for transferring patients from warfarin to ximelagatran, they should be strongly considered.

Which patients might require changing from ximelagatran (or an alternative DTI) to warfarin?

Patients who might need to be changed from ximelagatran to (or back to) warfarin will include those who develop a contraindication specifically to ximelagatran, but not to a strategy of anticoaglulation, those who develop a transient change in circumstances where data or custom might be interpreted as showing a preference for warfarin, or those where cost considerations favor generic warfarin. Progressive renal insufficiency or the unusual patient with persistent significant elevations of hepatic function tests during ximelagatan administration would be examples of the first group. Patients who are to undergo elective cardioversion might be an example of the second group if the physician involved does not use ximelagatran off-label for anticoagulation during the pre- and post-cardioversion period. Cost issues may become the determining factor for some self-pay patients and also for managed-care patients if ximelagatran is a noncovered agent whereas warfarin is fully covered. However, in circumstances where cost is a factor in the determination of which anticoagulant to use, one would hope that the total cost of care (i.e., the cost of the drug and of monitoring plus the differential medical costs for embolic events and bleeds due to their different anticipated incidences with each agent), would be appropriately considered.

How would one change from ximelagatran to warfarin?

Because it takes 6–60 h to inhibit the synthesis of the clotting proteins altered by warfarin while ximelagatran has anticoagulant effect in 2–5 h and is at steady state by 24 hours [40, 43, 44, 61–63], there will need to be some overlap of therapy when transferring a patient from ximelagatran to warfarin, and it may vary with whether or not warfarin loading is utilized. Using the model of overlap with heparin during warfarin loading seems reasonable. That is, one should begin warfarin before discontinuing ximelagatran, and discontinue ximelagatran when the INR approaches or reaches the therapeutic range (using a similar set of values as was discussed above in the section on switching from warfarin to ximelagatran).

Additional practical issues that will require consideration by clinicians upon the availability of ximelagatran (or an alternative DTI)

If ximelagatran (or an alternative DTI) is approved by the FDA and is widely accepted by clinicians for the anticoagulation of high-risk AF patients, several additional management issues are likely to become particular concerns for physicians and will have to be addressed. They will include the approach to the patient with new onset AF and the approach to conditions that require dose adjustments or assessment, such as:

- Temporary interruption of therapy for a procedure
- Management during a bleeding episode or following an acute stroke
- Changing renal function
- Missed doses
- Alterations in hepatic function studies
- Assessing dosing compliance.

New onset AF

The current approach to anticoagulation in a patient with new onset AF is usually dichotomized by a 48 h window [17]. If AF is known to be present for less than 48 h, cardioversion is generally carried out without anticoagulation. If, however, the duration of AF is longer than 48 h or its duration is uncertain, then current practice employs anticoagulation prior to elective cardioversion for a period of at least 3 weeks during which the INR is consistently >2.0, plus anticoagulation following cardioversion, or a strategy of transesophageal echocardiography (TEE) with immediate cardioversion (with postconversion anticoagulation) if atrial thrombus is absent, but delayed cardioversion following anticoagulation as above if atrial thrombus is detected [17].

The availability of ximelagatran, with its rapid onset of action, could alter the approach to new onset AF if data in this circumstance were available and it was used off-label in this setting. Since the onset of ximelagatran's effects is almost as rapid as with heparin, if the TEE were negative, then for new onset AF of >48 h duration, one might initiate ximelagatran, cardiovert, and continue on ximelagatran rather than having to initiate anticoagulation with a heparinoid plus warfarin, then discontinue the heparin compound when the INR reached 2.0, continue the warfarin for a month or more, and finally transfer the therapy to ximelagatran under an FDA approved indication. The latter is clearly less convenient but is consistent with currently available data, and will probably remain the officially sanctioned approach until a positive postmarketing phase 4 cardioversion trial is performed with ximelagatran. Alternatively, but still off-label, for new onset AF >48 h, one could initiate therapy with ximelagatran and cardiovert electively in 3 weeks. This would contrast with the approach of using warfarin without a TEE only in that with warfarin, the INR must be 2.0 or higher for 3 consecutive weeks prior to the cardioversion, which often requires 4–6 weeks in actuality because of the variability in warfarin requirements and the time it takes to achieve a stable INR value. Additionally, with new AF of recognized onset, one could initiate ximelagatran at the onset of symptoms. Full anticoagulation would be achieved within 24 h. The 48 h dichotomy period of unanticoagulated AF would become irrelevant for such patients, and cardioversion could then be performed as early as convenient, but would not have to be within the 48 h window. The role for TEE in such a circumstance would cease to exist. For AF without clear recognition of onset, TEE guided or delayed cardioversion would still be required.

Temporary interruption of therapy for a procedure

When an invasive procedure is to be performed in a patient taking warfarin, anticoagulation must be withheld for several days [64, 65] so as to eliminate the risk of excessive bleeding. In high-risk patients, heparin coverage is employed during the immediate pre- and postprocedure period of warfarin washout and reinitiation, holding the heparin only for the relatively short time it takes for elimination of heparin effect (i.e. 12 h or less). If ximelagatran were used instead of warfarin, the protocol would be much simpler. Since ximelagatran's effect is gone within 24 h, and its effects begin again approximately 2 h after reinitiation of therapy, one could hold ximelagatran 1 day before the procedure and restart it the night of or the day after the procedure (or when bleeding risk is felt to be acceptable). Heparin coverage would not be required. Additionally, one would avoid as long a period of subtherapeutic anticoagulation (2 days or more) as would follow warfarin discontinuation in the absence of heparin coverage.

Handling of ximelagatran during a bleeding event

As with the use of any anticoagulant, an acute bleeding event will usually signal the need to interrupt anticoagulation therapy. If the bleed were significant, ideally the effect of the agent being employed would be quickly reversible. This is the model of using vitamin K or fresh frozen plasma (FFP) to reverse warfarin's effects or protamine administration to reverse heparin's effects during such a circumstance. However, there is no direct "antidote" for ximelagatran. Accordingly, if bleeding occurs in a patient taking ximelagatran, ximelagatran should be discontinued, and the patient supported hemodynamically, with transfusion if necessary, until drug washout occurs (by 24 h) and/or the bleeding ceases. FFP can be employed, but because of the relatively large safety margin (see above) with achieved ximelagatran concentrations, FFP may not be effective. Importantly, ximelagatran, can be removed by dialysis and by charcoal hemofiltration, thus accelerating the termination of its anticoagulant action [66].

Ximelagatran dosing with renal dysfunction

Because ximelagatran is a renally excreted drug and its serum concentrations and actions increase substantially with significantly impaired renal function, patients with a creatinine clearance of <30 cc/min will require a modified dosing schedule. Possible responses would be to change to a once a day dose (i.e. 36 mg qd instead of bid) or to half the bid dose to 18 mg bid. It will be important to examine the package insert for the FDA instructions that are expected to be included with regard to this circumstance. Note, this circumstance would not be limited only to those with chronic renal disease but would also apply to those in whom renal function impairment is expected to be transient, as following an angiographic dye reaction. If one were uncertain as to whether the lower dose was sufficient, one could perform a thrombin time, as the thrombin time does have a roughly linear correlation with ximelagatran serum concentration. Of note, however, mildly elevated ximelagatran levels may not be of concern for short periods of time. In the ESTEEM trial of ximelagatran in acute coronary syndromes [54], where a wider dosing range was utilized than is used for AF (in combination with aspirin therapy), excessive short-term bleeding events and disconcerting hepatic impairment were not noted.

Handling of a patient who misses a dose of ximelagatran

One missed dose of ximelagatran does not have to be made up. The levels attained with the recommended 36 mg bid dosing regimen provide a margin of error that covers one missed dose (see section on assessing dosing compliance below). Missing more than one dose, however, will be associated with loss of adequate anticoagulant effect. In the event of a missed dose, the next dose can be taken early (with the dosing clock then being reset) or can be taken on time. Extra doses should be avoided.

Ximelagatran and hepatic dysfunction

The pharmacokinietics of ximelagatran in normal subjects and in liver-impaired patients appears to be similar [67]. The bioconversion of ximelagatran to melagatran has not been found to be altered in such subjects. Accordingly, except in patients with severe hepatic failure, it is unlikely that a dose adjustment of ximelagatran will be required. Nonetheless, after FDA approval of ximelagatran and its package insert, the clinician should consult the package insert to verify that specific recommendations have not been included upon the FDA's review of the total database experience with this agent. Of greater concern is the observation that in some patients, ximelagatran has been associated with the development of alterations in hepatic function tests, most notably the ALT level as was reviewed above in the description of the SPORTIF program results, and as was seen in the drug's other clinical trials [46–56]. Thus, although ximelagatran does not require monitoring of coagulation tests during its administration, and does not require a dosing adjustment in patients with hepatic dysfunction, ximelagatran will require monitoring of hepatic function tests during its administration. Because the increased enzyme levels occur predominantly during the first 2–6 months of exposure and such elevations have usually subsided with or without drug discontinuation [46–56], it is likely that monitoring will be required most frequently during this time period. In SPORTIF, the liver function testing protocol called for:

1 Baseline liver function testing (enzyme levels above twice normal excluded enrollment).
2 Laboratory testing monthly for the first 6 months, then every other month up to 1 year, then every 3 months.
3 If elevation of a hepatic function test was >3 times the upper level of normal, repeat testing was performed weekly until resolution or until determination of alternative cause.
4 Ximelagatran was discontinued per protocol if any level >5 times the upper level of normal was seen or if an increase between 3 and 5 times the upper level of normal persisted for 8 weeks, of if there was any associated clinical sign of hepatotoxicity.

Although what form the final recommendations will take in the package is not yet certain, is seems reasonable to assume that they will be similar to those used in the clinical trials since such guidelines appeared to protect against any clinically important adverse hepatic outcomes. Thus the clinician who prescribes ximelagatran should consult with, and follow, the recommendations for hepatic function testing that are ultimately included in the package insert.

Assessing compliance during treatment with ximelagatran

Coagulation tests are not used to monitor ximelagatran dosing or effectiveness. Coagulation tests, however, can be used to assess compliance [40, 43, 44, 66, 68]. Thrombin times, activated partial thromboplastin times (APTT), and the ACT are probably the most useful. Although melagatran's effects can increase the APTT, the relationship is highly variable to use the APTT to monitor therapy. The APTT will normalize if the last dose was missed (and thus may help in assessing patient compliance). The thrombin time is very sensitive to prolongation with melagatran and is too sensitive to use to assess whether serum concentrations are in the desired range. A normal thrombin time, however, can indicate that there is no meaningful level of the drug in the patient. Thrombin times are almost linearly related to the plasma melagatran concentration [66, 68]. While the thrombin time is not used for monitoring or to target dosing, it can confirm that the patient has been taking ximelagatran. Thrombin times lower than 100–125 s are usually associated with melagatran levels below the minimum effective level of approximately 0.05 micromol/l. The ACT is too sensitive to confirm that a dose has been recent, but it can confirm that ximelagatran has been taken. More specifically, the ACT will begin to become elevated at plasma melagatran concentrations as low as 0.03 micromol/l. At doses of 36 mg bid of ximelagatran, serum concentrations of melagatran will almost always remain above the 0.05 micromol/l concentration for almost 24 h after a dose (see the section on missed doses, above), and will remain above 0.03 micromol/l for somewhat longer. In contrast, the APTT begins to become elevated at melagatran serum concentrations approximating 0.05 micromol/l. Thus, it should be more than marginally elevated if the last dose had been taken, as the serum level should still be well above the 0.05 micromol/l range.

Concluding comments

From the material presented above, it should be clear to the reader that the availability of oral thrombin inhibition as an alternative to the use of warfarin will usher in a new and exciting era in chronic anticoagulation. This era should be one in which efficacy with regard to prevention of thromboembolic events is preserved but one in which lesser adverse events from therapy and fewer inconveniences for patients and physicians alike is achieved. Release of a new anticoagulant alternative to warfarin will not likely occur if these conditions are not met. Additionally, from the material presented above, it should be clear to the reader that the pharmacokinetic and pharmacodynamic profiles of warfarin and ximelagatran (or an alternative DTI) are significantly different such that the initiation of ximelagatran or any other new alternative into clinical practice will require the clinician to deal with this transition carefully and thoughtfully. Finally, it is hoped that the suggestions made above concerning the administration of ximelagatran will be useful guidelines for the clinician adopting this agent into his/her clinical practice.

References

1 Goldman ME, Pearce LA, Hart RG *et al.* Pathophysiologic correlates of thromboembolism in non-valvular atrial fibrillation: I. Reduced flow velocity in the left atrial appendage (The Stroke Prevention in Atrial Fibrillation [SPAF-III] study). *J Am Soc Echocardiol* 1999; **12**: 1080–1087.

2 Cai H, Li Z, Goette A *et al.* Downregulation of endocardial nitric oxide synthase expression and nitric oxide production in atrial fibrillation: potential mechanisms for atrial thrombosis and stroke. *Circulation* 2002; **106**: 2854 –2858.

3 Kamath S, Chin BS, Blann AD, Lip GY. A study of platelet activation in paroxysmal, persistent and permanent atrial fibrillation. *Blood Coag Fibrinolysis* 2002; **13**: 627 –636.

4 Kamath S, Blann AD, Caine GJ, Gurney D, Chin BS, Lip GY. Platelet P-selectin levels in relation to plasma soluble P-selectin and beta-thromboglobulin levels in atrial fibrillation. *Stroke* 2002; **33**: 1237–1242.

5 Roldan V, Marin F, Blann AD *et al.* Interleukin-6, endothelial activation and thrombogenesis in chronic atrial fibrillation. *Eur Heart J* 2003; **24**: 1373–1380.

6 Kamath S, Blann AD, Chin BS *et al.* A study of platelet activation in atrial fibrillation and the effects of antithrombotic therapy. *Eur Heart J* 2002; **23**: 1788–1795.

7 Li-Saw-Hee FL, Blann AD, Gurney D, Lip GY. Plasma von Willebrand factor, fibrinogen and soluble P-selectin levels in paroxysmal, persistent and permanent atrial fibrillation. Effects of cardioversion and return of left atrial function. *Eur Heart J* 2001; **22**: 1741–1747.

8 Al-Saady NM, Sopher M. Prothrombotic markers in atrial fibrillation: what is new? *Eur Heart J* 2001; **22**: 1635–1639.

9 Conway DS, Buggins P, Hughes E, Lip GY. Relationship of interleukin-6 and C-reactive protein to the prothrombotic state in chronic atrial fibrillation. *J Am Coll of Cardiol* 2004; **43**: 2075–2082.

10 Yamashita T, Sekiguchi A, Iwasaki YK *et al.* Thrombodulin and tissue factor pathway inhibitor in endocardium of rapidly paced rate atria. *Circulation* 2003; **108**: 2450–2452.

11 Wyse DG, Waldo AL, DiMarco JP *et al.* A comparison of rate control and rhythm control in patients with atrial fibrillation. *N Engl J Med* 2002; **347**: 1825–1833.

12 Van Gelder IC, Hagens VE, Bosker HA *et al.* A comparison of rate control and rhythm control in patients with recurrent persistent atrial fibrillation. *N Engl J Med* 2002; **347**: 1834–1840.

13 Gosselink AT, Crijns HJ, Hamer HP, Hillege H, Lie KI. Changes in left and right atrial size after cardioversion of atrial fibrillation: role of mitral valve disease. *J Am Coll Cardiol* 1993; **22**: 1666–1672.

14 Manning WJ, Silverman DI, Katz SE *et al.* Impaired left atrial mechanical function after cardioversion: relation to the duration of atrial fibrillation. *J Am Coll Cardiol* 1994; **23**: 1535–1540.

15 Pollak A, Falk RH. Aggravation of postcardioversion atrial dysfunction by sotalol. *J Am Coll Cardiol* 1995; **25**: 665–671.

16 Thomas L, Thomas SP, Hoy M, Boyd A, Schiller NB, Ross DL. Comparison of left atrial volume and function after linear ablation and after cardioversion for chronic atrial fibrillation. *Am J Cardiol* 2004; **93**: 165–170.

17 Fuster V, Ryden LE, Asinger RW *et al.* ACC/AHA/ESC Guidelines for the management of patients with atrial fibrillation: executive summary. A report of the American College of Cardiology/American Heart Association Task Force on Practice Guidelines and the European Society of Cardiology Committee for Practice Guidelines and Policy Conferences (Committee to Develop Guidelines for the Management of Patients with Atrial Fibrillation). Developed in collaboration with the North American Society of Pacing and Electrophysiology. *Circulation* 2001; **104**: 2118–2150.

18 Hart R, Halpern JL, Pearce LA *et al.* Lessons from the stroke prevention in atrial fibrillation trials. *Ann Intern Med* 2003; **128**: 8331–8838.

19 Connolly SJ. Prevention of vascular events in patients with atrial fibrillation: evidence, guidelines, and practice. *J Cardiovasc Electrophysiol* 2003; **14**: S52–S55.

20 Albers GW, Dalen JE, Laupacis A, Manning WJ, Petersen P, Singer DE. Antithrombotic therapy in atrial fibrillation. *Chest* 2001; **119**: 194S–206S.

21 Reiffel JA. Formulation substitution and other pharmacokinetic variability: under appreciated variables affecting antiarrhythmic drug efficacy and safety in clinical practice. *Am J Cardiol* 2000; **85**: 46D–52D.

22 Portnoi VA. The underuse of warfarin treatment in the elderly. *Arch Intern Med* 1999; **159**: 1374–1375.

23 Ono A, Fujita T. Stroke prevention in patients with atrial fibrillation. *J Clin Neurosci* 2003; **10**: 71–73.

24 Buckingham TA, Hatala R. Anticoagulants for atrial fibrillation: why is the treatment rate so low? *Clin Cardiol* 2002; **25**: 447–454.

25 Hohnloser SH, Connolly SJ. Combined antiplatelet therapy in atrial fibrillation: review of the literature and future avenues. *J Cardiovasc Electrophysiol* 2003; **4**: S60–S63.

26 Weitz JI, Hirsh J. New anticoagulant drugs. *Chest* 2001; **119**: 95S–107S.

27 AMADEUS. A safety and efficacy trial evaluating the use of SanOrg34006 compared to warfarin or acenocoumarol in patients with atrial fibrillation. 2004. www.clinicaltrials.gov

28 Bauer KA. Selective inhibition of coagulation factors: advances in antithrombotic therapy. *Semin Thromb Hemost* 2002; **28**: 15–25.

29 Heit JA. Mapping out the future in venous thromboembolism and acute coronary syndromes. *Semin Thromb Hemost* 2002; **28**: 33–39.

30 Nowak G. Clinical monitoring of hirudin and direct thrombin inhibitors. *Semin Thromb Hemost* 2001; **71**: 50–52.

31 Van Aken H, Bode C, Dariuis H *et al.* Anticoagulation: the present and future. *Clin Appl Thromb Hemost* 2001; **7**: 195–204.

32 Hauptmann J. Pharmacokinetics of an emerging new class of anticoagulant/antithrombotic drugs: a review of small-molecule thrombin inhibitors. *Eur J Clin Pharmacol* 2002; **57**: 751–758.

33 Smythe MA, Warkentin TE, Stephens JL *et al.* Venous limb gangerene during overlapping therapy with warfarin and a direct thrombin inhibitor for immune heparin-induced thrombocytopenia. *Am J Hematol* 2002; **71**: 50–52.

34 Rocha E, Panizo C, Lecumbern R. Inhibidores directos de la trombina: su papel en el tratamiento de la trombosis arterial y venosa. *Med Clin* (Barc). 2001; **116**: 63–75.

35 Weitz J, Crowther M. Direct thrombin inhibitors. *Thromb Res* 2002; **106**: V275–V284.

36 Eriksson BI, Arfwidsson AC, Frison L *et al.* A dose-ranging study of the oral direct thrombin inhibitor, ximelagatran, and its subcutaneous form, melagatran, compared with daltaprin in the prophylaxis of thromboembolism after hip or knee replacement: METHRO I. *Thromb Haemost* 2002; **87**: 231–237.

37 Heit J, Colwell CW, Francis CW *et al.* Comparison of the oral direct thrombin inhibitor ximelagatran with enoxaparin as prophylaxis against venous thromboembolism after total knee replacement. *Arch Intern Med* 2001; **161**: 2215–2221.

38 Francis CW, Davidson BL, Berkowitz SD *et al.* Ximelagatran versus warfarin for the prevention of venous thromboembolism after total knee arthroplasty. *Ann Intern Med* 2002; **137**: 648–655.

39 Eriksson BI, Agnelli G, Cohen AT *et al.* Direct thrombin inhibitor melagatran followed by oral ximelagatran in comparison with enoxaparin for prevention of venous thromboembolism after total hip or knee replacement: the METHRO III study. *Thromb Haemost* 2003; **89**: 228–296.

40 Eriksson UG, Bredberg U, Gislen K, Johanssson LC, Frison L, Ahnoff M, Gustafsson D. Pharmacokinetics and pharmacodynamics of ximelagatran, a novel oral direct thrombin inhibitor, in young healthy male subjects. *Eur J Clin Pharm* 2003; **59**: 35–43.

41 Nutescu EA, Wittkowsky AK. Direct thrombin inhibitors for anticoagulation. *Ann of Pharmacotherapy* 2004; **38**: 99–109.

42 Hrebickobca L, Nawarskas JJ, Anderson JR. Ximelagatran: a new oral anticoagulant. *Heart Dis* 2003; **5**: 397–408.

43 Gustafsson D, Elg M. The pharmacodynamics and pharmacokinetics of the oral thrombin ximelagatran and its active metabolite melagatran. *Thromb Res* 2003; **109**: 9–15.

44 Wolzt M, Wollbratt M, Svensson M, Wahlander K, Grind M, Eriksson UG. Consistent pharmacokinetics of the oral direct thrombin inhibitor ximelagatran in patients with non-valvular atrial fibrillation and in healthy subjects. *Eur J Clin Pharm* 2003; **59**: 537–43.

45 Petersen P, Grind M, Adler J *et al.* Ximelagatran versus warfarin for stroke prevention in patients with non-valvular atrial fibrillation: SPORTIF II: a dose guiding, tolerability and safety study. *J Am Coll Cardiol* 2003; **41**: 1445–51.

46 Halperin JL. Executive Steering Committee, SPORTIF III and V Study Investigators. Ximelagatran compared with warfarin for prevention of thromboembolism in patients with non-valvular atrial fibrillation. Rationale, objectives, and design of a pair of clinical studies and baseline patient characteristics (SPORTIF III and V). *Am Heart J* 2003; **146**: 431–438.

47 Olsson SB, Executive Steering Committee on behalf of the SPORTIF II Investigators. Stroke prevention with the oral direct thrombin inhibitor ximelagatran compared with warfarin in patients with non-valvular atrial fibrillation (SPORTIF III): randomized controlled trial. *Lancet* 2003; **362**: 1691–1698.

48 Cleland JG, Feemantle, N, Kaye G *et al.* Clinical Trials update from the American Heart Association meeting: Omega-3 fatty acids and arrhythmia risk in patients with an implantable defibrillator. ACTIV in CHF, VALIANT, the Hanover autologous bone marrow transplantation study, SPORTIF V, ORBIT and PAD and DEFINITE. *Eur J Heart Fail* 2004; **6**: 109–115.

49 Shulman S, Wahlander K, Lundstrom T, Clason SB, Eriksson H. THRIVE III Investigators. Secondary prevention of venous thromboemolism with the oral direct thrombin inhibitor ximelagatran. *N Eng J Med* 2003; **349**: 1713–1721.

50 Francis CW, Berkowitz SD, Comp PC *et al.* EXULT A Study Group. Comparison of ximelagatran with warfarin for the prevention of venous thromboembolism after total knee replacement. *N Eng J Med* 2003; **349**: 1703–1712.

51 Eriksson BI. Clinical experience of melagatran/ximelagatran in major orthopedic surgery. *Thromb Res* 2003; **109**: 23–29.

52 Eriksson BI, Agnelli G, Cohen AT *et al.* EXPRESS Study Group. The direct thrombin inhibitor melagatran followed by oral ximelagatran compared with enoxaparin for the prevention of venous thromboembolism after total hop or knee replacement. *J Thromb Haemost* 2003; **1**: 2490–2496.

53 Francis CW, Berkowitz SD, Comp PC *et al.* EXULT A Study Group. Comparison of ximelagatran with warfarin for the prevention of venous thromboembolism after total knee replacement. *N Eng J Med* 2003; **349**: 1703–1712.

54 Wallentin L, Wilcox RG, Weaver WD *et al.* ESTEEM Investigators. Oral ximelagatran for secondary prophylaxis after myocardial infarction. *Lancet* 2003; **362**: 789–797.

55 Eriksson H, Wahlander K, Gustafsson D *et al.* A randomized, controlled, dose-guiding study of the oral direct thrombin inhibitor ximelagatran compared with standard therapy for the treatment of acute deep vein thrombosis: THRIVE I. *J Thromb Haemosta* 2003; **1**: 41–47.

56 Petersen P, Grind M, Adler J, SPORTIF II Investigators. Ximelagatran versus warfarin for stroke prevention in patients with non-valvular atrial fibrillation. *J Am Coll Cardiol* 2003; **41**: 1445–1451.

57 Linder MW. Genetic mechanisms for hypersensitivity and resistance to the anticoagulant warfarin. *Clinic Chimica Acta* 2001; **308**: 9–15.

58 Physicians Desk Reference: Monthly prescribing guide. 2004 (5); 1995.

59 Tiseo PJ, Foley K, Friedhoff LT. The effect of multiple doses of donepezil HC1 on the pharmacokinetic and pharmacdynamic profile of warfarin. *Brit J Clin Pharmacol* **198**; 46: 45–50.

60 Turck D, Su CA, Heinzl G, Busch U, Bluhmki E, Hoffman J. Lack of interaction between meloxicam and warfarin in healthy volunteers. *Eur J Clin Pharmacol* 1997; **51**: 421–5.

61 Bovill EG, Mann KG. Warfarin and the biochemistry of the vitamin K dependent proteins. *Adv Exp Med Biol* 1987; **214**: 17–46.

62 Liao S, Palmer M, Fowler C, Nayak RK. Absence of an effect of levofloxacin on warfarin pharmacokinetics and anticoagulation in male volunteers. *J Clin Pharm* 1996; **36**: 1072–1077.

63 Yacobi A, Wingard LB Jr, Levy G. Comparative pharmacokinetics of coumarin anticoagulants. X. Relationship between distribution, elimination, and anticoagulant action of warfarin. *J Pharm Sci* 1974; **63**: 868–872.

64 Spandorfer J. The management of anticoagulation before and after procedure. *Med Clin North Am* 2001; **85**: 1109–1116.

65 Reiffel JA. Will direct thrombin inhibitors replace warfarin for preventing embolic events in atrial fibrillation? *Curr Opin Cardiol* 2004; **19**: 58–63.

66 Data on file. Astra-Zeneca Pharmaceutical, LP. www.astrazeneca.com

67 Wahlander K, Eriksson-Lepkowska M, Frison L, Fager G, Eriksson UG. No influence of mild-to-moderate hepatic impairment on the pharmacokinetics and pharmacodynamics of ximelagatran, an oral direct thrombin inhibitor. *Clin Pharmacokinetics* 2003; **42**: 755–64.

68 Gustafsson D, Elg M. The pharmacodynamics and pharmacokinetics of the oral direct thrombin inhibitor ximelagatran and its active metabolic melagatran. *Thromb Res* 2003; **109**: S9–S15.

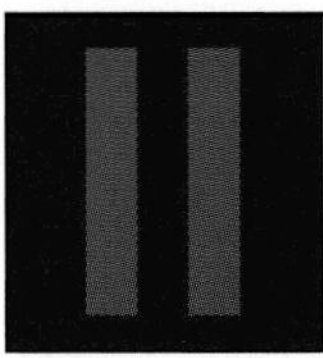

PART II

Future of antiarrhythmic therapy

CHAPTER 3

Principles of pharmacogenomics: Focus on arrhythmias

Dan M. Roden, MD

Genetics and variability in drug effects

The concept that drug therapy produces highly variable effects is well entrenched in the medical and lay communities, and the notion that genetic variants might contribute to this variability – the concept of "pharmacogenetics" – has been in place for decades [1]. Initial studies describing the role of DNA variants in modulating normal physiology or in drug responses focused on rare variants and extreme phenotypes. Such variants, which are often associated with congenital disease, are termed mutations. The sequencing of the first draft of the human genome, and the increasing appreciation of variants among individuals' genomes, has generated the much newer concept that multiple variants, acting together, may contribute to variability in drug action; this defines the more recent concept of "pharmacogenomics" [2–5]. These commoner variants, termed polymorphisms, are now increasingly well described and accessible through electronic databases. The most common type of polymorphism is a change in a single nucleotide, an SNP (single nucleotide polymorphism). SNPs, and other polymorphisms, may be located in coding or noncoding sequences and if in coding sequence may or may not alter function of the encoded protein in a discernible fashion. Polymorphisms in noncoding regions may nevertheless be functionally important, by altering the amount of protein generated by transcription of the gene in which they reside. Genomic science has also suggested one basis for variability in physiology or drug response across ethnicities. Some polymorphisms are detected in all ethnic groups and are termed "cosmopolitan"; others, however, are functionally important and occur predominantly (or exclusively) in a single ethnic group and thus may underlie ethnic-specific drug responses. A key question for genomic science is the extent to which individual polymorphisms, or combinations of polymorphisms, modulate normal physiology and its response to drugs.

Drug effects are mediated by their interactions with target and other proteins

Drugs interact with a series of proteins to generate their effects in patients. One group of molecules are the targets with which drugs interact to produce their desired and adverse effects. Our group has focused on pharmacogenetics and pharmacogenomics of drug-induced torsades de pointes; [5–7] the commonest culprit drugs are QT-prolonging antiarrhythmics. In this case, the molecular target producing the desired effect (QT prolongation) is the potassium channel encoded by the Human Ether-a-go-go Related Gene (*HERG*, also now known as *KCNH2*) that underlies the current known as I_{Kr}; HERG block is also the major molecular mechanism involved in generation of the adverse effect, Torsades. In many other cases, the molecular target involved in an adverse effect is dissimilar from that for the therapeutic effect. It is also important to recognize that drugs do not interact with their molecular targets in isolation, but rather as part of a complex biological system, which is often perturbed by disease. Thus, for example, the risk of marked QT prolongation during therapy with an I_{Kr} blocking drug is vanishingly small in a young, healthy male subject with a normal baseline QT interval, but is much higher in an elderly female with heart disease and QT prolongation at baseline. The difference likely reflects not simply differences in I_{Kr}, but rather differences in other components of the complex biology of cardiac repolarization that is well recognized to be perturbed by factors, such as female gender or congestive heart failure [8].

In addition, almost all drugs interact with a series of proteins that are involved in their absorption, distribution, metabolism, and excretion (processes collectively termed drug disposition). These proteins include not only enzymes responsible for drug biotransformation to metabolites (which sometimes are active), but also an increasingly well-appreciated role for specific transport molecules that function to move drugs into and out of cells where they can exert their pharmacologic effects [9, 10].

Having recognized that the normal function of many proteins modulates response to drug therapy in human beings, it follows that DNA variants, which modulate function of these proteins, may also contribute to variability in drug action. Indeed, viewed in this fashion, virtually all variability in drug actions will relate to genetic variant(s), environmental factors (including exposure to drugs), or a combination of the two. An excellent example of a "gene-by-environment" interaction has been provided by studies of patients with the Brugada Syndrome. Here, the ECG manifestations of the disease may be completely absent (despite a genetic defect) and only "exposed" by administration of a sodium-channel-blocking drug [11]. Similarly, there are data from the Cardiac Arrhythmia Suppression Trial (CAST) that suggest that transient myocardial ischemia strongly increases risk for sudden death during administration of sodium-channel-blocking drugs in the trial [12, 13].

Disease genetics and variable drug actions

An interesting corollary to the idea that genetic factors strongly modulate response to drug action is the concept that response to drug therapy may depend on the genetics of the disease being treated. This idea is particularly well established in oncology, where treatment for "cancer" is an increasingly antiquated concept that is being replaced by biology-specific treatments, such as imatinib (Gleevec) for chronic myelogenous leukemia [14]. In the same sense, identification of specific genetic lesions in rare diseases, such as the long QT syndromes, has had very important implications in terms of applying mutation-specific therapies: beta blockers for all forms (but especially LQT1) and sodium-channel blockers especially for LQT3 are examples [15, 16]. Similarly, many studies now support the concept that atrial fibrillation risk may include a prominent genetic component. This comes both from reports of large kindreds with familial atrial fibrillation, [17, 18] as well as population-based surveys that indicate a high incidence of positive family history among individuals with atrial fibrillation, particularly those with lone "atrial fibrillation" [19, 20]. Obviously, one mechanism underlying variability in response to pharmacotherapy for atrial fibrillation may be that this syndrome actually represents the clinical manifestation of multiple different molecular pathways. In this case, targeting specific pathways (once they are identified) holds out the hope of more specific therapies.

High-risk pharmacogenetics

The most high-profile examples in the field of pharmacogenetics come from clinical situations in which the action of a drug depends critically on normal function of a single protein. In such an instance, a DNA variant conferring aberrant function on that protein may produce extraordinary changes in drug action. One well described, but rather rare, example is a variant in the thiopurine methyltransferase (TPMT) gene that can result in the loss of enzymatic activity [21, 22]. TPMT plays a key role in the bioinactivation of azathioprine and 6-mercaptopurine. In patients who are homozygous for the defect and who receive these drugs, there is a very high incidence of potentially fatal bone marrow aplasia because of unexpected drug accumulation. Although this defect is relatively rare (1 in 300 individuals are homozygous null), it is nevertheless sufficiently common that many authorities recommend screening subjects who are to receive these agents prior to their administration. Further, increased enzymatic activity has been associated with decreased efficacy.

A more common example is the "poor metabolizer" (PM) genotype in the cytochrome P450 CYP2D6 [23]. Approximately 25% of Caucasian and African Americans carry one loss of function allele for this enzyme, and 7% are homozygous. Administration of drugs that are eliminated largely or exclusively by CYP2D6 can therefore result in very high plasma concentrations and exaggerated effects in PM subjects; examples include many antidepressants, some beta blockers (metoprolol, timolol), and propafenone. In PMs, plasma propafenone concentrations are much higher than in extensive metabolizers, and the pharmacologic effects are greater [24, 25]. These pharmacologic effects include bradycardia (due to the drug's beta-blocking action) as well as nonspecific side effects resulting in drug discontinuation. Another example of a drug in which CYP2D6 genotype determines response is the analgesic codeine. However, in this instance, metabolism of the drug results in generation of a potent active metabolite, morphine. Therefore, PM subjects actually have less pharmacologic effect than do extensive metabolizers. Flecainide is also metabolized by CYP2D6; however, flecainide also undergoes renal excretion of unchanged drug, so in most patients, CYP2D6 genotype has little influence on response to therapy. However, in the rare individual who is a poor metabolizer and who has renal dysfunction, flecainide may accumulate and has been implicated in proarrhythmia [26].

The marked increase in risk described above with certain TPMT and CYP2D6 substrates reflect the fact that elimination of culprit drugs is exclusively dependent upon these pathways, a situation we have previously termed "high-risk pharmacokinetics." The same logic applies to drug interactions with their molecular targets. Consider an example of an individual with subclinical LQT1 due to a loss of function mutation in the *KCNQ1* gene. As is now well recognized, many such individuals display normal QT intervals, presumably due to normal function of other important repolarizing mechanisms, notably a robust I_{Kr} (a situation we have previously termed "repolarization reserve" [8]). However, administration of an I_{Kr} blocking drug in such an individual runs a high risk of abrogating all normal repolarization mechanisms, and thus causing torsades de pointes.

Gene–gene interactions

Situations in which two DNA variants can interact to increase the likelihood for abnormal physiology (and presumably aberrant drug responses) are now increasingly well recognized. The variants can be located in the same or in different genes. A common polymorphism in the sodium channel seems to modulate the severity of the phenotype conferred by mutations in the same gene, through mechanisms that are now being worked out [27, 28]. The issue of flecainide metabolism is a situation in which two pathways interact. A second comes from studies of families with severe conduction disease and atrial standstill [29]. In one such kindred, a sodium-channel mutation was identified, but was not well associated with the clinical phenotype. Further investigation revealed the presence of a common polymorphism in the regulatory region of the connexin40 gene (*Cx40*), the region that controls the amount of protein synthesized. Only subjects with the variant *Cx40* and the sodium-channel mutation displayed the severe clinical phenotype, that is, this is an example of a gene–gene interaction.

Association studies: on to haplotypes

An increasingly common study design is one in which variant physiology or pharmacology is associated with a polymorphism in a specific gene. Often, these variants are selected based on physiologic rationale, or because *in vitro* studies suggest that the polymorphism produces alterations in some protein function that it could be linked to variant physiology in some logical fashion. Thus, we and others have associated variants in potassium- or sodium-channel genes in arrhythmia susceptibility, and these associations seem believable because of the statistics involved, as well as because of supporting *in vitro* studies [7, 30]. However, given the extraordinarily large number of polymorphisms in the human genome (certainly well over 10 million) the likelihood of false associations seems quite high. Indeed, one survey suggested that the vast majority of association studies were not reproducible [31, 32]. For this and many other reasons, research in the field has sought alternatives to searching for associations between variant physiology or pharmacology and DNA variants, polymorphism by polymorphism. One appealing approach is based on the concept of a haplotype map of the human genome. It is becoming increasingly clear that many polymorphisms are "linked," in the sense that knowledge of which polymorphism is present at one site provides information on which polymorphism is present at a second ("linked") site. When one polymorphism completely informs a second, the two sites are said to be in complete "linkage disequilibrium" (LD). Large segments of the human genome are now recognized to display strong LD, defining common "haplotype blocks." The National Human Genome Research Institute, along with collaborators worldwide, is defining haplotype structure for the human genome across ethnicities [33]. Thus, rather than interrogating tens of millions of polymorphic sites, researchers in this field may be able to relate specific haplotypes to specific physiologies or pharmacologies. One recent example is an association between a haplotype encompassing the regulatory region of the cardiac sodium channel and left bundle branch block [34]. This work identified a 20-kb block of conserved LD extending from 10 kb upstream of exon 1 (which is noncoding) to 10 kb into intron 1 defined by 9 frequent SNPs all with minor allele frequencies >10%. Within the block, 7 frequent haplotypes occurred with frequencies of 5–31. The hap3 haplotype had a minor allele frequency of 16% and uniquely included $\frac{3}{9}$ minor SNP alleles. This haplotype was significantly associated with the width of the QRS complex ($p = .0075$; QRS 93. 4 ms in wt/wt ($n = 474$), 96.3 ms in wt/hap3 heterozygotes ($n = 201$) and 100.8 ms in hap3/hap3 homozygotes ($n = 18$)). The effect appears attributable to left bundle branch block (LBBB prevalence 3/479 (0.6%) in wt/wt, 7/203 (3.4%) in wt/hap3 and 2/18 (11.1%) in hap3/hap3, odds ratio = 6.74 (1.81–25.1), p = .0011). Thus, these data provide support for the concept that variability in channel expression by polymorphisms in the regulatory region of the gene influences cardiac conduction even in normal individuals.

Summary

One important goal of genomics is to use polymorphism information to improve healthcare, by identifying patients at risk for disease or unusual drug responses and by identifying targets for new drug development. Many obstacles can be identified to such a vision: technologic, computational, ethical, and biologic to name a few [35–39]. Nevertheless, the field is very young; indeed, the first use of the term "pharmacogenomics" in PubMed occurred in 1997 [40]. Progress has been quite rapid, and thus there is some hope that important obstacles can be overcome to deliver this new science for better patient care.

Acknowledgements

Supported in part by grants from the United States Public Health Service (HL46681, HL49989, HL65962). Dr. Roden is the holder of the William Stokes Chair in Experimental Therapeutics, a gift from the Dai-ichi Corporation.

References

1 Kalow W. *Pharmacogenetics – Heredity and responses to drugs*. Philadelphia, PA: W.B. Saunders, 1962.
2 Evans WE, Relling MV. Pharmacogenomics: translating functional genomics into rational therapeutics. *Science* 1999; **286**: 487–491.
3 Kalow W. Pharmacogenetics, pharmacogenomics, and pharmacobiology. *Clin Pharmacol Ther* 2001; **70**: 1–4.
4 Johnson JA. Drug target pharmacogenomics: an overview. *Am J Pharmacogenomics* 2001; **1**: 271–281.
5 Roden DM. Cardiovascular Pharmacogenomics. *Circulation* 2003; **108**: 3071–3074.
6 Kanki H, Yang P, Xie HG *et al.* Polymorphisms in beta-adrenergic receptor genes in acquired long QT syndrome patients. *PACE* 2001; **24**: 606.
7 Yang P, Kanki H, Drolet B *et al.* Allelic variants in Long QT disease genes in patients with drug-associated Torsades de Pointes. *Circulation* 2002; **105**: 1943–1948.
8 Roden DM. Taking the idio out of idiosyncratic – predicting torsades de pointes. *PACE* 1998; **21**: 1029–1034.

9 Lee W, Kim RB. Transporters and renal drug elimination. *Annu Rev Pharmacol Toxicol* 2004; **44**: 137–166.
10 Marzolini C, Paus E, Buclin T *et al.* Polymorphisms in human MDR1 (P-glycoprotein): recent advances and clinical relevance. *Clin Pharmacol Ther* 2004; **75**: 13–33.
11 Alings M, Wilde A. "Brugada" syndrome: clinical data and suggested pathophysiological mechanism. *Circulation* 1999; **99**: 666–673.
12 Cardiac Arrhythmia Suppression Trial (CAST) Investigators. Increased mortality due to encainide or flecainide in a randomized trial of arrhythmia suppression after myocardial infarction. *N Engl J Med* 1989; **321**: 406–412.
13 Akiyama T, Pawitan Y, Greenberg H *et al.* Increased risk of death and cardiac arrest from encainide and flecainide in patients after non-Q-wave acute myocardial infarction in the Cardiac Arrhythmia Suppression Trial. *Am J Cardiol* 1991; **68**: 1551–1555.
14 Kantarjian H, Sawyers C, Hochhaus A *et al.* Hematologic and cytogenetic responses to imatinib mesylate in chronic myelogenous leukemia. *N Engl J Med* 2002; **346**: 645–652.
15 Priori SG. Inherited arrhythmogenic diseases: the complexity beyond monogenic disorders. *Circ Res* 2004; **94**: 140–145.
16 Priori SG, Aliot E, Blomstrom-Lundqvist C *et al.* Update of the guidelines on sudden cardiac death of the European Society of Cardiology. *Eur Heart J* 2003; **24**: 13–15.
17 Ellinor PT, Shin JT, Moore RK *et al.* Locus for atrial fibrillation maps to chromosome 6q 14–16. *Circulation* 2003; **107**: 2880–2883.
18 Brugada R, Tapscott T, Czernuszewicz GZ *et al.* Identification of a genetic locus for familial atrial fibrillation. *N Engl J Med* 1997; **336**: 905–911.
19 Darbar D, Herron KJ, Ballew JD *et al.* Familial atrial fibrillation is a genetically heterogeneous disorder. *J Am Coll Cardiol* 2003; **41**: 2185–2192.
20 Fox CS, Parise H, D'Agostino RB, Sr. *et al.* Parental atrial fibrillation as a risk factor for atrial fibrillation in offspring. *JAMA* 2004; **291**: 2851–2855.
21 McLeod HL, Krynetski EY, Relling MV *et al.* Genetic polymorphism of thiopurine methyltransferase and its clinical relevance for childhood acute lymphoblastic leukemia. *Leukemia* 2000; **14**: 567–572.
22 Black AJ, McLeod HL, Capell HA *et al.* Thiopurine methyltransferase genotype predicts therapy-limiting severe toxicity from azathioprine. *Ann Intern Med* 1998; **129**: 716–718.
23 Meyer UA, Zanger UM. Molecular mechanisms of genetic polymorphisms of drug metabolism. *Annu Rev Phamacol Toxicol* 1997; **37**: 269–296.
24 Siddoway LA, Thompson KAMKT, McAllister CB *et al.* Polymorphism of propafenone metabolism and disposition in man: clinical and pharmacokinetic consequences. *Circulation* 1987; **75**: 785–791.
25 Lee JT, Kroemer HK, Silberstein DJ *et al.* The role of genetically determined polymorphic drug metabolism in the beta-blockade produced by propafenone. *N Engl J Med* 1990; **322**: 1764–1768.
26 Evers J, Eichelbaum M, Kroemer HK. Unpredictability of flecainide plasma concentrations in patients with renal failure: relation to side effects and sudden death? *Ther Drug Monit* 1994; **16**: 349–351.
27 Viswanathan PC, Benson DW, Balser JR. A common SCN5A polymorphism modulates the biophysical effects of an SCN5A mutation. *J Clin Invest* 2003; **111**: 341–346.
28 Makielski JC, Ye B, Valdivia CR *et al.* A ubiquitous splice variant and a common polymorphism affect heterologous expression of recombinant human SCN5A heart sodium channels. *Circ Res* 2003; **93**: 821–828.
29 Groenewegen WA, Firouzi M, Bezzina CR *et al.* A cardiac sodium channel mutation cosegregates with a rare connexin40 genotype in familial atrial standstill. *Circ Res* 2003; **92**: 14–22.
30 Splawski I, Timothy KW, Tateyama M *et al.* Variant of SCN5A sodium channel implicated in risk of cardiac arrhythmia. *Science* 2002; **297**: 1333–1336.
31 Ioannidis JP, Ntzani EE, Trikalinos TA *et al.* Replication validity of genetic association studies. *Nat Genetics* 2001; **29**: 306–309.
32 Hirschhorn JN, Lohmueller K, Byrne E *et al.* A comprehensive review of genetic association studies. *Genet Med* 2002; **4**: 45–61.
33 The International HapMap Consortium. The International HapMap Project. *Nature* 2003; **426**: 789–796.
34 Pfeufer A, Bezzina CR, Jazilzadeh S *et al.* A common haplotype in the 5′ region of the SCN5A gene is strongly associated with ventricular conduction impairment. *Circulation* 2004; AHA Scientific Sessions.
35 Norbert PW, Roses AD. Pharmacogenetics and pharmacogenomics: recent developments, their clinical relevance and some ethical, social, and legal implications. *J Mol Med* 2003; **81**: 135–140.
36 Shah J. Economic and regulatory considerations in pharmacogenomics for drug licensing and healthcare. *Nat Biotechnol* 2003; **21**: 747–753.
37 Hoehe MR, Timmermann B, Lehrach H. Human inter-individual DNA sequence variation in candidate genes, drug targets, the importance of haplotypes and pharmacogenomics. *Curr Pharm Biotechnol* 2003; **4**: 351–378.
38 Amin AR. Pharmacogenomics: hype, hope, or metamorphosis of molecular medicine and pharmaceuticals. *Trends Pharmacol Sci* 2002; **23**: 583.
39 Rothstein MA, Epps PG. Ethical and legal implications of pharmacogenomics. *Nat Rev Genet* 2001; **2**: 228–231.
40 Marshall A. Genset-Abbott deal heralds pharmacogenomics era. *Nat Biotechnol* 1997; **15**: 829–830.

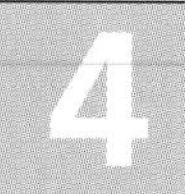

CHAPTER 4

The cardiac sodium-channel carboxy terminus: predicted and detected structure provide a novel target for antiarrhythmic drugs development

Robert S. Kass, PhD, *Joseph W. Cormier,* PhD, & *Ian W. Glaaser* PhD

Sodium-channel gating and molecular pharmacology

Sodium-channels in the heart: molecular determinants of inactivation

Voltage-gated Na^+ channels are integral membrane proteins [1, 2] that not only underlie excitation in excitable cells, but determine the vulnerability of the heart to dysfunctional rhythm by controlling the number of channels available to conduct inward Na^+ movement [3]. Na^+ channels open in response to membrane depolarization allowing a rapid selective influx of Na^+ that serves to further depolarize excitable cells and initiate multiple cellular signals [4]. Within milliseconds of opening, Na^+ channels enter a nonconducting inactivated state [5–12]. Channel inactivation is necessary to limit the duration of excitable cell depolarization, and disruption of inactivation by inherited mutations, which delays cellular repolarization, is associated with a diverse range of human diseases including myotonias [13], epilepsy and seizure disorders [14, 15], autism [16], and sudden cardiac death [17, 18].

The Na^+ channel α subunit, which forms the ion-conducting pore and contains channel gating components, consists of four homologous domains (I to IV) [19]. Each domain contains six α-helical transmembrane repeats (S1–S6), for which mutagenesis studies have revealed key functional roles [4]. Voltage-dependent inactivation of Na^+ channels is a consequence of voltage-dependent activation [20], and inactivation is characterized by at least two distinguishable kinetic components: an initial rapid component (fast inactivation) and a slower component (slow inactivation). Within milliseconds of opening, Na^+ channels enter a nonconducting inactivated state as the inactivation gate, the cytoplasmic loop-linking domains III and IV of the α subunit, occludes the open pore [5–9, 12, 21]. The residues that form a hydrophobic triplet (IFM) in the III–IV linker are involved in inactivation gating [7]. The IFM motif has been suggested to function as a "latch" that holds the inactivation gate shut. Cysteine scanning of the residues I1485, F1486, and M1487 in the human cardiac Na^+ channel revealed that these amino acids contribute to stabilizing the fast-inactivation particle [22] in analogy to the brain Na^+ channel [5, 23]. However, peptide-binding studies suggest that inactivation may not involve simple occlusive block of the inner mouth of the pore [24]. Glycine and proline residues that flank the IFM motif may serve as molecular hinges to allow closure of the inactivation gate like a hinged lid ("hinged-lid model") [7, 21].

In contrast with fast inactivation, evidence has accumulated describing slow inactivation of Na^+ channels as a current-dependent process. Slow inactivation is not affected when fast inactivation is prevented by protease treatment or when movement of the inactivation gate is blocked by specific antibodies [25], and therefore it is likely to be an independent gating process. It has been shown that transposition of all four cardiac isoform P-loops into the human skeletal muscle isoform (hSkM1) backbone conferred heart isoform-like slow-inactivation properties on the chimeric construct, suggesting a role for the P-loops in slow inactivation [26, 27].

The outer pore region of the Na^+-channel protein contains highly conserved aspartate, glutamate, lysine, and alanine residues (the "DEKA" ring), which are thought to form the channel selectivity filter [28, 29]. Selectivity in sodium channels is likely due to a single file ion permeation process in analogy to selectivity of L-type calcium channels which contain an outer pore EEE motif [30, 31]. Mutations in the sodium-channel selectivity filter have been shown to affect gating as well as permeation and most of the effects to date have implicated slow inactivation in this process. Changes in flexibility of the P-loops may affect slow inactivation. Also, a single residue in the D-II P-loop of the cardiac Na^+ channel (I891) has been shown to regulate the steady-state availability of slow inactivation. Tomaselli *et al.* [27, 32] found that mutation of a residue in the external pore mouth of the Na^+ channel not only reduces single-channel conductance but also accelerates the activation kinetics of the channel. Moreover, there are reports that mutations in the DEKA ring enhance the entry of Na^+ channels into an ultra-slow inactivated state [33]. Thus slow inactivation of sodium channels resembles C-type inactivation of potassium channels [34].

Na-channel block by local anesthetics is linked to channel inactivation

Blockade of voltage-dependent Na^+ channels has long been recognized as a therapeutic approach to the management of many cardiac arrhythmias, but with considerable risk of toxic side effects [35]. The discovery that mutant forms of Na^+ channels linked to inherited human cardiac arrhythmias might make distinct targets for Na^+-channel blocking drugs [36–41] has stimulated reinvestigation of the molecular determinants of Na^+-channel blockade in the heart.

Voltage-dependent block of Na^+ channels by local anesthetics and related drugs has been well described within the framework of the modulated receptor hypothesis which proposes that allosteric changes in a drug receptor occur when changes in voltage induce changes in channel conformation states (Figure 4.1) (states) [42, 43]. Extensive mutagenesis experiments have been performed with several different drugs in many sodium-channel isoforms in an effort to define the molecular determinants of drug binding. While a clear consensus has not been reached regarding precisely where drug binds and there is certainly variability in drugs, isoforms, and how the data is interpreted, the current evidence strongly suggests that most drugs tested bind in the pore of the channel on the intracellular side of the selectivity filter. Furthermore, mutagenesis studies by several groups find specific amino acid residues that contribute to drug binding on the S6 segment of

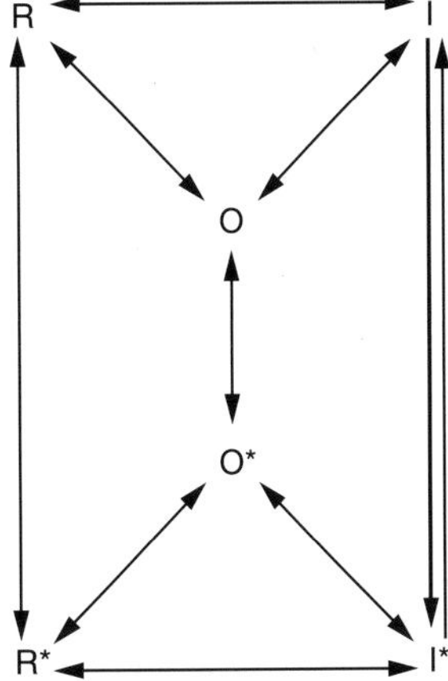

Figure 4.1 Modulated receptor hypothesis scheme for preferential binding to inactivated channels. R is the rested, O is the open, and I is the inactivated state of sodium channels without drug bound. The drug bound channel states are represented as R*, O*, and I*. The thicker arrow for the transition from I to I* represents the higher affinity for the inactivated state.

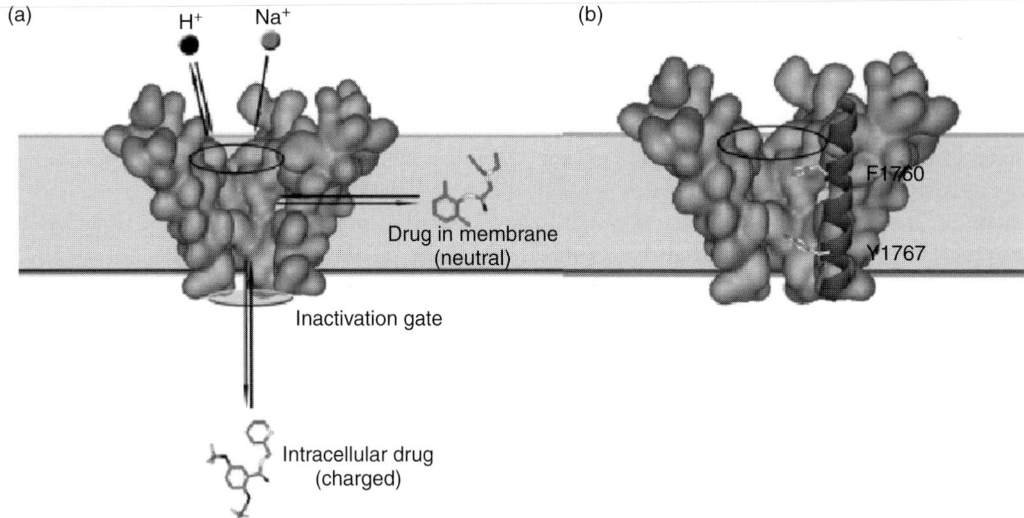

Figure 4.2 Drug access pathways and molecular determinants of drug binding. Schematic of the modulated receptor hypothesis. Two pathways exist for drug block. The hydrophilic pathway (vertical arrows) is the likely path for charged drug and requires channel openings. The hydrophobic pathway (horizontal arrows) is the likely pathway for neutral drug through the membrane. (a) Extracellular Na^+ and H^+ can reach bound drug molecules through the selectivity filter. (b) Structural determinants of drug binding. Globular representation of the sodium-channel membrane associated regions. The helical representation of domain IV S6 is shown with side chains for the primary structural determinants of drug binding, F1760 and Y1767. The selectivity filter is represented as a black ellipse.

domains I, III, and IV. The most dramatic effects on drug binding can be attributed primarily to two aromatic residues on DIV S6 , a phenylalanine at position 11760 (F1760) and a tyrosine at position 1767 (Y1767) using NaV 1.5 numbering, that are conserved among sodium-channel isoforms [44–47] (Figure 4.2).

Thus targeting sodium channels as a therapeutic approach to manage arrhythmias has been interrelated to an understanding of the molecular basis of sodium-channel inactivation. However, despite the importance of modulation of drug block by voltage-dependent conformational states of the channel, this basic approach has been formulated around the concept of occluding the channel pore and, in an all-or-none manner, reducing the number of channels that are available to conduct impulses. This approach has led to the finding that pore block of sodium channels often results in more arrhythmic activity, even in unaffected patients, than no channel block at all [48–52]. As a result, it is clearly important to define novel sodium-channel targets that may be useful to control channel activity, perhaps through allosteric control of channel gating in contrast to all-or-none pore block [53].

Disease-related mutations reveal a critical role of the carboxy-terminal (C-T) domain

As described above, fast Na^+-channel inactivation is due to rapid block of the inner mouth of the channel pore by the cytoplasmic linker between domains III and IV that occurs within milliseconds of membrane depolarization [5, 7, 25, 54]. NMR analysis of this inactivation linker (gate) in solution has revealed a rigid helical structure that is positioned such that it can block the pore, providing a structural explanation of the functional studies [55] and a biological mechanism of inhibiting channel conduction.

Disease associated mutations that disrupt inactivation may result in an increase in experimentally detectable sustained tetrodotoxin (TTX)-sensitive current (I_{sus}) [56, 57] which, though only a fraction ($<1\%$) of the peak current elicited in response to depolarization, is sufficient to account for disease phenotype: delay in repolarization [58–60]. The disruption of inactivation by mutation of the IFM motif resembles, to a certain extent, the effects of some disease-associated mutations on Na^+-channel inactivation. Some mutations, such as the ΔKPQ deletion mutation [61], occur in the III–IV linker region and promote inactivation-free gating modes [61]. Unexpectedly, however, mutations in other regions of the channel, notably the C-T domain, can also destabilize inactivation and promote an inactivation deficient gating mode [62–64] (Figure 4.3). These findings raised the possibility that the carboxy-terminal domain of the cardiac sodium channel may play a more important role than previously thought in regulating the inactivated state of the channel: a possibility that has required insights into the possible structural basis of these interactions.

Structural basis of Na-channel modulation: Importance of computational methodology

Despite a wealth of experimental evidence documenting the functional consequences of the disease-linked mutations in ion channels, understanding the physical mechanisms affected by the mutations at the structural level has been lacking. This is due in large part to the difficulty in obtaining structural information with high-resolution experimental techniques such as x-ray crystallography and multidimensional NMR methods in integral membrane proteins. Computational methods that predict three-dimensional structures from amino acid sequences have become increasingly accurate and have provided insights into structure–function relationships for proteins without structural information [66–68]. Although

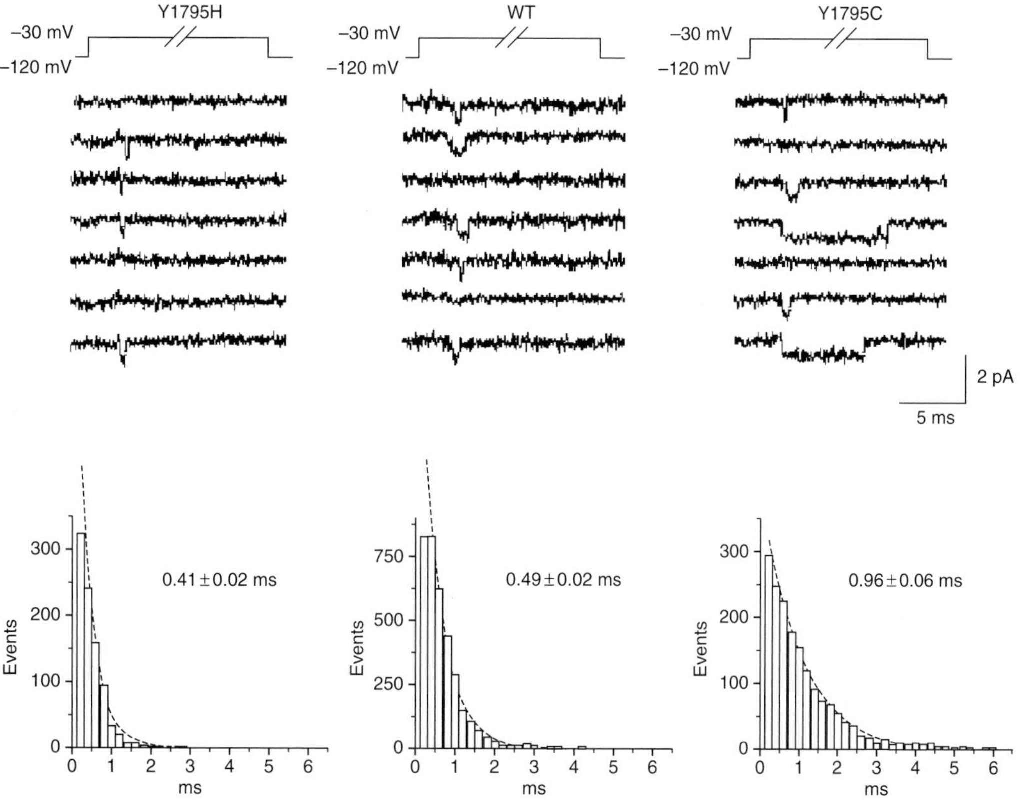

Figure 4.3 Inherited mutations of the Nav1.5 carboxy-terminal domain alter channel gating. Single-channel recordings of a Brugada mutant (Y1795H, left) and an LQT-3 mutant (Y1795C) channel reveal mutation-induced changes in channel mean open times (lower histograms). (Reprinted from *J Gen Physiol* [72], with permission.)

the information required to generate a protein structure is expected to be embedded in its amino acid sequence, current computational methodologies that unravel how three-dimensional information is mapped onto a linear sequence predict low-resolution structures at best, when close homologous structural templates from protein structural databases are absent.

A model of the Nav1.5 carboxy-terminal structure

This approach was taken to estimate the structure of the carboxy-terminal domain of the cardiac sodium-channel α subunit (Nav 1.5). Amino acid sequence comparison of the C-terminus of several human isoforms of the sodium channel reveals a conserved proximal region of about 140 residues, and a less conserved distal half of about 100 residues, depending on the specific gene (Figure 4.4) [69]. The proximal region is highlighted by a concentration of glutamic and aspartic acid residues, comprising the acid rich domain. Additionally, there is a conserved IQ motif that has been suggested to be a calmodulin-binding domain in some isoforms. The distal region contains a PY motif that is a binding site for ubiquitination proteins, and is therefore involved in protein trafficking. Homology modeling of the C-terminus predicts that the proximal half contains six helical structures, while the distal half consists of unstructured peptide (Figure 4.5).

Experimental measurement of C-T secondary structure is consistent with model predictions

Circular dichroism, which probes protein secondary structure, confirmed the basic prediction of the homology modeling: the C-terminus consists of α-helical structure, concentrated in the proximal half, and loop regions, predominantly in the distal portion [69]. The homology model of the C-terminus suggests that the first four helices (H1–H4) form two E–F hands (see Figure 4.6), a structural motif typically used exclusively by calcium-binding proteins. The loops between E–F hand pairs, however, do not

```
                   Acidic Rich Domain
SCN5A (1773) ENFSVATEES TEPLSEDDFD MFYEIWEKFD PEATQFIEYS VLSDFADALS EPLRIAKPNQ ISLINMDLPM VSGD
SCN2A (1777) ENFSVATEES AEPLSEDDFE MFYEVWEKFD PDATQFIEFA KLSDFADALD PPLLIAKPNK VQLIAMDLPM VSGD
SCN8A (1767) ENFSVATEES ADPLSEDDFE TFYEIWEKFD PDATQFIEYC KLADFADALE HPLRVPKPNT IELIAMDLPM VSGD
SCN9A (1750) ENFSVATEES TEPLSEDDFE MFYEVWEKFD PDATQFIEFS KLSDFAAALD PPLLIAKPNK VQLIAMDLPM VSGD
SCN4A (1599) ENFNVATEES SEPLGEDDFE MFYETWEKFD PDATQFIAYS RLSDFVDTLQ EPLRIAKPNK IKLITLDLPM VPGD
                           H1                  H2                  H3

                                                                               IQ Motif
SCN5A (1847) RIHCMDILFA FTKRVLGESG EMDALKIQME EKFMAANPSK ISYEPITTTL RRKHEEVSAM VIQRAFRRHL LQRS
SCN2A (1851) RIHCLDILFA FTKRVLGESG EMDALRIQME ERFMASNPSK VSYEPITTTL KRKQEEVSAI IIQRAYRRYL LKQK
SCN8A (1841) RIHCLDILFA FTKRVLGDSG ELDILRQQME ERFVASNPSK VSYEPITTTL RRKQEEVSAV VLQRAYRGHL ARR-
SCN9A (1824) RIHCLDILFA FTKRVLGESG EMDSLRSQME ERFMSANPSK VSYEPITTTL KRKQEDVSAT VIQRAYRRYR LRQN
SCN4A (1673) KIHCLDILFA LTKEVLGDSG EMDALKQTME EKFMAANPSK VSYEPITTTL KRKHEEVCAI KIQRAYRRHL LQRS
                  H4                    H5                         H6

                                                                   PY Motif
SCN5A (1921) LKHASFLFRQ QAGSGLSEED APEREGLIAY VMSENFSRPL GPPSSSSISS TSFPPSYDSV TRATSDN--- LQVR
SCN2A (1925) VKKVSSIYKK DKGK--ECDG TPIKEDTLID KLNENS---- TPEKTDMTPS TTSPPSYDSV TKPEKEK--- FEKD
SCN8A (1914) ----GFICKK TTSN-KLENG GTHRE----- ---------- ---KKESTPS TASLPSYDSV TKPEKEKQQR AEEG
SCN9A (1898) VKNISSIYIK DGDR---DDD LLNKKDMAFD NVNENS---- SPEKTDATSS TTSPPSYDSV TKPDKEK--- YEQD
SCN4A (1947) MKQASYMYRH SHDG--SGDD APEKEGLLAN TMSKMYG--- -HENGNSSSP SPEEKGEAGD AGPTMGLMPI SPSD

SCN5A (1992) GSDYSHSEDL ADFPPSPDRD RESIV
SCN2A (1990) KSEK--EDKG KDIRESKK-- -----
SCN8A (1965) RRER--AKRQ KEVRESKC-- -----
SCN9A (1962) RTEK--EDKG KDSKESKK-- -----
SCN4A (1815) TAWPPAPPPG QTVRPGVKES LV---
```

Figure 4.4 Human sodium-channel homology. Sequence alignment of the SCN5AC terminus and the C-terminus of four other human voltage-gated sodium channels: SCN2A, the brain isoform; SCN8A, also from the central nervous system; SCN9A, the peripheral nervous system; and SCN4A, found in skeletal muscle. Colored letters distinguish homology: identical (red), conserved (blue), similar (purple), weakly similar (green), and nonhomologous (black). Alignment gaps are denoted by a dash. The six computed C-terminus helices are shown by shaded bars below the sequences. Conserved domains and motifs are surrounded by boxes and labeled accordingly. (Reprinted from *J Biol Chem* [69], with permission.)

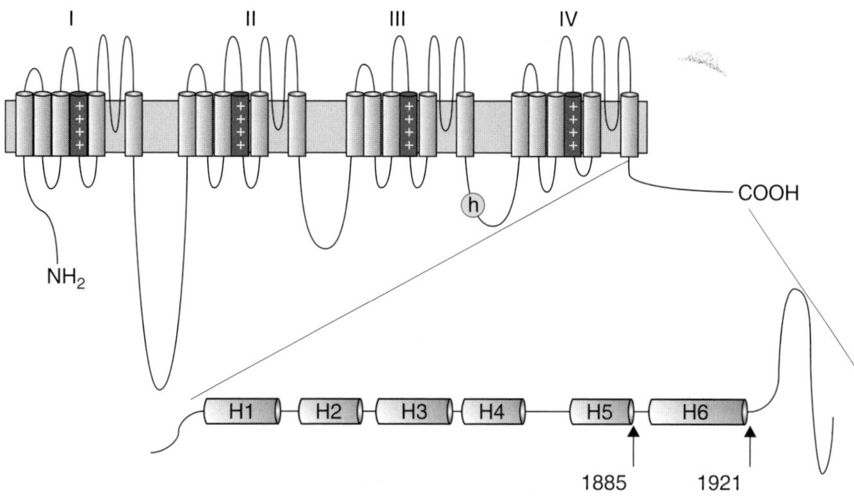

Figure 4.5 Schematic of the voltage-gated sodium-channel α subunit. The protein consists of four domains each comprised six transmembrane helices and a pore-forming region. The fourth helix (red) in each domain contains a series of positively charged residues and is the putative voltage sensor required for activation. The putative inactivation gate consisting of hydrophobic residues (IFM) is indicated by the circled h (yellow). The C-terminal region is detailed to give relative size and sequence position of the six predicted α-helices, H1–H6.

contain the necessary residues for divalent cation chelation. This implies that although the proximal half of the C-terminus is predicted to contain these E–F hand-like structures, they are not expected to be a calcium sensor for the channel.

Further experimental tests of model-predicted structure: identification of partner cysteines in an LQT-3 mutant channel. One set of experimental test of the model focused on understanding the structural basis for the unique effects of an inherited C-terminal mutation (Y1795C) that is associated with variant 3 of the long-QT syndrome (LQT-3) and has pronounced effects on the entry of Na^+ channels into a nonconducting inactivated state (see Figure 4.3) [60, 65]. The model structure of the C-terminal domain described above which was predicted to have a calmodulin-like fold with one pair of E–F-hands packed against each other as in calmodulin also precisely predicted the location of a potential cysteine partner for this LQT-3-mutated channel. Experimental evidence indicated that the naturally occurring mutation, in which a cysteine replaces a tyrosine at position (Y1795C), enables the formation of disulfide bonds with a partner cysteine in the channel. Using the predictions of the model, the cysteine at position 1850 of the channel was identified as the putative cysteine partner in the formation of a disulfide bond with the mutated C1795. This model prediction was using mutagenesis and pharmacology [70]. The implication of this experimental work was that the tertiary structure predicted for the C-terminus must be a reasonable model for the first half of the sodium-channel C-terminal domain (Figure 4.7).

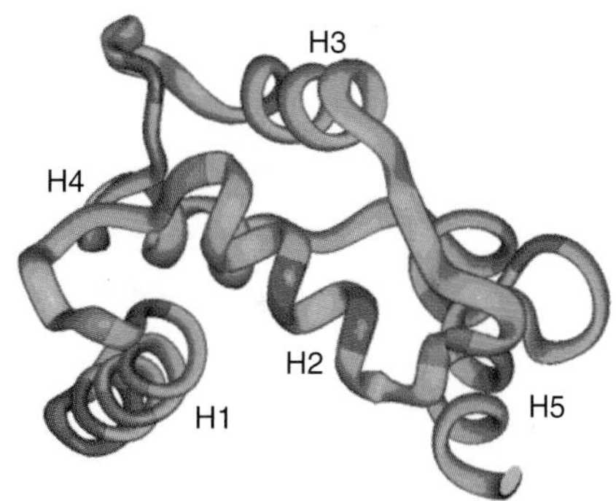

Figure 4.6 Homology model of the sodium-channel proximal C-terminus. Predicted structure of the first-half of the C-terminus SCN5A (residues 1785–1885). The backbone structure is shown with aspartic acid residues in red and glutamic acid residues in magenta. The sixth predicted helix, H6, cannot be accurately determined with confidence, and is not shown in the model. The sequence regions assigned to H1–H6 are shown in Figure 4.4.

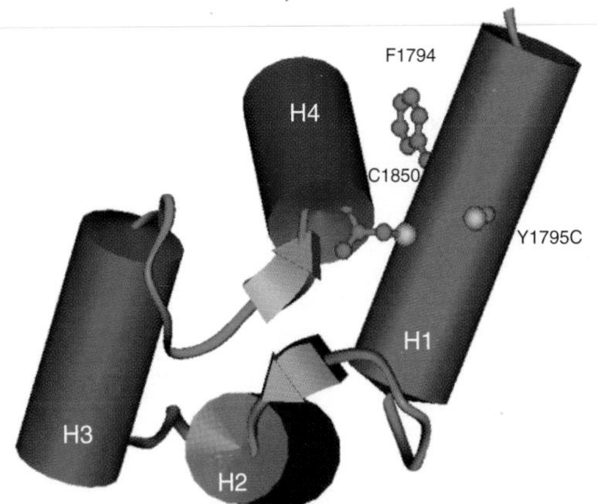

Figure 4.7 Predicted spatial relationship between two residues in the C-terminus. The helix barrels H1–H2 show the first EF hand structural motif in the model presented in Figure 4.6; the H3–H4 helix barrels show the second EF hand structural motif. Three-dimensional ball-and-stick models show the predicted positions of the residues Y1795C and C1850 in the structural model. The sulfur atoms in the cysteines are colored in yellow. These two atoms are separated by 4 Å in the model structure. Residue F1794 that appears from the back of H1 helix is also shown in ball-and-stick model. (Reprinted from *Biophys J* [70], with permission.)

Functional roles of C-T domain structures

Does the structured C-T domain underlie important structural control of channel gating in general, and control of inactivation in particular? To address this question, functional experiments were carried out in which the predicted distal unstructured region was deleted (1921stop mutation) or in which deletion of this region was accompanied by deletion of the predicted sixth helix of the proximal half of the C-terminus (1885stop). Deleting the distal, unstructured region (1921stop) shows no differences from the function of the wild-type channel (Figure 4.8). However, deleting the predicted sixth helix (H6), as well as the distal region (1885stop) shows significant changes in channel inactivation, but no discernable changes in activation, consistent with the idea of the C-terminus' role in channel inactivation. The 1885stop truncation results in a large sustained macrosopic sodium-channel current that is caused by an increase in channel bursting during prolonged

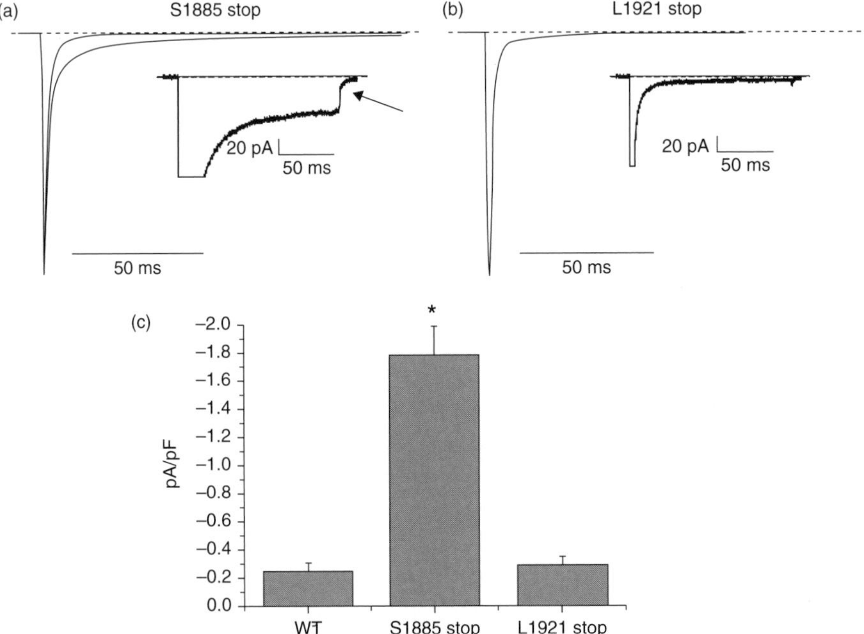

Figure 4.8 Truncation of H6 enhances maintained sodium-channel current. A and B, averaged and normalized TTX-sensitive traces recorded upon a prolonged depolarizing step (150 ms at −10 mV) reveal changes in inactivation caused by H6 truncation. The panels show superimposed averaged WT and (a) S1885stop and (b) L1921 stop currents along with insets of nonnormalized currents at high gain. (C) summary of the effects of C-terminus truncation on average current density measured at the end of 150 ms for each construct. *, significantly different from WT. (Reprinted from *J Biol Chem* [69], with permission.)

depolarization. This mutation additionally slows the channel's recovery from inactivation, as well as shifts the steady-state inactivation curve in the hyperpolarizing direction, both of which seem contradictory to the increased sustained current observed, and consistent with stabilization of a closed inactivated channel state. These pivotal experiments demonstrated a definitive role of the C-T domain in controlling channel inactivation and pointed clearly to the proximal structured half of the C-T domain as a critical structural component in stabilizing the inactivated state of the channel during prolonged depolarization. Suppression of channel bursting during prolonged depolarization decreases inward current during the cardiac action potential plateau (tends to shorten action potential duration (APD)) whereas enhancement of sodium-channel bursting would prolong APD (as in LQT-3 mutations) hence the possibility exists that the structured C-T domain may represent a novel sodium-channel target to regulated channel activity in an allosteric, as opposed to pore block, manner. What may be the basis for this control of inactivation?

III–IV linker and C-T interactions

Recent work in which biochemical and functional experiments were combined directly addressed the question whether or not the C-terminus may have a direct structural role in the control of channel inactivation, and, if so, how the C-T domain affects stabilization of the inactivated Na^+ channel. The conclusion from this work is that the cardiac sodium-channel inactivation gate is a molecular complex, providing additional structural insight into the role of the carboxy-terminal domain in regulating channel activity. Experimental data support the view that the III–IV linker interacts directly with the carboxy-terminal domain of the channel to stabilize inactivated channels [71].

In these experiments, biochemical evidence was presented for direct physical interaction between the C-T domain of the channel and the III–IV linker inactivation gate. It was shown that the full-length C-T domain, as well as a truncated construct in which the distal unstructured region is deleted, bind to the III–IV linker, but that truncation of the predicted sixth helix uncouples the C-terminus from the III–IV linker (Figure 4.9). These biochemical

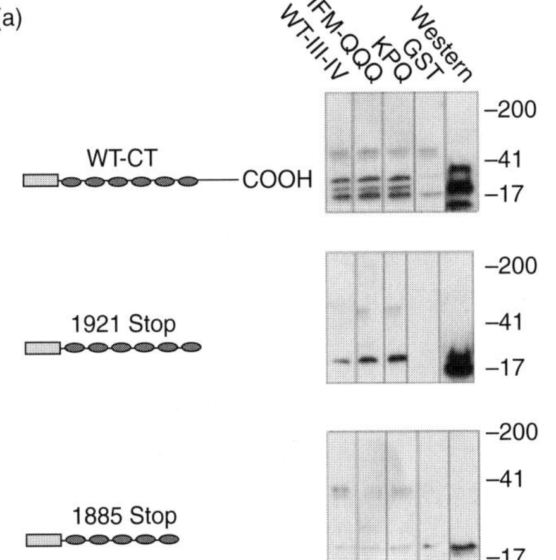

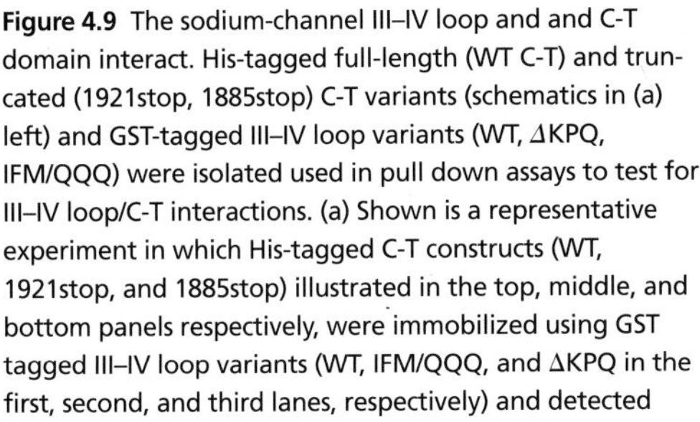

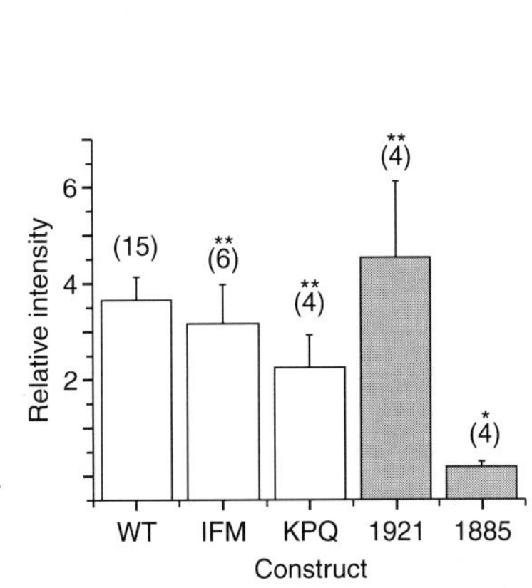

Figure 4.9 The sodium-channel III–IV loop and and C-T domain interact. His-tagged full-length (WT C-T) and truncated (1921stop, 1885stop) C-T variants (schematics in (a) left) and GST-tagged III–IV loop variants (WT, ΔKPQ, IFM/QQQ) were isolated used in pull down assays to test for III–IV loop/C-T interactions. (a) Shown is a representative experiment in which His-tagged C-T constructs (WT, 1921stop, and 1885stop) illustrated in the top, middle, and bottom panels respectively, were immobilized using GST tagged III–IV loop variants (WT, IFM/QQQ, and ΔKPQ in the first, second, and third lanes, respectively) and detected using an anti-His monoclonal antibody. The control lane (GST alone, fourth lane) indicates specificity of the reactions. The last lane is a Western blot detecting the His-tagged C-T in the bacterial lysates. (b) Histogram of scanned pull downs normalized to total protein and corrected for background and total GST loaded. Open bars correspond to interactions between His-tagged full length C-T construct and labeled III–IV linker variants. Filled bars correspond to wild type III–IV loop interacting with 1921stop and 1885stop C-T constructs. **, n.s. versus WT ; *, $p < .007$ versus WT. (Reprinted from *J Gen Physiol* [71], with permission.)

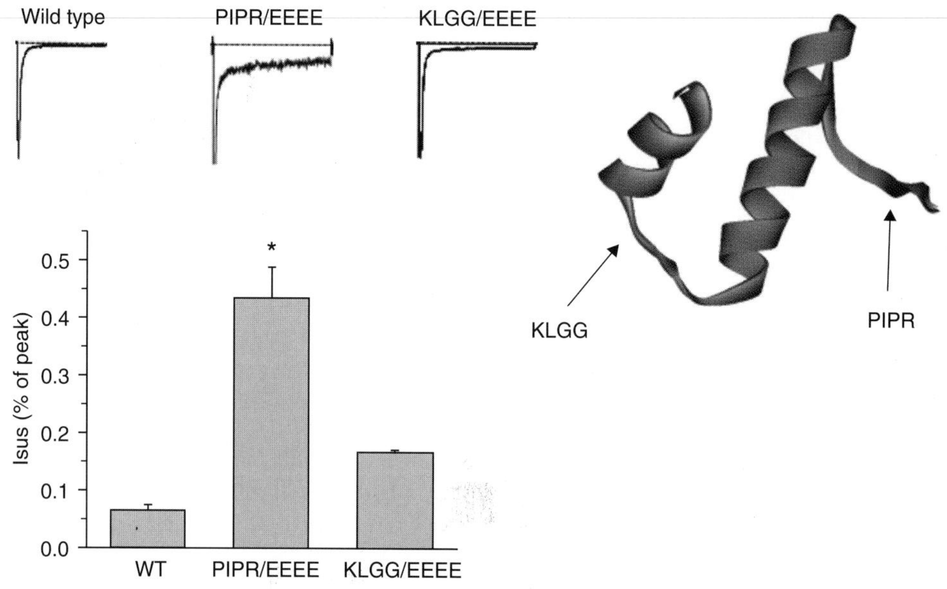

Figure 4.10 Disruption of III–IV linker/C-T domain interactions destabilizes inactivation. Mutations of two motifs of the III–IV linker (PIPR and KLGG), shown independently to disrupt III–IV linker/C-T interactions, increase sustained Na^+ current (upper traces, lower bar graphs). (Reprinted from *J Gen Physiol* [71], with permission.)

data are remarkably consistent with a role of the C-terminal/III–IV linker in stabilization of the inactivated state. Further, using glutamate scanning of the III–IV linker peptide, a region on the linker was suggested to be the motif that coordinates III–IV linker/C-T interactions and this motif was found to be distinct from the III–IV linker motif previously identified as the region that coordinates binding of the inactivation gate to the inner mouth of the channel pore (Figure 4.10). These data provided strong evidence that the inactivation gate of the voltage-dependent Na^+ channel is a molecular complex that consists of the III–IV linker and the C-terminal domain of the channel, and that this interaction underlies the stabilization of the inactivated state by the C-T domain during prolonged depolarization. Uncoupling of this complex destabilizes inactivation and increases the likelihood of channel reopening during prolonged depolarization.

Summary and future directions

Investigation into the molecular basis of inherited cardiac arrhythmias caused by mutations of the α subunit of the principal cardiac sodium channel (Nav1.5) have led to an appreciation of the role of the carboxy-terminal domain of the channel in regulating channel gating. Theoretical and experimental structural analysis of the channel C-T domain provides strong evidence for a highly structured region of the channel and that interactions between the C-T domain and the channel inactivation gate are necessary to control channel activity that directly affects action potential, and hence QT, duration in the heart. This structured region thus provides a novel target against which to develop drugs that have the potential to regulate the activity of this key cardiac ion channel, not by blocking the conduction pore, but by regulating, in an allosteric manner, channel gating.

References

1 Catterall WA. Structure and function of voltage-gated ion channels. *Annu Rev Biochem* 1995; **64**: 493–531.
2 Catterall WA. Molecular properties of sodium and calcium channels. *J Bioenerg Biomembr* 1996; **28**: 219–230.
3 Rivolta I, Abriel H, Kass RS. Ion channels as targets for drugs. In: Sperelakis N, ed. *Cell Physiology Sourcebook*. Academic Press, New York, 2001: 643–652.
4 Catterall WA. From ionic currents to molecular mechanisms: the structure and function of voltage-gated sodium channels. *Neuron* 2000; **26**: 13–25.

5 Stuhmer W, Conti F, Suzuki H *et al.* Structural parts involved in activation and inactivation of the sodium channel. *Nature* 1989; **339**: 597–603.

6 Patton DE, West JW, Catterall WA, Goldin AL. Amino acid residues required for fast Na(+)-channel inactivation: charge neutralizations and deletions in the III-IV linker. *Proc Natl Acad Sci USA* 1992; **89**: 10905–10909.

7 West JW, Patton DE, Scheuer T, Wang Y, Goldin AL, Catterall WA. A cluster of hydrophobic amino acid residues required for fast Na(+)-channel inactivation. *Proc Natl Acad Sci USA*. 1992; **89**: 10910–10914.

8 McPhee JC, Ragsdale DS, Scheuer T, Catterall WA. A mutation in segment IVS6 disrupts fast inactivation of sodium channels. *Proc Natl Acad Sci USA* 1994; **91**: 12346–12350.

9 McPhee JC, Ragsdale DS, Scheuer T, Catterall WA. A critical role for transmembrane segment IVS6 of the sodium channel alpha subunit in fast inactivation. *J Biol Chem* 1995; **270**: 12025–12034.

10 Kellenberger S, West JW, Catterall WA, Scheuer T. Molecular analysis of potential hinge residues in the inactivation gate of brain type IIA Na^+ channels. *J Gen Physiol* 1997a; **109**: 607–617.

11 Kellenberger S, West JW, Scheuer T, Catterall WA. Molecular analysis of the putative inactivation particle in the inactivation gate of brain type IIA Na^+ channels. *J Gen Physiol* 1997b; **109**: 589–605.

12 McPhee JC, Ragsdale DS, Scheuer T, Catterall WA. A critical role for the S4-S5 intracellular loop in domain IV of the sodium channel alpha-subunit in fast inactivation. *J Biol Chem* 1998; **273**: 1121–1129.

13 Yang N, Ji S, Zhou M *et al.* Sodium channel mutations in paramyotonia congenita exhibit similar biophysical phenotypes *in vitro. Proc Natl Acad Sci USA*. 1994; **91**: 12785–12789.

14 Kearney JA, Plummer NW, Smith MR *et al.* A gain-of-function mutation in the sodium channel gene Scn2a results in seizures and behavioral abnormalities. *Neuroscience* 2001; **102**: 307–317.

15 Lossin C, Wang DW, Rhodes TH, Vanoye CG, George AL, Jr. Molecular basis of an inherited epilepsy. *Neuron* 2002; **34**: 877–884.

16 Weiss LA, Escayg A, Kearney JA *et al.* Sodium channels SCN1A, SCN2A and SCN3A in familial autism. *Mol Psychiatry*. 2003; **8**: 186–194.

17 Keating MT, Sanguinetti MC. Molecular and cellular mechanisms of cardiac arrhythmias. *Cell* 2001; **104**: 569–580.

18 Kass RS, Moss AJ. Long QT syndrome: novel insights into the mechanisms of cardiac arrhythmias. *J Clin Invest* 2003; **112**: 810–815.

19 Sato C, Ueno Y, Asai K *et al.* The voltage-sensitive sodium channel is a bell-shaped molecule with several cavities. *Nature* 2001; **409**: 1047–1051.

20 Aldrich RW, Corey DP, Stevens CF. A reinterpretation of mammalian sodium channel gating based on single channel recording. *Nature* 1983; **306**: 436–441.

21 Kellenberger S, Scheuer T, Catterall WA. Movement of the Na^+ channel inactivation gate during inactivation. *J Biol Chem* 1996; **271**: 30971–30979.

22 Deschenes I, Trottier E, Chahine M. Cysteine scanning analysis of the IFM cluster in the inactivation gate of a human heart sodium channel. *Cardiovasc Res* 1999; **42**: 521–529.

23 Sheets MF, Kyle JW, Hanck DA. The role of the putative inactivation lid in sodium channel gating current immobilization. *J Gen Physiol* 2000; **115**: 609–620.

24 Tang L, Kallen RG, Horn R. Role of an S4-S5 linker in sodium channel inactivation probed by mutagenesis and a peptide blocker. *J Gen Physiol* 1996; **108**: 89–104.

25 Vassilev P, Scheuer T, Catterall WA. Inhibition of inactivation of single sodium channels by a site-directed antibody. *Proc Natl Acad Sci USA* 1989; **86**: 8147–8151.

26 Balser JR, Nuss HB, Chiamvimonvat N, Perez-Garcia MT, Marban E, Tomaselli GF. External pore residue mediates slow inactivation in mu 1 rat skeletal muscle sodium channels. *J Physiol* 1996; **494**(Pt 2): 431–442.

27 Vilin YY, Makita N, George AL, Jr, Ruben PC. Structural determinants of slow inactivation in human cardiac and skeletal muscle sodium channels. *Biophys J* 1999; **77**: 1384–1393.

28 Heinemann SH, Terlau H, Stuhmer W, Imoto K, Numa S. Calcium channel characteristics conferred on the sodium channel by single mutations. *Nature* 1992; **356**: 441–443.

29 Perez-Garcia MT, Chiamvimonvat N, Marban E, Tomaselli GF. Structure of the sodium channel pore revealed by serial cysteine mutagenesis. *Proc Natl Acad Sci USA* 1996; **93**: 300–304.

30 Yang J, Ellinor PT, Sather WA, Zhang JF, Tsien RW. Molecular determinants of $Ca2^+$ selectivity and ion permeation in L-type $Ca2^+$ channels [see comments]. *Nature* 1993; **366**: 158–161.

31 Sather WA, Yang J, Tsien RW. Structural basis of ion channel permeation and selectivity. *Curr Opin Neurobiol* 1994; **4**: 313–23.

32 Tomaselli GF, Chiamvimonvat N, Nuss HB *et al.* A mutation in the pore of the sodium channel alters gating. 1995; **68**: 1814–1827.

33 Hilber K, Sandtner W, Kudlacek O *et al.* The selectivity filter of the voltage-gated sodium channel is involved in channel activation. *J Biol Chem* 2001; **276**: 27831–27839.

34 Liu Y, Jurman ME & Yellen G. Dynamic rearrangement of the outer mouth of a K^+ channel during gating. *Neuron* 1996; **16**: 859–867.

35 Rosen MR, Hoffman BF, Wit AL. Electrophysiology and pharmacology of cardiac arrhythmias v. cardiac

antiarrhythmic effects of lidocaine. *Am Heart J* 1975; **89**: 526–536.

36 An RH, Bangalore R, Rosero SZ, Kass RS. Lidocaine block of LQT-3 mutant human Na^+ channels. *Circ Res* 1996; **79**: 103–108.

37 Wang DW, Yazawa K, Makita N, George AL, Bennett PB. Pharmacological Targeting of Long QT Mutant Sodium Channels. *J Clin Invest* 1997; **99**: 1714–1720.

38 Dumaine R, Wang Q, Keating MT *et al.* Multiple mechanisms of Na^+ channel linked long-QT syndrome. *Circ Res* 1996; **78**: 916–924.

39 Dumaine R, Kirsch GE. Mechanism of lidocaine block of late current in long Q-T mutant Na^+ channels. *Am J Physiol* 1998; **274**: H477–H487.

40 Nagatomo T, January CT, Makielski JC. Preferential block of late sodium current in the LQT3 DeltaKPQ mutant by the class I(C) antiarrhythmic flecainide. *Mol Pharmacol* 2000; **57**: 101–107.

41 Viswanathan PC, Bezzina CR, George AL, Jr., Roden DM, Wilde AA, Balser JR. Gating-dependent mechanisms for flecainide action in SCN5A-linked arrhythmia syndromes. *Circulation* 2001; **104**: 1200–1205.

42 Hille B. Local anesthetics: hydrophilic and hydrophobic pathways for the drug-receptor reaction. *J Gen Physiol* 1977; **69**: 497–515.

43 Hondeghem LM, Katzung BG. Time- and voltage-dependent interactions of antiarrhythmic drugs with cardiac sodium channels. *Biochim Biophysi Acta* 1977; **472**: 373–398.

44 Ragsdale DS, McPhee JC, Scheuer T, Catterall WA. Molecular determinants of state-dependent block of Na^+ channels by local anesthetics. *Science* 1994; **265**: 1724–1728.

45 Ragsdale DS, McPhee JC, Scheuer T, Catterall WA. Common molecular determinants of local anesthetic, antiarrhythmic, and anticonvulsant block of voltage-gated Na^+ channels. *Proc Natl Acad Sci USA* 1996; **93**: 9270–9275.

46 Li HL, Galue A, Meadows L, Ragsdale DS. A molecular basis for the different local anesthetic affinities of resting versus open and inactivated states of the sodium channel. *Mol Pharmacol* 1999; **55**: 134–141.

47 Weiser T, Qu Y, Catterall W A, Scheuer T. Differential interaction of R-mexiletine with the local anesthetic receptor site on brain and heart sodium channel alpha-subunits. *Mol Pharmacol* 1999; **56**: 1238–1244.

48 Benhorin J, Merri M, Alberti M *et al.* Long QT syndrome. New electrocardiographic characteristics. *Circulation* 1990; **82**: 521–527.

49 Pratt CM, Moye LA. The Cardiac Arrhythmia Suppression Trial: background, interim results and implications. *Am J Cardiol* 1990; **65**: 20B–29B.

50 Woosley RL. CAST: implications for drug development. *Clin Pharmacol Ther* 1990; **47**: 553–556.

51 Lazzara R. From first class to third class: recent upheaval in antiarrhythmic therapy – lessons from clinical trials. *Am J Cardiol* 1996; **78**: 28–33.

52 Roden DM. Ionic mechanisms for prolongation of refractoriness and their proarrhythmic and antiarrhythmic correlates. *Am J Cardiol* 1996; **78**: 12–16.

53 Liu H, Clancy C, Cormier J, Kass R. Mutations in cardiac sodium channels: clinical implications. *Am J Pharmacogenomics* 2003; **3**: 173–179.

54 Vassilev PM, Scheuer T, Catterall WA. Identification of an intracellular peptide segment involved in sodium channel inactivation. *Science* 1988; **241**: 1658–1661.

55 Rohl CA, Boeckman FA, Baker C, Scheuer T, Catterall WA, Klevit RE. Solution structure of the sodium channel inactivation gate. *Biochemistry* 1999; **38**: 855–861.

56 Clancy CE, Kass RS. Defective cardiac ion channels: from mutations to clinical syndromes. *J Clin Invest* 2002; **110**: 1075–1077.

57 Clancy CE, Rudy Y. Na(+) channel mutation that causes both Brugada and long-QT syndrome phenotypes: a simulation study of mechanism. *Circulation* 2002; **105**: 1208–1213.

58 Clancy CE, Rudy Y. Linking a genetic defect to its cellular phenotype in a cardiac arrhythmia. *Nature* 1999; **400**: 566–569.

59 Nuyens D, Stengl M, Dugarmaa S *et al.* Abrupt rate accelerations or premature beats cause life-threatening arrhythmias in mice with long-QT3 syndrome. *Nat Med* 2001; **7**: 1021–1027.

60 Clancy CE, Tateyama M, Kass RS. Insights into the molecular mechanisms of bradycardia-triggered arrhythmias in long QT-3 syndrome. *J Clin Invest* 2002; **110**: 1251–1262.

61 Bennett PB, Yazawa K, Makita N, George AL. Molecular mechanism for an inherited cardiac arrhythmia. *Nature* 1995; **376**: 683–685.

62 Wei J, Wang DW, Alings M *et al.* Congenital long-QT syndrome caused by a novel mutation in a conserved acidic domain of the cardiac Na^+ channel. *Circulation* 1999; **99**: 3165–3171.

63 Baroudi G, Chahine M. Biophysical phenotypes of SCN5A mutations causing long QT and Brugada syndromes. *FEBS Lett* 2000; **487**: 224–228.

64 Veldkamp MW, Viswanathan PC, Bezzina C *et al.* Two distinct congenital arrhythmias evoked by a multidysfunctional Na(+) channel. *Circ Res* 2000; **86**: E91–E97.

65 Rivolta I, Clancy CE, Tateyama M, Liu H, Priori SG, Kass RS. A novel SCN5A mutation associated with long QT-3: altered inactivation kinetics and channel dysfunction. *Physiol Genomics* 2002; **10**: 191–197.

66 Yang AS, Honig B. An integrated approach to the analysis and modeling of protein sequences and structures. II. On the relationship between sequence and structural

similarity for proteins that are not obviously related in sequence. *J Mol Biol* 2000; **301**: 679–689.

67 Yang AS. Structure-dependent sequence alignment for remotely related proteins *Bioinformatics* 2002; **18**: 1658–1665.

68 Yang AS, Wang LY. Local structure-based sequence profile database for local and global protein structure predictions *Bioinformatics* 2002; **18**: 1650–1657.

69 Cormier JW, Rivolta I, Tateyama, M, Yang AS, Kass RS. Secondary structure of the human cardiac Na^+ channel C terminus. Evidence for a role of helical structures in modulation of channel inactivation *J Biol Chem* 2002; **277**: 9233–9241.

70 Tateyama M. Liu H. Yang AS, Cormier JW, Kass RS. Structural effects of an LQT-3 mutation on heart Na^+ channel gating. *Biophys J* 2004; **86**: 1843–1851.

71 Motoike HK, Liu H, Glaaser IW, Yang AS, Tateyama M, Kass RS. The Na^+ channel inactivation gate is a molecular complex: a novel role of the COOH-terminal domain. *J Gen Physiol* 2004; **123**: 155–165.

72 Liu H, Tateyama M, Clancy CE, Abriel H, Kass RS. Channel openings are necessary but not sufficient for use-dependent block of cardiac $Na^{(+)}$ channels by flecainide: evidence from the analysis of disease-linked mutations. *J Gen Physiol* 2002; **120**: 39–51.

5

CHAPTER 5

Embryonic stem-cell-derived cardiomyocytes as a model for arrhythmia

J. Hescheler MD, PhD, *M. Halbach,* MD, *Z.J. Lu, H. Bohlen,* PhD, *B.K. Fleischmann,* MD, *&* *M. Reppel,* MD

Introduction

Heart failure and arrhythmias are the leading causes of morbidity and mortality in developed countries and is in essence, a myocyte-deficiency disease. In recent years, the understanding that regenerative processes exist at the level of the myocardium has placed stem cell research into the center of cardiology. Instead of heart transplantation, advances in cellular biology have improved the development of tissue engineering techniques using embryonic heart tissue as a new therapeutic paradigm that have already been proved in principle for animal heart failure models [1–3]. Through these cellular therapies, the concept of "growing" heart muscle and vascular tissue and manipulating the myocardial cellular environment has revolutionized the approach to treatment of heart disease. Clinically, adult hematopoietic stem cells are the most familiar of adult stem cells, with a capacity to create not merely various blood lineages, but also other cell types including cardiomyocytes. However, approaches in humans that favored the use of undifferentiated progenitor cells from bone marrow could recently *not* prove transdifferentiation into intact cardiomyocytes [4]. Therefore, the use of embryonic stem (ES) cell-derived cardiomyocytes indeed serves as the most promising tool for cell replacement strategies. It may also prove interesting for the treatment of certain forms of arrhythmias.

Generation of ES-cell-derived cardiomyocytes

In general, stem cells are defined by their capacity to keep (1) the potential to proliferate *in vitro* in a (2) undifferentiated and (3) pluri/multipotent state, thereby maintaining a relatively normal and stable karyotype even with continual passaging (self-renewal) (Figure 5.1). The most prominent stem cells are of course, the earliest formed during development, named embryonic stem (ES) cells, which occur within the inner cell mass of the blastocyst and are the origin of all cells within our body. Obviously, during their further development, the mammalian organisms keep a certain pool of undifferentiated cells that hold a certain regenerative potential of the organs. It is not yet unequivocally clarified what the properties of these adult stem cells are, but it is mostly assumed that they are in the genetic state of committed cells, that is, progenitor cells that are already genetically determined to become a certain organotypic cell. Human ES cells evoke especially intense scientific interest, given their rise to specialized human cells. The crucial and innovative finding that human ES cells can indeed form heart muscle *in vitro* has now been confirmed independently for multiple ES cell lines. Cardiac myocytes derived from human ES cells, human ES cell differentiation into the cardiac lineage and their potential suitability for clinical grafting *in vivo* have been recently reviewed [5–8].

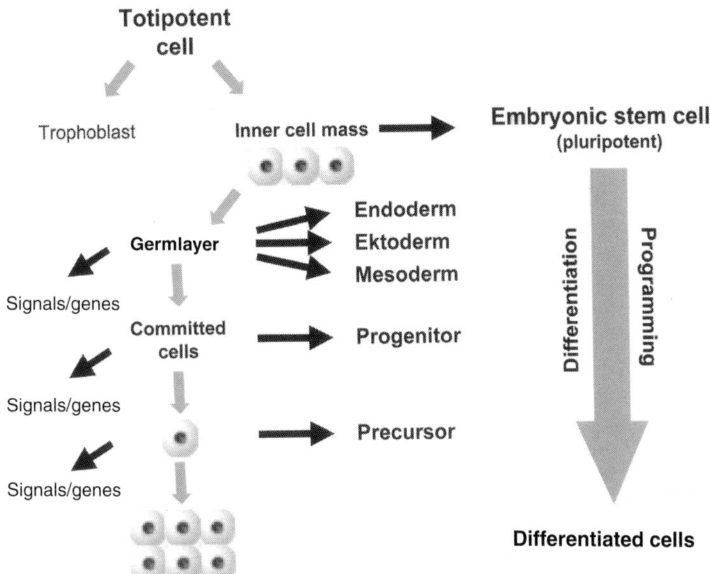

Figure 5.1 Embryonic development is reproduced by ES cells. All tissues within the organism develop from pluripotent stem cells of the inner cell mass within the blastocyst. During the physiological development signaling cascades are activated leading to the developmental dependent activation of transcription factors and organotypic genes. It is well accepted that the ES cells in culture are the only cell type that can reproduce this step-by-step development.

In vitro, ES cells spontaneously differentiate into derivatives of all three primary germ layers (Figure 5.2), the endoderm, ectoderm, and mesoderm [9, 10]. The procedure includes (1) 2 days culture of a defined number of ES cells (ca. 400 cells) in "hanging drops" as embryoid bodies, (2) 5 days culture in bacteriological dishes, (3) plating of 7 days old ("7d") embryoid bodies onto adhesive substrates. In the developing outgrowths of embryoid bodies (from "7 + 1 d" to "7 + 7 d") cardiomyocytes appear beside other cell types as spontaneously contracting cell clusters. The clusters increase in size during further development up to the terminal differentiation stage (from "7 + 9 d" to "7 + 18 d"). Single cardiomyocytes are enzymatically prepared from beating areas of embryoid body outgrowths [11]. Immunofluorescence labeling using monoclonal antibodies suggests a certain morphological development of the ES cell aggregate: First, an outer ring of endodermal alpha-fetoprotein positive cells is formed surrounding the inner cells that are differentiating into the ectodermal derivative. When plated, the third layer, that is, the mesodermal cells, develop in the contact zone between endoderm and ectoderm presumably under the influence of endodermal differentiation factors [9].

Application of microelectrode arrays

Microelectrode arrays (MEAs) find broad application in the study of excitable multicellular preparations. We cultivated mouse and human ES cells' differentiated aggregates with beating clusters of cardiomyocytes on MEAs allowing for the first time long-term recordings on a single preparation. With the differentiating ES cell aggregates and the MEA we were also able to continuously monitor the spatial and temporal structure and dynamics of electrical activity of the developing cardiac structure. Measurement of extracellularly recorded field potentials (FPs) hereby provides detailed information about the origin and spread of excitation in the heart. A similar analytical approach for cardiac FPs advanced the analysis of excitation spread and arrhythmic activity in multicellular preparations, such as developmental differentiation tissue of mouse ES cells, multicellular preparations of isolated native embryonic cardiomyocytes, or the

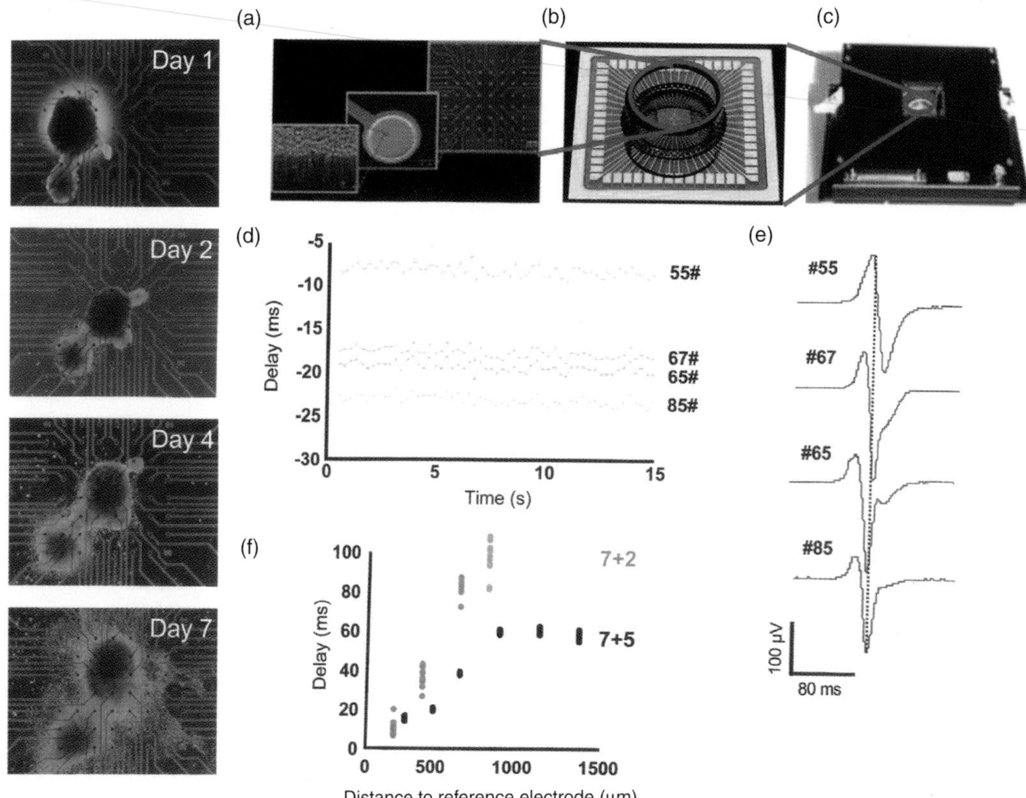

Figure 5.2 Mapping of cardiac clusters derived from the hES cell system. When ES cells are differentiated within defined protocols they develop in a morphologically determined manner that is different to the development of an embryo. The formation of narrow tissue strands in hES cell clusters is demonstrated (left). Using a MEA system (a–c) cardiac excitation and conduction delay can be calculated shown for murine ES-cell-derived cardiomyocytes during differentiation (f) and native murine heart tissue (e, d) For further details see text.

embryonic heart *in toto*. The use of substrate-integrated MEAs (Multi Channel Systems, Reutlingen, Germany) allows recording of FPs at a high signal to noise ratio. The possibility to electrically stimulate the tissue further expands the range of applications and bioassays. It may thus facilitate the evaluation of drug research providing detailed information about the interplay of the complex cardiac network, and might improve the predictability of physiological and pathophysiological conditions or antiarrhythmic drug effects in embryonic heart tissue.

In order to obtain information on the interaction of these various types of cardiomyocytes, single cell measurements by patch clamp are unfeasible but more integrative techniques need to be applied. We therefore cultivated ES cells differentiated aggregates with beating clusters of cardiomyocytes on MEAs allowing for the first time long-term recordings on a single preparation [12]. Although the signal recorded with an extracellular electrode reflects local changes of the membrane potential, currents generated in the electrically connected neighboring tissue influence it [13, 14]. These currents include active voltage-dependent currents and passive capacitive currents compensating inward currents at membrane areas of electrically coupled neighboring cells. In the case of extensively coupled cardiac myocytes, the extracellular electrode can be considered small in comparison to the structurally compact signal-generating compartment. This allows the simplification that the extracellular signal reflects local currents only. The approximation is further improved in recordings with substrate-integrated electrodes where electrogenic structures are located only on one side of the electrode. Nevertheless, interpretations of FPs can be based only on the assumption of a locally homogenous cell population.

MEA recordings of rhythmic and arrhythmic cell models

Besides the analysis of the beating frequency and the velocity of excitation spread by means of the FP, developmental changes of FP parameters that are proportionally related to the duration of the action potential (AP) upstroke and AP duration have previously been investigated. With the repeated, comparative analysis of these parameters within the same specimen of wild type and genetically manipulated preparations, the importance of individual components for the developmental or pathophysiological change of spontaneous electrophysiological properties can be revealed. Using murine ES-cell-derived cardiomyocytes the average number of electrodes detecting electrical activity increased sevenfold during the first 10 days of culture. During the increase of the beating aggregate, the beating frequency increased from initially 1 to 5 Hz. The time course of the functional development of the cardiomyocyte structure within the embryoid body compares well with that of the developing embryonic mouse heart [15], where electrical as well as contractile activity start at 8.5 days postcoitum, when myocardium is still added to the heart tube [16]. The electrophysiological basis of the increased beating frequency could depend on multiple factors. In isolated ES-cell-derived cardiomyocytes, intracellular Ca^{2+} oscillations as well as ATP-dependent K^+ channels, I_{to}, and the pacemaker current (I_f) have been described to play an important role in the development of pacemaker activity [11]. The developmental increase in frequency could therefore be based on either a switch between the major mechanisms of pacemaker activity or an increased current density of the responsible current component as described for I_f in ES-cell-derived cardiomyocytes [17]. Besides an increase of the beating frequency, we observed within the area of differentiating cardiac myocytes (1) an increase of FP rise time (FP_{rise}), (2) a decrease of the FP duration (FP_{dur}), and (3) an increase of the propagation velocity. These parameters relate to the following changes of the intrinsic electrophysiological properties described for isolated ES cells and cardiac cells isolated from embryonic mice. First, all FPs recorded at the time of onset of visible beating, that is, days 7 + 1 or 7 + 2, exhibited a homogenous shape with a long FP_{rise} and prolonged FP_{dur}. This result corresponds to the slow rise times described for APs recorded from the embryonic chicken [18] and from isolated ES cells up to day 7 + 3 in culture [19]. The potentials were similar to those recorded from the origin of excitation in embryoid bodies at later stages of development. These data indicate that all cells are functionally homogeneous and pacemaker-like at the onset of beating and that no fast voltage-activated depolarizing currents such as Na^+ current are involved in the generation of the AP, consistent with the findings in isolated ES-cell-derived cardiomyocytes [11].

Currently, the MEA technology is attracting increased interest owing to the academic need to characterize several electrophysiological features of ES-cell-derived cardiac tissue in order to provide the basis for cardiomyoplasty with improved safety and selectivity. As the MEA technology detects beating frequency, rhythmicity, and ion-channel activity, the MEA biosensor system is an ideal *in vitro* system to monitor both acute and chronic effects of drugs and to perform functional studies under physiological or induced pathophysiological conditions. By simultaneous recording at different locations, a spatial map of the excitation pathway and propagation velocities as well as of drug effects can be generated. Like sotalol-induced QT interval prolongation, drug-induced alterations of the depolarization and repolarization phase of the heart are of major concern in antiarrhythmic therapy. As has been shown for APs, the extracellular recorded FPs allow a partial reconstruction of the kinetics and time course of the underlying ion-channel activities. In particular, the duration of APs in ventricular myocytes, influenced among others by the activity of voltage-dependent Ca^{2+} channels, are closely related to the QT interval on ECGs. In a recent study, different substances with a reported QT interval prolonging effect, including E4031, amiodarone, quinidine, and sotalol, were used to study the applicability of the MEA system to study QT prolongation [20]. Since these substances evoked a significant prolongation of the FP duration, the MEA biosensor is an ideal tool to study drug toxicity with focus on effects on proarrhythmicity in three-dimensional cardiac tissue.

In a previous study taking murine EBs as a model, activity consisted of regular beating with a frequency of 0.5–5 Hz [21]. However, many EBs spontaneously developed complex activity patterns, obviously due to intermittent propagation block between the pacemaker site and the site of recording. A comparable block could also be induced in regularly beating embryoid bodies by nimodipine (NDP, 20–200 nM) and reversed upon washout. The stepwise decrease of the frequency often occurred before the pacemaker frequency was affected. To exclude that the NDP-induced complex rhythm patterns could already occur at the single cell level, perforated patch clamp recordings were performed on enzymatically isolated ES-cell-derived cardiomyocytes. Upon NDP application, current clamp recordings showed a smooth decline of the AP frequency up to a complete stop. These data demonstrate that in ES-cell-derived cardiomyocytes, NDP acts on the pacemaker activity as well as on AP propagation. Frequently, beating activity of a cell cluster is depressed by failure of AP propagation before pacemaker activity is affected.

Human ES cells

In line with the murine ES cell system, human ES cells APs exhibit three major types: nodal-like, embryonic atrial-like, and embryonic ventricular-like. Observations of beating human EBs in culture reveal distinct patterns of beating, (1) continuous beating or (2) arrhythmic, episodic beating. In ~40% episodic burst-like pattern activity has been observed in a recent study [22]. The duration of active periods and pauses varied from EB to EB, and there were parallels in the duration of spontaneous electrical activity and pauses for the respective EBs. However, other studies observed more regular beating patterns.

While there are also clear differences between mouse and human embryonic stem (hES) cells with regard to the onset of beating and its frequency development during differentiation, the effects of standard stimulators of the β-adrenergic and muscarinic signaling cascade, are both comparable to that of the mouse ES cell system [5]. This is of major importance since it demonstrates that cardiac myocytes derived from hES cells are physiologically intact and show, beside basic electrophysiological properties, also the respective functionally active hormonal receptors as well as the receptor-related signaling cascades. Cardiac mapping based on FP measurements serves as an ideal tool since it allows to measure frequency modulation and ionic-channel regulation of ES-cell-derived cardiac preparations online and in parallel [5]. This was also demonstrated in a recent report by the characterization of intrinsic AP parameters during simultaneous recording of APs and FPs in native murine embryonic cardiomyocytes [23]. As has been described for other models, not only different AP and FP morphologies representing atrial, ventricular, or pacemaker-like potentials, but also a linear relationship between AP and FP rise time as well as a linear relationship between AP and FP durations was demonstrated. In line with these similarities between APs and FPs, it was shown that individual ion channels, that is, Na^+ and voltage-dependent Ca^{2+} channels, contribute to individual FP morphologies. Thus, the development of the hES cell system and new technologies for cardiac mapping in ES-cell-derived tissue may broaden our understanding of the genesis of physiological cardiac excitation and the initiation of pathophysiological conditions, for example, arrhythmia.

References

1 Robbins J. Gene targeting. The precise manipulation of the mammalian genome. *Circ Res* 1993; **73**(1): 3–9.

2 Roell W, Fan Y, Xia Y *et al.* Cellular cardiomyoplasty in a transgenic mouse model. *Transplantation* 2002; **73**(3): 462–465.

3 Roell W, Lu ZJ, Xia Y *et al.* Transplantation of transgenic embryonic cardiomyocytes in a mouse model. *Ptlugers Arch* 2002; **441**: 153.

4 Nygren JM, Jovinge S, Breitbach M *et al.* Bone marrow-derived hematopoietic cells generate cardiomyocytes at a low frequency through cell fusion, but not transdifferentiation. *Nat Med* 2004; **10**(5): 494–501.

5 Reppel M, Boettinger C, Hescheler J. Beta-adrenergic and muscarinic modulation of human embryonic stem cell-derived cardio-myocytes. *Cell Physiol Biochem* 2004; **14**: 187–196.

6 Kehat I, Amit M, Gepstein A *et al.* Development of cardiomyocytes from human ES cells. *Methods Enzymo* 2003; **365**: 461–473.
7 Kehat I, Gepstein L. Human embryonic stem cells for myocardial regeneration. *Heart Fail Rev* 2003; **8**: 229–236.
8 Gepstein L. Derivation and potential applications of human embryonic stem cells. *Circ Res* 2002; **91**(10): 866–876.
9 Wobus AM, Wallukat G, Hescheler J. Pluripotent mouse embryonic stem cells are able to differentiate into cardiomyocytes expressing chronotropic responses to adrenergic and cholinergic agents and Ca^{2+} channel blockers. *Differentiation* 1991; **48**(3): 173–182.
10 Wobus AM, Holzhausen H, Jakel P, Schoneich J. Characterization of a pluripotent stem cell line derived from a mouse embryo. *Exp Cell Res* 1984; **152**: 212–219.
11 Maltsev VA, Rohwedel J, Hescheler J *et al.* Embryonic stem cells differentiate *in vitro* into cardiomyocytes representing sinusnodal, atrial and ventricular cell types. *Mech Dev* 1993; **44**: 41–50.
12 Banach K, Halbach MD, Hu P *et al.* Development of electrical activity in cardiac myocyte aggregates derived from mouse embryonic stem cells. *Am J Physiol Heart Circ Physiol* 2003; **284**(6): H2114–H2123.
13 Yamamoto M, Honjo H, Niwa R *et al.* Low-frequency extracellular potential recorded from the sinoatrial node. *Cardiovasc Res* 1998; **39**(2): 360–372.
14 Sprossler C, Denyer M, Britland S *et al.* Electrical recordings from rat cardiac muscle cells using field-effect transistors. *Phys Rev E Stat Phys Plasmas Fluids Relat Interdiscip Topics* 1999; **60**: 2171–2176.
15 Phoon CK, Aristizabal O, Turnbull DR. 40 MHz Doppler characterization of umbilical and dorsal aortic blood flow in the early mouse embryo. *Ultrasound Med Biol* 2000; **26**(8): 1275–1283.
16 Fishman MC, Chien KR. Fashioning the vertebrate heart: earliest embryonic decisions. *Development* 1997; **124**: 2099–2117.
17 Abi-Gerges N, Ji GJ, Lu ZJ *et al.* Functional expression and regulation of the hyperpolarization activated non-selective cation current in embryonic stem cell derived cardiomyocytes. *J Physiol* 2000; **523** (Pt 2): 377–389.
18 Fuj ii S, Hirota A, Kamino K. Optical recording of development of electrical activity in embryonic chick heart during early phases of cardiogenesis. *J Physiol* 1981; **311**: 147–160.
19 Maltsev VA, Rohwedel J, Hescheler J *et al.* Embryonic stem cells differentiate *in vitro* into cardiomyocytes representing sinusnodal, atrial and ventricular cell types. *Mech Dev* 1993; **44**(1): 41–50.
20 Meyer T, Boven KH, Gunther E *et al.* Micro-electrode arrays in cardiac safety pharmacology: a novel tool to study QT interval prolongation. *Drug Saf* 2004; **27**: 763–772.
21 Igelmund P, Fleischmann BK, Fischer IR *et al.* Action potential propagation failures in long-term recordings from embryonic stem cell-derived cardiomyocytes in tissue culture. *Pflugers Arch* 1999; **437**(5): 669–679.
22 He JQ, Ma Y, Lee Y *et al.* Human embryonic stem cells develop into multiple types of cardiac myocytes: action potential characterization. *Circ Res* 2003; **93**(1): 32–39.
23 Halbach M, Egert U, Hescheler J *et al.* Estimation of action potential changes from field potential recordings in multicellular mouse cardiac myocyte cultures. *Cell Physiol Biochem* 2003; **13**: 271–284.

6

CHAPTER 6

Gene and cell therapy for sinus and AV nodal dysfunction

Peter Danilo Jr., PhD, *Steven Girouard*, PhD, *Peter R. Brink*, PhD, *Ira S. Cohen*, MD, PhD, *Richard B. Robinson*, PhD, *&* *Michael R. Rosen*, MD

Introduction

In this chapter we will first consider the current status of treatment for sinoatrial and atrioventricular (AV) nodal disease and then provide a brief overview regarding gene and cell therapies.

The clinical setting: electronic pacemakers for the treatment of sinus and of AV nodal dysfunction

Fully implanted electronic pacemakers have been used clinically since 1960 [1] to treat an ever-increasing number of abnormalities of impulse formation and conduction, including sinus node dysfunction and high degree AV block [2]. The earliest pacemakers were functionally simple, fixed-rate, nonprogrammable devices incapable of sensing intrinsic electrical activation. These devices rapidly depleted their batteries and were prone to mechanical failures of the leads that attach the pulse generator to the heart [1]. In addition, early pacemakers presented the medical community with an apparent dilemma associated with the cost of technological advances in the treatment of cardiovascular disease; that is, there was a gap between the need for treatment and the wherewithal in terms of skills and dollars to provide it. These growing pains were overcome, however; it is estimated that the worldwide market for pacemakers is now greater than 900 000 devices/year [3]. Advances in electronics fabrication, programmable logic, computer memory and battery design, and lead technologies have resulted in modern pacemaker systems that are small, highly reliable, and employ sophisticated, sensor-driven logic to control heart rate and impulse timing in a more physiologic manner.

Yet, despite advances in component technology, sensor development and pacing algorithms challenges remain. Batteries still have a finite life span, and it is not uncommon for patients to outlive their device resulting in one or more pulse generator replacements. For pediatric or young adult patients this can mean numerous device replacements with the additional challenge that the system must allow for the demands of growth. Each device replacement requires surgical intervention that carries a finite risk of infection of the surgical site and lead tract [4]. Lead extractions resulting from infection or mechanical failure (a typical lead will flex >100 000 times/day) carry a relatively high morbidity and mortality compared with the implant procedure itself.

Finally, and of importance with regard to quality of life, even the most sophisticated rate-responsive pacemakers are not perfectly responsive to metabolic and emotional demands nor do they truly mimic intrinsic activation patterns of the atria and ventricles. Rate-responsive pacemakers employ complex algorithms and sensors that estimate systemic demand based on inputs such as activity and respiratory rate [5], however, these devices are not responsive to neural input and circulating neurohormones. Based on clinical observations [6, 7], future trends in pacing may attempt to minimize the paced beats and restore more normal ventricular conduction patterns.

Thus, while technology advances have created a durable treatment for impulse formation and conduction abnormalities, pacemakers are not a permanent cure and do not completely replace the normal function of an intact sinus or AV node. It is for these reasons that pacemaker technology would benefit from an evolution to a curative, biological solution.

Gene and cell therapy

Experimental gene therapy generally employs plasmids or viral vectors to insert genes into cells. For these approaches, the genes selected encode molecules whose modulation is thought to have therapeutic potential. Regrettably, naked plasmids have a low transfection rate and employing viruses for gene delivery is accompanied by problems including an increased risk of infection and/or neoplasia, depending on the viral vector used. In addition, plasmids and some viral vectors provide an episomal transfection: that is, the transfected gene does not become a permanent part of the cell's machinery.

Stem cells that may or may not have been genetically modified provide an alternative approach for transporting genes to target cells or tissues. The major focus of stem cell therapy for nearly a decade has been on functional replacement of myocytes lost to cardiac failure or to myocardial infarction [8–11]. Embryonic stem cells, myocytes derived from skeletal or cardiac muscle, and stem cells obtained from autologous bone marrow have been applied or injected directly into the myocardium to improve the mechanical function of the heart [12–14]. Yet, until recently, little information has been available on the use of gene or stem cell therapy for the treatment of arrhythmias in general, much less sinus or AV nodal dysfunction.

Gene and cell therapies of sinus node and AV nodal dysfunction

Within the past decade, efforts have begun to manipulate cardiac function by reversing cardiac disease without reliance on electrical or mechanical devices. Genetic manipulation of cell function was an initial and obvious means to attempt such modulation of cardiac function. Although admittedly mixed, the history of gene therapy for cystic fibrosis provided one catalyst for believing that gene therapy approaches to other diseases might be of benefit [15]. The general strategy involves insertion of the gene of interest into cells using a plasmid or a viral vector (most often a modified, nonreplicating virus). The goal is to change the expression and/or function of specific cell proteins and, ultimately, the physiology of the cells themselves and the tissues in which they reside. Providing a pacemaker when intrinsic pacemaker activity is dysfunctional and providing a substitute AV node when its nodal physiology is depressed are two settings in which genetic manipulation may prove successful. Certainly, proof of concept has been provided for the former [16], and tantalizing advances in tissue repair have been obtained [17] that relate to the latter.

Cell therapies, chiefly using embryonic or adult-derived cells, are another approach to the same goal. Investigators have explored the use of embryonic stem cells, which are pluripotent and have the property of differentiating into cells of any organ, although almost all work thus far has been *in vitro* [10]. More recently, genetically modified adult-derived mesenchymal stem cells have been used [9, 11, 18]. These are multipotent and can differentiate into cell types of mesenchymal tissues, such as bone, cartilage, connective tissue, and smooth muscle.

Although the stem cell field is rife with discovery there are major problems that are not based on science. Discovery derives from the fact that we are in the early phases of learning how to communicate with them, how to modify them and benefit from their potential, and how to identify their potential for pathologic sequellae. The nonscientific problems are political, religious, and ethical in origin. On the one hand, scientists with a need to know the why and wherefore of these cells' physiology are in partnership with physicians with a need to apply new and better therapies for disease. On the other hand, in the United States and some other countries, governmental constraints have been placed on many efforts at embryonic stem cell discovery.

Requisites of gene and cell therapies of sinus and AV node dysfunction

Any form of genetic or cellular manipulation used to treat sinus or AV nodal dysfunction must not only provide the primary activity of the tissue replaced (e.g. pacemaking or propagation) but also should be responsive to endogenous autonomic control. When genes are delivered to native cardiocytes *in situ*, they are likely to be incorporated in cells that have intact adrenergic and cholinergic receptors and the respective signal transduction pathways. This observation highlights a major advantage of gene therapy, that is, one is attempting to modify a single protein in an otherwise fully functional cell. If the cell is not fully or appropriately functional, additional genes may need to be incorporated in any construct, and this adds to the complexity of gene therapy.

Stem cells present a unique subset of issues: some have autonomic receptors and appear to have intact coupling systems [19–21]; but for most, there are unresolved questions regarding the presence and function of such systems and the extent to which this depends on the state and pathway of differentiation. Suffice it to say that when administered, a stem cell must either have an intact and functional autonomic transduction system, or must couple effectively to cells (e.g. myocytes) that not only have but can share such a system. If neither possibility exists, then the stem cell must be engineered to incorporate such a system.

The site of administration of genes or cells is also critical to their ultimate functioning in the heart. Genes or cells must be placed where they (1) have electrical access to the normal pathways of conduction, thereby optimizing contraction, (2) are least likely to induce arrhythmias, and (3) have an adequate blood supply. Diseased myocardium or conducting tissue could present barriers to the effectiveness of any form of therapy; that is, an impulse may be initiated normally by a biological pacemaker and if the implant is incorrectly placed, be unable to gain access to the bulk myocardium.

An additional problem with regard to cell therapies is the need to ensure that they couple tightly to target cells (most likely myocytes) to which they are to deliver a signal. The synchrony of contraction of native adult and transplanted fetal myocytes has been demonstrated [22]; and more recently data have become available indicating that mesenchymal stem cells make gap junctional proteins and demonstrate both the passage of current and of small molecules to adjacent myocytes, providing evidence for appropriate coupling [23]. Yet, the ability to provide pacemaker function with gene or cell therapies depends not only on coupling but on a balance between coupling and isolation. For example, in the SA node, pacemaker cells must remain relatively depolarized compared with surrounding tissue yet coupled sufficiently to initiate a cardiac impulse by depolarizing surrounding atrial myocardium.

When a site appropriate for gene or cell therapy is identified, a simple and effective means of delivery must be available, optimally avoiding surgical procedures. Catheter-based delivery systems to insert gene constructs have been used experimentally in animals with some success [24–26]. Although these systems are now operative, fine tuning is needed with regard to minimization of tissue damage [26] as well as optimal dose of the construct to be given. Additional problems associated with either gene or cell therapies are immune responses, concurrent infections, and the potential for neoplasia. In the case of cell therapies, there are two additional issues. We must learn the extent to which the cells administered will/will not further differentiate (and if they do differentiate, into what cell type and with what change in effectiveness of delivering their message). We must also determine whether the cells remain where administered or migrate elsewhere and, if so, with what consequences

Determinants of pacemaker function – building a biological pacemaker

All parts of the cardiac specialized conducting system have the property of automaticity, but the primary pacemaker in the normal heart, and the prototype for any biological pacemaker is the sinoatrial node (Figure 6.1). The rate of impulse initiation by subsidiary pacemakers diminishes as one proceeds from SA node distally through the conducting system [27]. The pacemaker current is referred to as I_f is a *h*yperpolarization activated, cyclic *n*ucleotide gated current that is determined

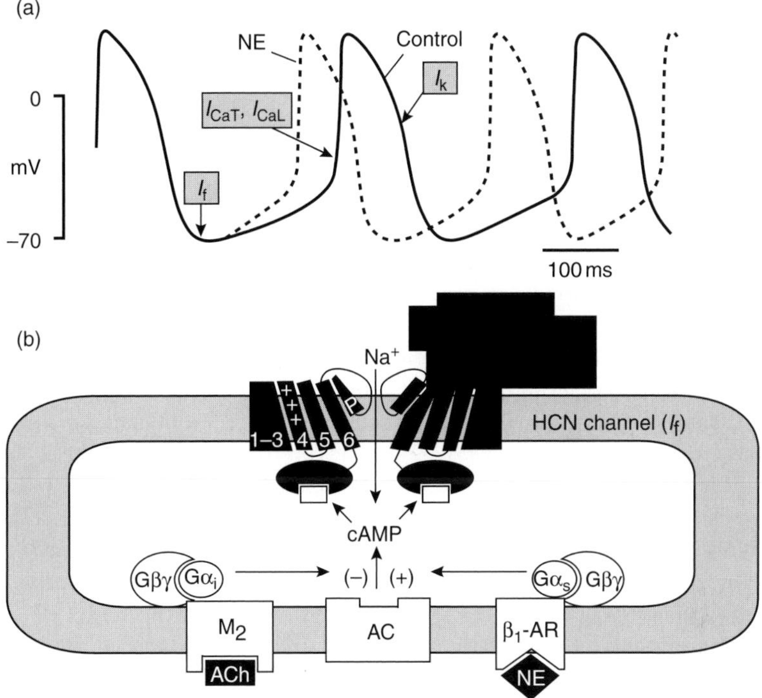

Figure 6.1 The ion channels responsible for cardiac automaticity. (a) Solid trace: sinus node action potential – the pacemaker potential is initiated by If, the "funny current" which initiates phase 4 depolarization. Both T- and L-type calcium channels may contribute to the latter portion of phase 4, and repolarization is the result of a delayed rectifier current, I_K. On exposure to catecholamine (broken trace) the slope of phase 4 increases and with this, so does spontaneous rate. (b) The figure shows the diagrammatic representation of the pacemaker, or HCN (for *h*yperpolarization activated, cyclic *n*ucleotide gated) channel. The channel has six transmembrane spanning domains and four repeats of it occur in the cell membrane. Critical to channel function are the Na entry that occurs on hyperpolarization, and the cyclic nucleotide binding sites near the carboxyterminus that – on cyclic AMP binding – cause a positive shift in activation, resulting in an increase in spontaneous rate. Binding of catecholamine to beta-adrenergic receptors results in a GTP-regulatory protein-transduced increase in adenylyl cyclase function to metabolize ATP to cyclic AMP. This makes available increased cAMP for binding to its site on the channel. Muscarinic stimulation by acetylcholine antagonizes this process, and can result in a brake on impulse initiation. (Reprinted from Biel *et al*. Cardiac HCN channels: structure, function, and modulation. *Trends Cardiovasc* 2002; **12**: 206–221 by permission.)

by four isoforms of the pacemaker gene, HCN (the isoforms being HCN1–4). The predominant isoform in sinus node is HCN4, the predominant one in ventricular myocardium is HCN2. HCN3 is not present in heart. Each isoform has different characteristics with regard to activation kinetics and cyclic AMP gating that influences the magnitude of current and the rate at which it is generated.

Although a family of ion channels determine the pacemaker rate of any tissue, the key to impulse initiation is seen in the interaction between inward sodium current, carried by I_f, and repolarizing current, especially that carried by the inward rectifier, I_{K1}. There is little I_{K1} in SA node and a great deal in ventricular myocardium [28]. Since a large outward current would oppose the depolarizing effect of I_f, the large I_{K1} in myocardium in part explains the minimal to absent automaticity that is expressed by this tissue.

Gene therapy of pacemaker function

Initial proof of concept regarding the use of gene therapy to fabricate biological pacemakers came from studies of beta-2 adrenergic receptor overexpression. The hypothesis was that modulation of beta-adrenergic receptors can influence cardiac pacemaker function by changing the response to endogenous neurohumors. Thus, Edelberg *et al.* [29, 30] injected a plasmid containing the cDNA from cloned beta-2 adrenergic receptors into swine atria. Although the effect was short-lived, they found that intrinsic pacemaker rate was increased, as was its response to isoproterenol, showing that it is possible to enhance pacemaker function using gene transfer techniques.

A direct approach to genetic modulation of ion channels has relied on using replication deficient adenoviruses to insert genetic material. Proof of concept here was provided by Miake, *et al.* [31, 32] who used an adenoviral vector carrying a dominant negative construct to inhibit I_{K1}, the inward rectifier current in guinea pig ventricle. Injection of the modified Kir gene into the left ventricular cavity resulted in automaticity of isolated myocytes and idioventricular rhythms *in vivo*. They also showed that by inhibiting I_{K1} action potential duration in the plateau voltage range was increased, terminal repolarization was prolonged, and the QTc interval on ECG was increased [32]. This result not only demonstrates the benefits of reducing outward current as a means of increasing pacemaker rate, but highlights a potential proarrhythmic effect, that is, the excess QT prolongation. A further drawback to this approach is that preliminary data suggest that rather than a single inward current being responsible for the pacemaker potential here, several inward currents may be contributory in an as yet incompletely defined fashion [33].

We have used overexpression of pacemaker current I_f to build biological pacemakers [16, 26, 34]. In principle, this approach is straightforward in that I_f activates at diastolic potential ranges and therefore would have little effect on action potential duration. Moreover, it is modulated by autonomic neurohumors. Of the four known isoforms of the HCN gene encoding I_f, three have been shown to exist in the heart. All are activated by hyperpolarization and all bind cyclicAMP. Of these three isoforms, HCN2 exhibits a strong response to cAMP and relatively fast kinetics.

Qu *et al.* [16] transfected rat ventricular myocytes in culture with HCN2 to increase spontaneous rate. Patch clamp experiments showed an increase in I_f of 100 times compared with nontransfected cells. To test whether HCN2 could also function to modulate rate *in vivo*, the adenoviral construct was injected directly into the left atrial myocardium of dogs [34]. Pacemaker activity was observed during vagal stimulation (to suppress sinus node automaticity) and originated near the site of injection of the viral construct. Atrial myocytes isolated from these sites showed at least a 100-fold increase in pacemaker current as compared to controls.

Subsequent experiments [26] were designed to deliver HCN directly into the proximal left ventricular specialized conducting system (Figure 6.2). The construct was injected directly into left bundle branches using a fluoroscopically guided catheter. In these animals during vagal stimulation, prior HCN2 injection was associated with escape rhythms originating from the region of injection at approximately 60 beats/min. Cells and tissue isolated from injection sites displayed biophysical (increased I_f) and immunohistochemical evidence of overexpressed HCN2 as well as increased automaticity during microelectrode studies.

These results all support the concept that biological pacemaking using gene therapy is a functional reality. The major obstacles to overcome relate to the fact that injecting plasmids gives a low transfection rate and transient expression of function, and both the plasmids and the replication-deficient adenoviruses are episomal, having no effect to permanently transform the genome. To make this approach feasible in the long-term requires the use of viruses (e.g. retroviruses) whose potential for inflammation, infection, and malignant transformation render them unfit in any risk/benefit analysis. Hence, the identification of the appropriate vector and a strategy for genomic incorporation of the construct are pressing needs if the field is to advance.

Stem cell therapy of pacemaker function

Embryonic stem cells

Embryonic stem cells have the potential to differentiate into cells typical of any tissue, taking on the functional characteristics of that tissue. Kehat *et al.* [13] induced human embryonic stem cells to differentiate into embryoid bodies some of which

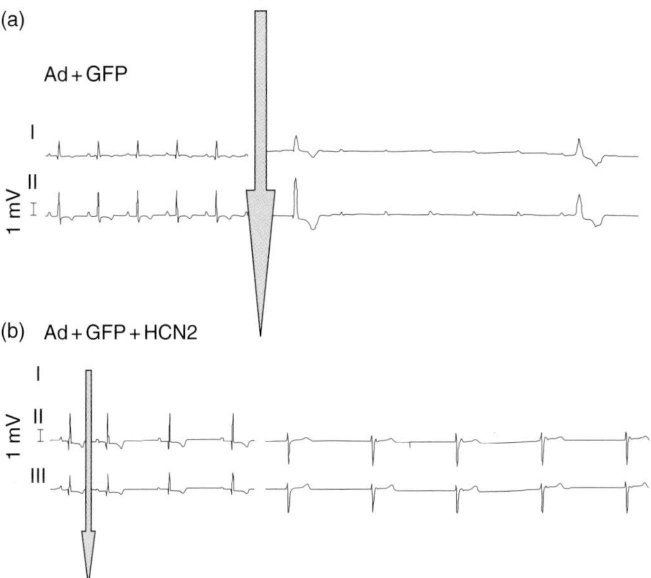

Figure 6.2 Effects of direct injection into canine left bundle branch of adenovirus + GFP (green fluorescent protein) or adenovirus + GFP + HCN2. In both parts, vagal stimulation (vertical arrow) was used to allow emergence of idioventricular rhythm. (a) The figure shows a slow idioventricular rhythm (although not shown, initial escape time was 22 s). (b) The figure shows emergence of a more rapid rhythm having a rate of about 60/min. Escape time (duration of break between traces) was 5 s. (Reprinted from *Circulation* [26], with permission.)

displayed functional characteristics of cardiac myocytes. Among the properties demonstrated was the ability to beat spontaneously, the presence of intercalated disks, positive staining with cardiacspecific antibodies, and excitability and responsiveness to adrenergic and cholinergic stimuli. Electrograms recorded from areas of contracting cells displayed sharp upstrokes and slow repolarization, a configuration similar to that recorded from cardiac tissues. Using the calcium sensing dye, fura-2AM, calcium transients were recorded that were synchronous with contraction.

Igelmund *et al.* [35] found that myocytes derived from murine embryonic stem cells had functional Na channels blocked by tetrodotoxin as determined from extracellular electrogram recordings. He *et al.* [14] found that human embryonic stem-cell-derived embryoid bodies in culture-displayed action potentials are similar to those found in SA nodal, atria, and ventricles. These cells had arrhythmic potential in that early after depolarizations (EADs) and delayed after depolarizations (DADs) could be elicited. Zhang *et al.* [36] found that mouse-derived embryoid bodies could differentiate into cardiocytes with action potentials typical of nodal, atrial, and ventricular tissues. They also found that EADs and DADs could arise from ventricular-type cells. Thus, although it is possible to have stem cells differentiate into potentially useful cardiac cells with action potentials similar to those found in native tissues, further study is needed to determine their arrhythmogenic potential in the *in situ* heart and to learn how to drive them to become and remain a specific cardiac cell type, such as SA nodal.

Adult mesenchymal stem cells

Adult mesenchymal stem cells, often derived from bone marrow, can differentiate into cell lines including skeletal muscle, bone, and other connective tissues. We have used them as a platform for gene therapy because of their ready availability, the lack of any governmental restrictions or social taboos, and the observation that they may be "immunopriviliged," that is, of low likelihood to elicit significant immune responses in host tissue [37]. Heubach *et al.* [38] using patch clamp techniques found outward currents including a Ca-activated potassium current, a clofilium-sensitive current, and, less frequently, inward L-type Ca currents. No other inward currents were demonstrated. Potapova *et al.* [21] used electroporation to load adult human mesenchymal stem cells (hMSCs) with the pacemaker gene, HCN2. Transfection efficacy approached 50% and the technique required no reliance on a viral vector. Patch clamp experiments demonstrated that the cells now expressed I_{HCN2}, the analog of I_f (Figure 6.3). This current increased on application of isoproterenol and demonstrated accentuated antagonism to acetylcholine.

For stem cells to be useful, they must be capable of coupling with cells in the tissues in which they have been implanted. That is, in contrast to myocytes virally transfected with pacemaker genes, nondifferentiated hMSCs containing the pacemaker gene, HCN2, cannot spontaneously depolarize to provide pacemaker function. In fact, all they can do is generate a current in response to hyperpolarization: they generate no action potential on their own. This highlights the importance of their coupling to the myocytes: the hMSC provides the current or driver, the coupled myocyte provides the hyperpolarized membrane potential to initiate the driver, as well as the action potential, itself. In other words, the coupled cells act as a single functional unit.

The hMSCs did, in fact, form gap junctions with cardiocytes, as was demonstrated *in vitro* and *in vivo* [21]. Injection of hMSCs into the canine left ventricular epicardium initiated idioventricular rhythms originating from the site of stem cell injection over a 5–10 day period after administration. Figure 6.4 shows a representative experiment. That this result was due to the pacemaker function of stem cells was suggested by other experiments showing that hMSCs lacking the pacemaker gene, HCN2, did not demonstrate I_f *in vitro* and were not associated with ectopic ventricular sites *in vivo* [21]. Moreover, the rhythms that originated in the hearts that had received HCN2-loaded hMSCs were pace mapped to the site of injection. Finally, histological and immunocytochemical studies clearly demonstrated the presence of hMSCs at the site of injection and gap junctions between hMSCs and adjacent myocytes (Figure 6.5) [21].

These studies demonstrate the potential therapeutic use of hMSCs in fabricating biological

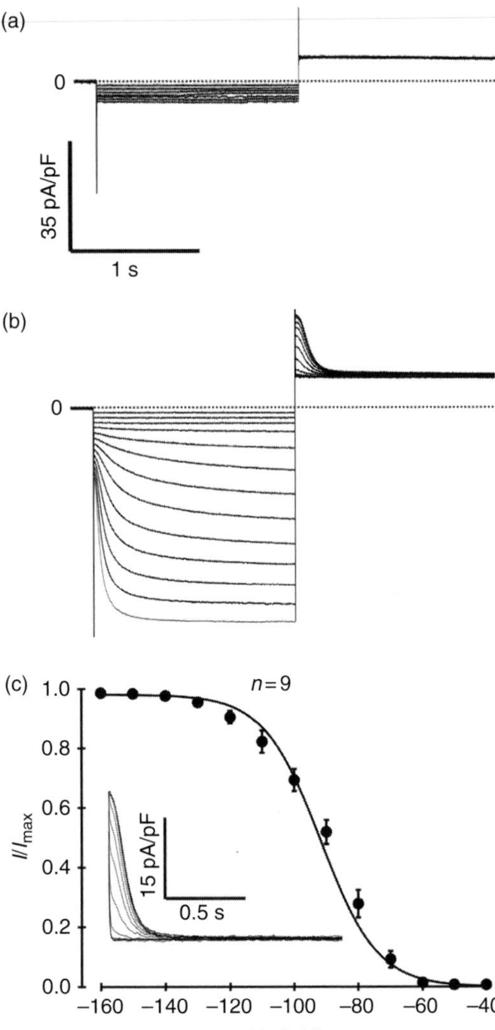

Figure 6.3 Functional expression of I_f in human mesenchymal stem cells transfected with the HCN2 gene. (a) The figure shows that I_f is not expressed in nontransfected cells. (b) The figure shows expression of I_f in transfected cells. (c) The figure shows normalized tail currents of I_f fit by the Boltzman distribution. Midpoint is −92 mV, slope = 8.8 mV. I_f was fully activated near −140 mV. Inset of (c) shows representative tail currents used to construct I_f activation curves. (Reprinted from *Circ Res* [21], by permission.)

pacemakers. They do not deal in any depth with immune responses of the recipient or possible de-differentiation or maturation of the stem cells, or the possibility of their migrating to other sites in the body.

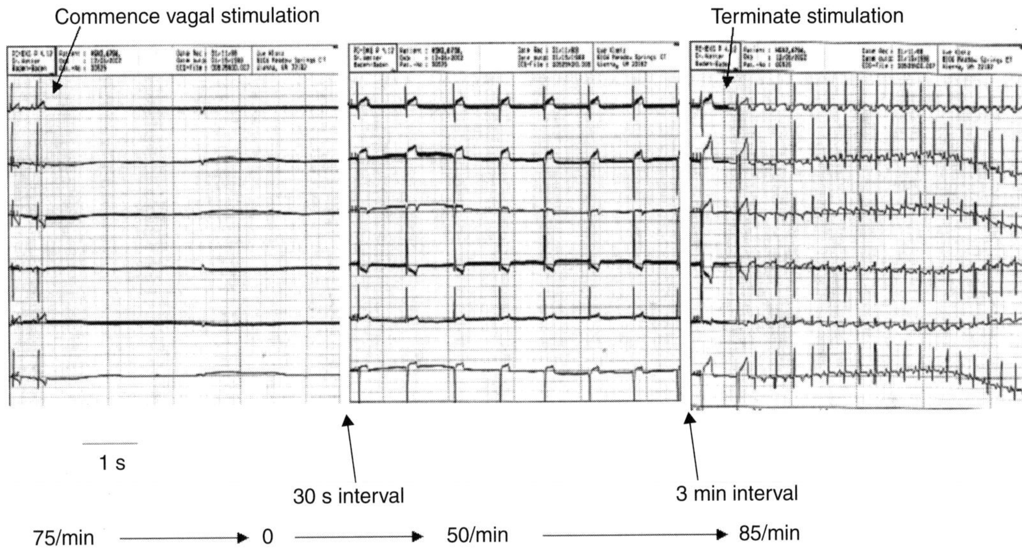

Figure 6.4 Pacemaker function in canine heart *in situ*. Top to bottom: ECG leads, I, II, III, AVR, AVL, AVF. Left panel: last 2 beats in sinus rhythm and onset of stimulation of cervical vagus nerves (arrow) causing sinus arrest in a dog studied 7 days after implanting HCN2 transfected hMSCs in left ventricular anterior wall epicardium. Middle panel: during continued vagal stimulation, an idioventricular escape focus emerges, having a regular rhythm. Right panel: on cessation of vagal stimulation (arrow), there was a postvagal sinus tachycardia. (Reprinted from *Circ Res* [21], by permission.)

Building a biological AV node

Building a biological AV node represents an attempt to correct high-degree AV block, which is a major indication for electronic pacemaker therapy. In this instance, one would be treating a patient with normal sinus node function and either a congenital or acquired form of heart block. Current therapy is usually an AV sequential pacemaker via which the sinus node drives the ventricles through an electrical circuit. The intent of the biological therapy would be to permit normal sinus node function to drive the heart via a cell-based AV bypass tract having the function of an AV node.

The AV node is a complex structure, which transmits impulses from atria to ventricles. Because of its small size and relative inaccessibility to dissection it has been less well-characterized electrophysiologically and biophysically than other structures of the heart. Hoffman *et al.* [39]. recorded membrane potentials from intact nodes and Kokobun, *et al.* [40]. recorded membrane currents from AV nodal cells. More recently, AV nodal

Figure 6.5 Immunostaining for Cx43 in a region of stem-cell-injected myocardium in the interface between stem cells and muscle cells. DAPI staining shows nuclei, which are densely packed in an area largely comprised of stem cells and loosely packed in a region of myocytes. The bright green fluorescence is connexin43 staining, indicating the presence of gap junctions. White arrows point to gap junctions from stem cell to stem cell; red arrows, from stem cell to muscle cell; purple arrows, from muscle cell to muscle cell. (Reprinted from *Circ Res* [21], by permission.)

cells have been isolated from rabbit hearts and normal action potentials and ion currents recorded [41, 42]. In the node, proper, it is clear that the action potential is largely Ca-dependent and slowly propagating. In addition the small diameter of the cells contributes to the slow conduction velocity.

To date, efforts to modulate conduction of the cardiac impulse in general and to create an artificial AV node in particular have met with only partial success. Camelliti *et al.* [43] and Gaudesius *et al.* [44] report that fibroblasts couple to myocytes and provide synchronization of contraction via electrotonic interactions. Other groups including our own are working to engineer heart cells with the capability of propagating impulses at the appropriate velocity from atrium to ventricle. This approach requires tissue engineering, including the use of genes and/or cells to provide function lost to disease. (See Reference 45 for a review on the biophysics of tissue engineering.) Relevant examples of tissue engineering are "artificial" bone and skin applied when original tissue loss is so extensive that normal healing takes too long or is not possible.

A successful attempt to modulate AV nodal function via gene therapy was reported by Murata, *et al.* [46]. They demonstrated focal Ca channel blockade resulting in a prolongation of AH and PR intervals and the downregulation of AV conduction. The challenge now would be to use alternative approaches whereby the function of the same target channel is upregulated as a means to enhance AV conduction. In a preliminary communication Kizana *et al.* [17] reported the possibility that fibroblasts could be made electrically conductive by gene transfer thereby providing a potential means of overcoming AV block.

Conclusions

The use of gene therapy to modulate and restore cardiac function has reached a clinically imaginable and in some instances applicable threshold. Data thus far indicate the feasibility of this approach to pacemaker activity as a therapeutic modality, although many questions remain to be answered. How can we fine-tune interactions between genetically modified and normal cells? Will anchoring strategies be required to keep stem cells where they are needed? Will these constructs and cells maintain their characteristics or will they lose the ability to function as they were designed or, in fact, will they become detrimental? Will we be able to prevent neoplastic activity arising from viral constructs and stem cells? Similarly, can inflammation and immune responses to this therapeutic modality be minimized? As answers to these questions are obtained, the utility and application of gene and cell therapies as therapeutic tools will be further defined and, we believe, brought to fruition clinically.

Acknowledgments

The research presented was supported by USPHS-NHLBI grants HL-28958, HL-67101, HL-20558, and GM-55263 and by Guidant Corporation. The authors wish to thank Laureen Pagan and Eileen Franey for their careful attention to the preparation of the manuscript.

References

1 Kirk Jefferey. Machines in Our Hearts. The Johns Hopkins University Press, Baltimore, MD, 2001.

2 Hayes DL, Naccarelli GV, Furman S *et al.* NASPE training requirements for cardiac implantable electronic devices: selection, implantation, and follow-up. *PACE* 2003; **7**: 1556–1562.

3 Reicin G, Miksic M. Hospital supplies and medical Technology. Notes from 8th Annual CRM Conference. Morgan Stanley Industry Overview. September 8, 2004.

4 Cohen MI, Bush DM, Gaynor JW, Vetter VL, Tanel RE, Rhodes LA. Pediatric pacemaker infections: twenty years of experience. *J Thorac Cardiovasc Surg* 2002; **124**(4): 821–827.

5 Freedman RA, Hopper DL, Mah J, Hummel J, Wilkoff BL. Assessment of pacemaker chronotropic response: implementation of the Wilkoff mathematical model. *PACE* 2001; **12**: 1748–1754.

6 Wilkoff BL, Cook JR, Epstein AE *et al.* Dual-chamber pacing or ventricular backup pacing in patients with an implantable defibrillator: the Dual Chamber and VVI Implantable Defibrillator (DAVID) Trial. *JAMA* 2002; **288**(24): 3115–3123.

7 Sweeney MO, Hellkamp AS, Ellenbogen KA *et al.* Adverse effect of ventricular pacing on heart failure and atrial fibrillation among patients with normal baseline QRS duration in a clinical trial of pacemaker therapy for sinus node dysfunction. *Circulation* 2003; **107**(23): 2932–2937.

8 Sakai T, Ling Y, Payne TR, Huard J. The use of ex vivo gene transfer based on muscle-derived stem cells for cardiovascular medicine. *Trends Cardiovasc Med* 2002; **12**: 115–120.

9 Orlic D, Hill JM, Arai AE. Stem cells for myocardial regeneration. *Circ Res* 2002; **91**: 1092–1102.

10 Caspi O, Gepstein L. Potential applications of human embryonic stem cell-derived cardiomyocytes. *Ann NY Acad Sci* 2004; **1015**: 285–298.

11 Mathur A, Martin JF. Stem cells and repair of the heart. *Lancet* 2004; **364**: 183–192.

12 Klug MG, Soonpa MH, Koh GY, Field LF. Genetically selected cardiomyocytes from diffentiating embryonic stem cells form stable intracardiac grafts. *J Clin Invest* 1996; **98**: 216–224.

13 Kehat I, Kenyagin-Karsenti D, Snir M *et al.* Human embryonic stem cells can differentiate into myocytes with structural and functional properties of cardiocytes. *J Clin Invest* 2001; **108**: 407–414.

14 He H, N Y, Lee Y, Thornton JA, Kamp TJ. Human embryonic stem cells develop into multiple types of cardiac myocytes. Action potential characteristics. *Circ Res* 2003; **93**: 21–39.

15 Ratko TA, Cummings JP, Blebera J, Mautszewski KA. Clinical gene therapy for nonmalignant disease. *Am J Med* 2003; **115**: 560–569.

16 Qu J, Barbuti A, Protas L, Santoro B, Cohen IS, Robinson RB. HCN2 overexpression in newborn and adult ventricular myocytes. Distinct effects on gating and excitability. *Circ Res* 2001; **89**: e8–e14.

17 Kizana E, Allen DG, Ross DL, Alexander IE. Fibroblasts can be rendered electrically conductive by genetic modification: toward a biological therapy for heart block. *Circulation* 2003; **108**: 183.

18 Strauer BE, Brehm M, Zeus T *et al.* Repair of infracted myocardium by autologous intracoronary mononuclear bone marrow transplantation in humans. *Circulation* 2002; **106**: 1913–1916.

19 Hakuno D, Fukuda K, Makino S *et al.* Bone marrow-derived regenerated cardiomyocytes (CMG cells) express functional adrenergic and muscarinic receptors. *Circulation* 2002; **105:** 380–386.

20 Fukuda K. Reprogramming of bone marrow mesenchymal stem cells into cardiomyocytes. *C R Biol* 2002; **325:** 1027–1038.

21 Potopova I, Plotnikov A, Lu Z *et al.* Human mesenchymal stem cells as a gene delivery system to create cardiac pacemakers. *Circ Res* 2004; **94**: 952–959.

22 Rubart M, Pasumarthi KBS, Nakajima H, Soonpa MH, Nakajima HO, Field LJ. Physiological coupling of donor and host cardiomyocytes after cellular transplantation. *Circ Res* 2003; **92**: 1217–1224.

23 Valiunas V, Doronin S, Valiuniene L *et al.* Human mesenchymal sem cells make cardiac connexins and form functional gap junctions. *J Physiol* 2004; **555**: 617–626.

24 Vale PR, Losordo DW, Tkebuchava T, Chen D, Milliken CE, Isner JM. Catheter-based myocardial gene transfer utilizing nonfluoroscopic electromechanical left ventricular mapping. *J Am Coll Cardiol* 1999; **34**: 246–254.

25 Losordo DW, Vale PR, Hendel RC *et al.* Phase 1–2 placebo-controlled, double-blind, dose-escalating trial of myocardial vascular endothelial growth factor 2 gene transfer factor by catheter delivery in patients with chronic myocardial ischemia. *Circulation* 2002; **105**: 2012–2018.

26 Plotnikov AN, Sosunov EA, Qu J *et al.* Biological pacemaker implanted in canine left bundle branch provides ventricular escape rhythms that have physiologically acceptable rates. *Circulation* 2004; **109**: 506–512.

27 Vassalle M, Yu H, Cohen IS. Pacemaker channels and cardiac automaticity. In: Zipes DP Jalife J, eds. *Cardiac Electrophysiology: From Cell to Bedside.* 3rd edn. WB Saunders, Philadelphia, PA, 2000; 94–103.

28 Noma A, Nakayama T, Kurachi Y, Irisawa H. Resting K conductances in pacemaker and non-pacemaker cells of the rabbit. *Jap J Physiol* 1984; **34**: 245–254.

29 Edelberg JM, Aird WV, Rosenberg RD. Enhancement of murine cardiac chronotropy by the molecular transfer of the human beta2 adrenergic receptor cDNA. *J Clin Invest* 1998; **101**: 337–343.

30 Edelberg JM, Huang DT, Josephson ME, Rosenberg RD. Molecular enhancement of porcine cardiac chronotropy. *Heart* 2001; **86**: 559–562.

31 Miake J, Marban E, Nuss HB. Gene therapy: biological pacemaker created by gene transfer. *Nature* 2002; **419**: 132–133.

32 Miake J, Marban E, Nuss HB. Functional role of inward rectifier current in heart probed by Kir2.1 overexpression and dominant-negative suppression. *J Clin Invest* 2003; **111**: 1529–1536.

33 Silva J, Rudy Y. Mechanism of pacemaking in $I(k_1)$-downregulated myocytes. *Circ Res* 2003; **92**: 261–263.

34 Qu J, Plotnikov AN, Danilo P Jr. *et al.* Expression and function of a biological pacemaker in canine heart. *Circulation* 2003; **107**: 1106–1109.

35 Igelmund P, Fleischmann BK, Fischer IR *et al.* Action potential propagation failures in long-term recordings from embryonic stem cell-derived cardiomyocytes in tissue culture. *Pflugers Arch* 1999; **437**: 669–679.

36 Zhang YM, Hartzell C, Narlow M, Dudley SC. Stem cell-derived cardiomyocytes demonstrate arrhythmic potential. *Circulation* 2002; **106**: 1294–1299.

37 Liechty KW, MacKenzie TC, Shaaban AF *et al.* Human mesenchymal stem cells engraft and demonstrate site-specific differentiation after in utero transplantation in sheep. *Nature Med* 2000; **6**: 1282–1286.

38 Heubach JF, Graf EM, Leutheuser J *et al.* Electrophysiological properties of human mesenchymal stem cells. *J Physiol* 2003; **554**: 659–672.

39 Hoffman BF, Paes de Carvalho A, de Mello WC, Cranfield PF. Electrical acitivity of single fibers of the atrioventricular node. *Circ Res* 1959; **7**: 11–18.

40 Kokobun S, Nishimura M, Noma NA, Irisawa H. Membrane currents in the rabbit atrioventricular node cell. *Pflugers Arch* 1982; **393**: 15–22.

41 Hancox JC, Levi AJ, Lee CO, Heap P. A method for isolating rabbit atrioventricular node myocytes which retain normal morphology and function. *Am J Physiol* 1993; **265**: H755–H7666.

42 Munk AA, Adjemian RA, Zhao J, Ogbaghebriel A, Shrier A. Electrophysiological properties of morphologically distinct cells isolated from the rabbit atrioventricular node. *J Physiol* 1996; **493**: 801–818.

43 Camelliti P, Green CR, LeGrice I, Kohl P. Fibroblast network in rabbit sinoatrial node. Structural and functional identification of homogeneous and heterogenous cell coupling. *Circ Res* 2004; **94**: 828–835.

44 Gaudesius G, Miragoli M, Thomas SP, Rohr S. Coupling of cardiac electrical activity over extended distances by fibroblasts of cardiac origin. *Circ Res* 2003; **93**: 421–428.

45 Curtis A, Riehle M. Tissue engineering: the biophysical background. *Phys Med Biol* 2001; **46**: R47–R65.

46 Murata M, Cingolani E, McDonald AD, Donahue JK, Marban E. Creation of a genetic calcium channel blocker by triggered gem gene transfer in the heart. *Circ Res* 2004; **95**: 398–405.

7

CHAPTER 7

Gene therapy for cardiac tachyarrhythmias

J. Kevin Donahue, MD, *Amy D. McDonald*, BS
Alexander Bauer, MD, *Kan Kikuchi*, PhD, & *Tetsuo Sasano* MD

An explosion in availability and ease of use for techniques related to the identification, characterization, and manipulation of genetic material has provoked intense interest in gene therapy for numerous diseases. The promise of genetic therapies is twofold: improved specificity of action could reduce side effects relative to pharmacotherapy, and a more directed response to an underlying problem (e.g. replacement of under active genes or dominant-negative suppression of overactive genes) might increase therapeutic potency. Interest in molecular electrophysiology was sparked with the connection of sodium and potassium channel mutations to a specific disease state, the long-QT syndrome [1, 2]. Around the same time, intense research focused on development of gene transfer methods that might one day translate gene discoveries into therapeutics [3–5].

In this review, we will focus on the development of gene transfer techniques for treatment of cardiac tachyarrhythmias. Work in this field proceeds along three lines: (1) identification of proteins and their related genes, with actions that affect the electrical substrate, (2) characterization of the function of these proteins and of the underlying electrophysiological substrate in health and disease, and (3) development of gene transfer techniques in ways that could be applied to eventual clinical use. Here, we will briefly review the current state of gene transfer technology and the application of the available technology to treatment of atrial, atrioventricular (AV) nodal, and ventricular substrates.

Gene therapy technology

Technical advances in the field of myocardial gene therapy have come at what most people would characterize as a frustrating pace. Original gene transfer methods were restricted to direct injection of plasmid-based vectors directly into the myocardium [6]. Using this method, gene transfer efficiency was low, affecting only a small number of cells in a confined space. The poor results were related in part to the delivery technique and to the function of the available gene transfer vectors. Improved delivery methods have been slow in coming. An early study characterized the physical factors relevant to gene transfer efficiency during coronary perfusion [7]. Virus and receptor concentrations, temperature, contact time, coronary flow rate, and avoidance of inhibitors to the attachment interaction (e.g. adenoviral antibodies, red blood cells, nonionic contrast media) affected the overall percentage of cells expressing the transgene in an isolated whole heart model. Further improvements came with the identification of catheters and needles that did not inactivate the adenoviral vectors, [8] the documentation of increased efficacy using coronary veins rather than coronary arteries for vector perfusion [9], and the demonstration that enhancement of microvascular permeability could dramatically increase the efficiency of gene transfer [10, 11]. The current state of the field is that genes can be transferred to approximately half of the cells in narrowly confined regions of large animal hearts

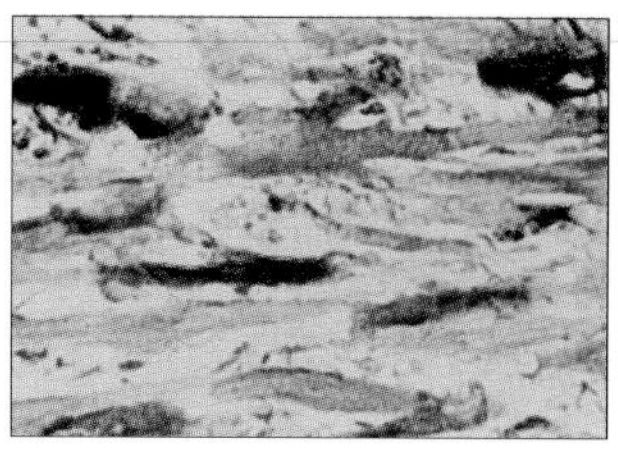

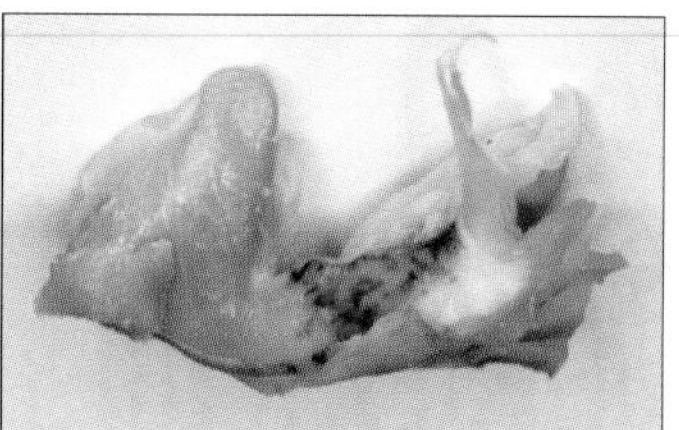

Figure 7.1 Example showing gene transfer to ~50% of cells in the AV node. An adenovirus encoding the reporter gene β-galactosidase was perfused through the AV nodal artery after pretreatment with vascular endothelial growth factor and nitroglycerin. Blue cells (left) are expressing the reporter gene, indicating successful gene transfer. Typical for this type of delivery, the pattern of gene transfer is heterogeneous, as noted in the gross specimen (right). (Reproduced from *Nature Med* [12], with permission.)

or to ~80% of cells broadly in small mammal hearts (Figure 7.1) [12, 13].

Gene transfer vectors most commonly used for cardiovascular applications include plasmid DNA, adenoviruses, and adeno-associated viruses (AAVs). Plasmids were the original vectors used because they are easy to produce and manipulate. Little sustained interest has been generated in the use of plasmid vectors for cardiac electrophysiological applications, however, because the efficiency of gene uptake is extremely poor, inflammatory reactions occur after plasmid delivery, and the ability to sustain gene expression after plasmid-mediated gene transfer has not been demonstrated [14].

Recombinant adenoviruses are the most commonly used gene transfer vectors for myocardial research. The majority of published work used so-called early generation vectors that have deletions of the E1 and E3 genes. Deletion of E1 is sufficient to render the virus incapable of replication, and the E3 deletion was performed primarily to increase the space for insertion of the transgene. With these deletions, early generation vectors could accommodate up to ~10 kb of genetic material. Early generation adenovirus vectors attach to cardiac myocytes with reasonable efficacy, but biodistribution is broad due to the ubiquitous expression of the adenoviral receptor, inflammatory reactions to the vector are a major problem, and transgene expression is limited to 3–4 weeks with these early generation adenoviruses [15].

Fully deleted adenoviral vectors solve some of the problems found with the early generation vectors. These viruses, also called helper-dependent, gutted, or gutless, have been deleted of all adenoviral genes. Production of these vectors requires coinfection with helper viruses or plasmids that carry the relevant adenoviral genes, causing the problem that all gutted adenoviruses are contaminated at low levels with these helper viruses. The gutted viruses have capacity for over 30 kb of genetic material, and they appear capable of sustained gene expression when tissue-specific promoters are used to drive the transgene [16]. Problems with the initial immune response to the adenoviral particle and the broad biodistribution remain [17]. In addition, the gutted vectors are considerably more difficult to produce than their earlier generation counterparts.

Adeno-associated viruses are related to adenoviruses in name only, having been originally isolated from adenovirus-infected tissues [18]. AAV is a small, single-strand DNA virus dependent on coinfection by other viruses to complete its life cycle. The viral genome contains only two genes, encompassing ~5 kb of space. Like adenoviruses, the receptor for AAV is ubiquitously expressed, so gene transfer is efficient but the biodistribution is broad. The major advantage of AAV seems to be its stealth abilities, with minimal immune response and an ability to sustain gene expression in a variety of tissues. The major disadvantages of AAV are the small genetic size, the need for synthesis of the second, complementary DNA strand prior to gene expression (taking 2–4 weeks for peak effect), and the need for helper viruses or plasmids to produce the vector [14].

In spite of technical limitations, gene transfer techniques for treatment of cardiac arrhythmias has already been shown to affect the ventricular response rate to atrial fibrillation (AF) [12], the automaticity of atrial and ventricular myocytes (covered elsewhere in this book) [19, 20], and ventricular repolarization [21, 22]. In the remaining sections of this review, we will briefly discuss the underlying pathophysiological substrate for atrial, AV nodal, and ventricular tachyarrhythmias, and the available gene therapy literature for treatment of these diseases.

Atrial arrhythmias

The mechanisms for generation of atrial arrhythmias include focal areas of either abnormal automaticity and zones of slow conduction allowing creation of reentrant circuits. Focal mechanisms are responsible for many atrial tachycardias. Reentrant mechanisms play a role in atrial flutter, sinus node reentry, and macro-reentrant atrial tachycardias. At the current time, these arrhythmias are most effectively treated with radiofrequency ablation [23].

Atrial fibrillation is a complex rhythm that likely includes focal and macro-reentrant mechanisms. Pulmonary vein firing has been shown to cause so-called lone AF [24], and it may play an important role in the more common type of AF associated with structural heart disease. The mechanism of these pulmonary vein firings, micro-reentrant circuits, abnormal automaticity, or triggered activity, remains a matter of controversy. Multicircuit intraatrial reentry has long been thought to play a dominant role in sustaining AF [25]. The lack of knowledge of the underlying mechanisms responsible for AF will limit the ultimate use of gene-transfer technologies because selecting a gene target will require some understanding of what functional alteration will eliminate or prevent the fibrillation. On the other hand, gene transfer techniques may play a role in answering these fundamental questions because gene-transfer-induced alterations of the underlying substrate can be evaluated for their ability to prevent AF or to cardiovert already existent AF.

To date, the lone literature report of atrial-directed gene therapy is a recent paper describing a method for atrial gene transfer [26]. In that article, we reported the ability to transfer genes transmurally to all atrial walls that have epicardial access (Figure 7.2(a)). The gene transfer vector is complexed

(a)

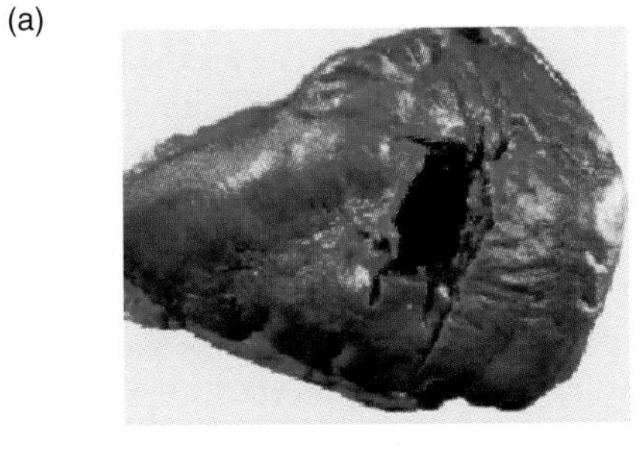

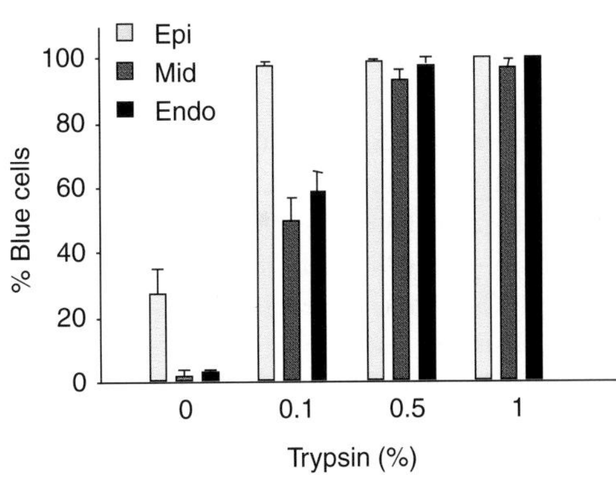

(b)

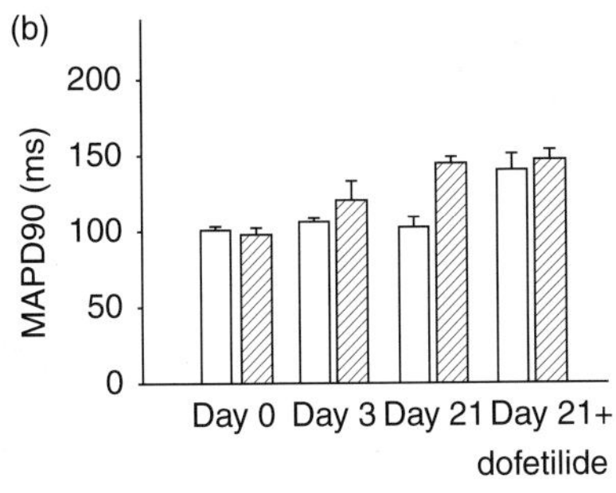

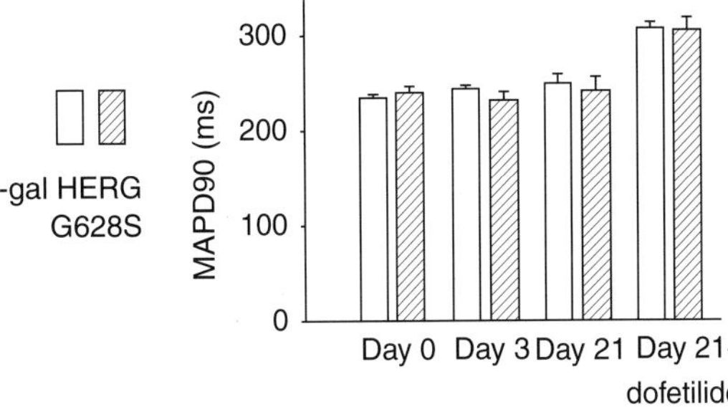

Figure 7.2 (a) Gene transfer efficacy using the atrial gene painting method. The left panel shows an example of an atrium 3 days after painting with a solution containing adenoviruses encoding β-galactosidase (see Reference 26 for details of delivery). The right panel shows quantification of gene transfer. For solutions containing 0.5–1% trypsin, complete transmural gene transfer was observed. (b) Changes in left atrial (right) and left ventricular action potential duration after gene transfer with a dominant negative mutation of KCNH. (Reproduced from *Circulation* [26], with permission.)

in a gel matrix and painted onto the atrial epicardial surface. The inclusion of trypsin in the mixture allows transmural penetration of the vector, but the concentration of trypsin is dilute enough so that atrial structure and tensile strength are not affected. Specificity of the technique is afforded by the control provided by direct application with a paintbrush. No ventricular gene transfer was noted when evaluated using the β-galactosidase reporter gene, and no electrophysiological changes in the ventricles were noted when the atria were painted with a knockout mutation of the I_{Kr} channel. We documented the antiarrhythmic potential of this technique by demonstrating prolongation of atrial repolarization after I_{Kr} knockout (Figure 7.2(b)), but use of the method with an atrial tachyarrhythmia model has not yet been reported.

AV nodal gene therapy

Atrioventricular nodal arrhythmias include AV nodal reentrant tachycardia (AVNRT), AV reciprocating tachycardia (AVRT), and the rapid ventricular response to atrial fibrillation. AVNRT and AVRT are most effectively treated by radiofrequency ablation, being among the first arrhythmias treated with that technology. The success rate is far in excess of 90% and complications are rare [23]. Often, pharmacological methods can effectively suppress AV nodal conduction to control the heart rate in AF. Calcium channel blockers, β-adrenergic receptor blockers, and digoxin have long histories in this role. Problems arise when the pharmacological agents are not effective, or when their common side effects are not tolerated [27]. In those situations, the only currently available therapy is radiofrequency ablation of the AV node, with implantation of a ventricular pacemaker to sustain the heart rate. Recent data suggests that right ventricular pacing has negative hemodynamic effects, in particular when heart failure coexists with right ventricular pacing [28]. These data suggest that biventricular pacing is a more appropriate replacement of the AV node, adding complexity and expense to the procedure.

We recently showed the ability to suppress AV nodal conduction with gene transfer of $G\alpha_{i2}$, an α subunit of the G protein family responsible for intracellular signaling of cholinergic and purinergic receptor events. In the original report, we found a 20% reduction in ventricular rate comparing the $G\alpha_{i2}$ group to controls [12]. Even in the setting of adrenergic stimulation, a 16% reduction in heart rate was found in these normal pigs. The underlying AV nodal function had suggestions of conduction slowing and increased refractoriness, with a 12% increases in AH interval on intracardiac recording and a 10% increase in AV nodal effective refractory period during programmed stimulation. For these original studies, the AF was acutely induced and self-limited, and the physiological effects of gene transfer were evaluated in anesthetized animals.

A follow-up report showed that the model plays a critical role in evaluating the functional effects of the transgene. In the follow-up, we adapted the burst pacing, persistent AF model initially reported in goats [29]. Atrial burst pacemakers were implanted into the pigs 3 weeks prior to the date of gene transfer. After 5–10 days, the animals sustained atrial fibrillation without continual bursting by the pacemaker. Unlike the goat model, the pigs had incredibly fast ventricular response rates to AF. The awake, normally functioning pigs had an average ventricular rate of 265 beats per minute (bpm), compared with an average sinus rhythm rate of 120 bpm. The rapid heart rate was sufficient to cause a tachycardiomyopathy in the animals [30]. Ejection fraction fell from a normal 70% to below 30%, and four-chamber dilation occurred. Cellular evidence of hypertrophy, myocyte disorganization, and rampant apoptosis accompanied the dilation and decrease in function. In that background, we tested the ability of diltiazem, esmolol, or digoxin to reduce heart rate, and found that none of the conventional pharmacological agents had any significant effect. AV nodal gene transfer of the wild-type $G\alpha_{i2}$ used in the acute studies was also insufficient. With the wild-type protein, we observed a 12% reduction in heart rate during sedation, but the combination of arousal and the hyperadrenergic state from the underlying heart failure was sufficient to overcome this effect. A constitutively active mutant $G\alpha_{i2}$ (Q205L)[31] sustained a 15–25% reduction in heart rate in spite of the adrenergic overdrive of heart failure or the waking state (Figure 7.3). We found that this level of heart rate reduction had physiological relevance,

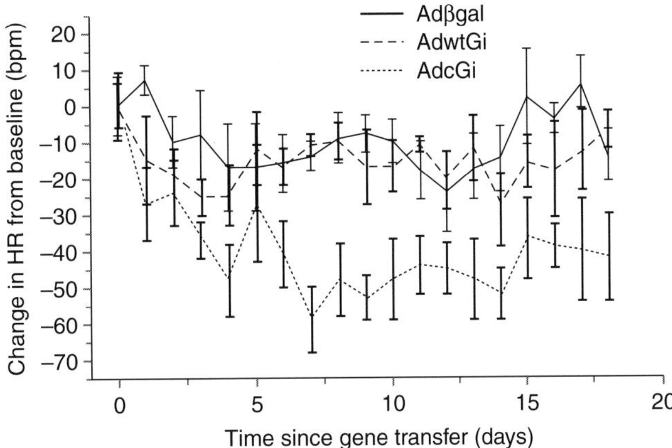

Figure 7.3 Daily heart rate measurements in animals after gene transfer with Adβgal (reporter encoding β-galactosidase), AdwtGi (wild type Gα_{i2}) or AdcGi (constitutively active mutant of Gα_{i2}). (Reproduced from *Circulation* [32], with permission.)

since the ejection fraction was near normal 2 weeks after gene transfer. In addition, no adverse effects were noted in this limited study [32].

Gene therapy for ventricular tachyarrhythmias

Life-threatening ventricular arrhythmias most commonly occur in the setting of ischemia, infarction, or heart failure. All of these conditions have been extensively reviewed [33, 34], and the reader is referred to those excellent works for a more detailed discussion than is possible in this limited review. In general, initiation and maintenance of ventricular arrhythmias requires either slowing of conduction or abnormalities in repolarization. To date, no literature report has focused on the possibilities for gene transfer to modify the slow conduction zone associated with ventricular arrhythmias. More information is available regarding the possibilities of altering repolarization.

Hoppe *et al.* [22] documented the ability to alter ventricular repolarization and refractory period in a guinea pig model using adenovirus vectors injected directly into the myocardium. Like other direct injection models, concerns regarding this work included the localized, heterogeneous gene transfer limited to the area around the injection needle track and the inflammatory and fibrotic response accompanying myocardial injection of adenoviruses [3, 35]. In spite of these limitations, Hoppe showed that action potential duration shortened with overexpression of KCNH, encoding the α subunit of the I_{Kr} current. Dominant negative knockout of this current prolonged repolarization. In contrast, a more modest effect on action potential duration was observed with overexpression of KCNE1, encoding minK, the β subunit most closely aligned with the I_{Ks} current, but knockout of this subunit had a much more pronounced effect on repolarization and generation of cellular afterpotentials.

Ennis *et al.* [21] analyzed the effect of combined calcium handling and potassium channel gene transfer. The underlying concern for this work was that potassium channel overexpression mediated effects on repolarization could have the beneficial effect on arrhythmia vulnerability but also a detrimental effect on contractility. In particular, the concern was most pronounced in heart failure, where decreased efficiency of cytoplasmic calcium handling might increase contractility but also might play a role in the ventricular arrhythmias associated with heart failure. Ennis transferred the sarcoplasmic reticular calcium ATPase pump (SERCA) along with the Kir 2.1 potassium channel responsible for the I_{K1} current. The potassium channel shortened repolarization, but in the presence of the calcium pump myocyte contractility was preserved.

Kodirov *et al.* [36] extended the findings of the above investigators to a disease model. They evaluated the possibility of rescuing a long-QT transgenic mouse, where a truncation mutation of the Kv 1.1 channel created the long-QT phenotype in the mouse line. Direct injection of adenovirus vectors encoding the Kv 1.5 channel into the mouse ventricular myocardium caused a reduction in the QT interval. In addition to showing the possibility of correcting a disease state with gene transfer, Koderov also demonstrated that it is not necessary to transfer the gene to all cells in the myocardium. There is currently controversy in the field about the proarrhythmic and antiarrhythmic potential of gene transfer. Koderov, Ennis, and Hoppe show that alterations in the electrical phenotype are possible with gene-transfer to a minority of myocytes. These data are consistent with the known cell-to-cell electrical communication between myocytes. The concerns focus on the effects of gene-transfer-induced heterogeneity under conditions where this communication is reduced, such as ischemia. Further investigation is required to answer these concerns.

Conclusion

The field of myocardial gene transfer is still in its infancy. Problems related to controlling transgene expression, improving delivery techniques, increasing target specificity, and reducing inflammation are essential for widespread adoption of this technology into clinical practice. Already, significant advances have occurred. The principle that gene therapy is a viable option for cardiac arrhythmias has been established. The use of the technology as a research tool to evaluate the mechanisms and potential treatments of tachyarrhythmias is gaining momentum. With continued work on the remaining problems, there is hope that this tool will eventually join pharmacotherapy, ablation, and implantable devices as a viable option for patients with cardiac arrhythmias.

Acknowledgments

The authors thank the National Institutes of Health, the American Heart Association, and the Deutschen Forschungsgemeinschaft for financial support and St. Jude Medical Inc. and Medtronic Inc. for equipment donations that contributed to the data discussed in this chapter.

References

1 Curran M, Splawski I, Timothy K, Vincent G, Green E, Keating M. A molecular basis for cardiac arrhythmia: HERG mutations cause long QT syndrome. *Cell* 1995; **80**: 795–803.

2 Wang Q, Curran M, Splawski I *et al.* SCN5A mutations associated with an inherited cardiac arrhythmia, long QT syndrome. *Cell* 1995; **80**: 805–811.

3 Guzman RJ, Lemarchand P, Crystal R, Epstein SE, Finkel T. Efficient gene transfer into myocardium by direct injection of adenovirus vectors. *Circ Res* 1993; **73**(6): 1202–1207.

4 Kass-Eisler A, Falck-Pedersen E, Elfenbein DH, Alvira M, Buttrick PM, Leinwand L. The impact of developmental stage, route of administration and the immune system on adenovirus-mediated gene transfer. *Gene Therapy* 1994; **1**: 395–402.

5 Kirshenbaum L, MacLellan WR, Mazur W, French B, Schneider MD. Highly efficient gene transfer into adult ventricular myocytes by recombinant adenovirus. *J Clin Invest* 1993; **92**: 381–387.

6 Lin H, Parmacek M, Morle G, Bolling S, Leiden J. Expression of recombinant genes in the myocardium *in vivo* after direct injection of DNA. *Circulation* 1990; **82**(6): 2217–2221.

7 Donahue J, Kikkawa K, Johns D, Marban E, Lawrence J. Ultrarapid, highly efficient viral gene transfer to the heart. *Proc Natl Acad Sci USA* 1997; **94**: 4664–4668.

8 Marshall D, Palasis M, Lepore J, Leiden J. Biocompatibility of cardiovascular gene delivery catheters with adenovirus vectors: an important determinant of the efficiency of cardiovascular gene transfer. *Mol Ther* 2000; **1**: 423–429.

9 Boekstegers P, von Degenfeld G, Giehrl W *et al.* Myocardial gene transfer by selective pressure-regulated retroinfusion of coronary veins. *Gene Ther* 2000; **7**(3): 232–240.

10 Donahue J, Kikkawa K, Thomas AD, Marban E, Lawrence J. Acceleration of widespread adenoviral gene transfer to intact rabbit hearts by coronary perfusion with low calcium and serotonin. *Gene Therapy* 1998; **5**: 630–634.

11 Nagata K, Marban E, Lawrence J, Donahue J. Phosphodiesterase inhibitor-mediated potentiation of adenovirus delivery to myocardium. *J Mol Cell Cardiol* 2001; **33**: 575–580.

12 Donahue J, Heldman A, Fraser H *et al.* Focal modification of electrical conduction in the heart by viral gene transfer. *Nature Med* 2000; **6**: 1395–1398.

13 Ikeda Y, Gu Y, Iwanaga Y *et al.* Restoration of deficient membrane proteins in the cardiomyopathic hamster by *in vivo* cardiac gene transfer. *Circulation* 2002; **105**(4): 502–508.

14 Robbins P, Tahara H, Ghivizzani S. Viral vectors for gene therapy. *Trends Biotechnol* 1998; **16**: 35–40.

15 Kaneda Y. Gene therapy: a battle against biological barriers. *Curr Mol Med* 2001; **1**(4): 493–499.

16 Chen HH, Mack LM, Kelly R, Ontell M, Kochanek S, Clemens PR. Persistence in muscle of an adenoviral

vector that lacks all viral genes. *Proc Natl Acad Sci USA* 1997; **94**(5): 1645–1650.

17 Liu Q, Muruve D. Molecular basis of the inflammatory response to adenovirus vectors. *Gene Ther* 2003; **10**(11): 935–940.

18 Brandon F, McLean I Jr. Adenoviruses. *Adv Virus Res* 1962; **13**: 157–193.

19 Miake J, Marban E, Nuss H. Biological pacemaker created by gene transfer. *Nature* 2002; **419**: 132–133.

20 Qu J, Plotnikov A, Danilo PJ *et al.* Expression and function of a biological pacemaker in canine heart. *Circulation* 2003; **107**(8): 1106–1109.

21 Ennis I, Li R, Murphy A, Marban E, Nuss H. Dual gene therapy with SERCA1 and Kir 2.1 abbreviates excitation without suppressing contractility. *J Clin Invest* 2002; **109**(3): 393–400.

22 Hoppe U, Marban E, Johns D. Distinct gene-specific mechanisms of arrhythmia revealed by cardiac gene transfer of two long QT disease genes, HERG and KCNE1. *Proc Natl Acad Sci USA* 2001; **98**(9): 5335–5340.

23 Calkins H, Yong P, Miller J *et al.* Catheter ablation of accessory pathways, atrioventricular nocal reentrant tachycardia, and the atrioventricular junction: final results of a prospective, multicenter clinical trial. *Circulation* 1999; **99**: 262–270.

24 Jais P, Haissaguerre M, Shah D *et al.* A focal source of atrial fibrillation treated by discrete radiofrequency ablation. *Circulation* 1997; **95**(3): 572–576.

25 Moe G. Evidence for reentry as a mechanism of cardiac arrhythmias. *Rev Physiol Biochem Pharmacol* 1975; **72**: 55–81.

26 Kikuchi K, McDonald A, Sasano T, Donahue J. Targeted modification of atrial electrophysiology by homogeneous transmural atrial gene transfer. *Circulation.* 2005; **111**(3): 264–70.

27 Natale A, Zimerman L, Tomassoni G *et al.* AV node ablation and pacemaker implantation after withdrawal of effective rate-control medications for chronic atrial fibrillation: effect on quality of life and exercise performance. *PACE* 1999; **22**: 1634–1639.

28 Wilkoff B, Cook J, Epstein A *et al.* Dual-chamber pacing or ventricular backup pacing in patients with an implantable defibrillator: the Dual Chamber and VVI Implantable Defibrillator (DAVID) Trial. *JAMA* 2002; **288**(24): 3115–3123.

29 Wijffels M, Kirchhof C, dorland R, Allessie M. Atrial fibrillation begets atrial fibrillation. A study in awake chronically instrumented goats. *Circulation* 1995; **92**(7): 1954–1968.

30 Bauer A, McDonald A, Donahue J. Pathophysiological findings in a model of atrial fibrillation and severe congestive heart failure. *Cardiovasc Res* 2004; **61**(4): 764–770.

31 Wong Y, Federman A, Pace A *et al.* Mutant alpha subunits of Gi2 inhibit cyclic AMP accumulation. *Nature* 1991; **351**(6321): 63–65.

32 Bauer A, McDonald AD, Peller L, Rade JJ, Miller JM, Heldman AW, and Donahue JK. Physiologically-relevant heart rate control in persistent atrial fibrillation. *Circulation* 2004; **110**: 3115–3120.

33 Tomaselli G, Marban E. Electrophysiological remodeling in hypertrophy and heart failure. *Cardiovasc Res* 1999; **42**: 270–283.

34 Janse M. Electrophysiology of arrhythmias. *Arch Mal Coeur Vaiss* 1999; **92**(S1): 9–16.

35 Kass-Eisler A, Falck-Pedersen E, Alvira M *et al.* Quantitative determination of adenovirus-mediated gene delivery to rat cardiac myocytes *in vitro* and *in vivo*. *Proc Natl Acad Sci USA* 1993; **90**(12): 11498–11502.

36 Kodirov S, Brunner M, Busconi L, Koren G. Long-term restitution of 4-aminopyridine-sensitive currents in Kv1DN ventricular myocytes using adeno-associated virus-mediated delivery of Kv1.5. *FEBS Lett* 2003; **550**(1–3): 74–78.

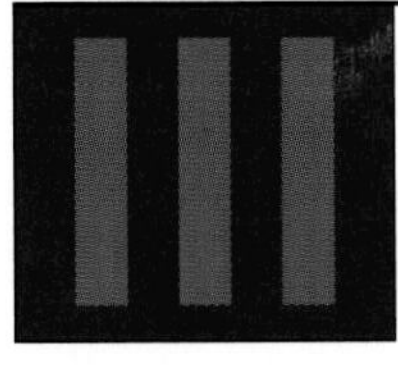

PART III

Monitoring, noninvasive mapping, risk assessment, and external defibrillation

8

CHAPTER 8

New developments in noninvasive rhythm monitoring, implantable hemodynamic monitoring, functional status monitoring, and noninvasive mapping

Jonathan Weinstock, MD, *Munther K. Homoud,* MD, *Mark S. Link,* MD, *& N.A. Mark Estes III,* MD

Despite considerable advances in the care of cardiac patients, there remain areas which pose significant challenges. Among these are noninvasive remote arrhythmia monitoring, accurate functional status data on patients with cardiac disease, remote continuous hemodynamic monitoring, and noninvasive arrhythmia mapping. This chapter will review novel emerging technologies that may, in the future, assist practitioners achieve these goals.

Mobile cardiac outpatient telemetry

Remote monitoring of patients with suspected cardiac arrhythmias with Holter monitoring is limited in the length of time of recorded data. Loop or event recorders are unable to detect asymptomatic arrhythmias, and are not practical for the detection of infrequent episodes. A recently developed mobile cardiac outpatient telemetry (MCOT) system (CardioNet, Inc., San Diego, CA) overcomes some of the obstacles of more traditional outpatient noninvasive electrocardiographic monitoring, and more closely simulates current inpatient telemetry monitoring. The system consists of three surface electrodes attached to a small lightweight sensor that can be worn by the patient. This transmits a two channel electrocardiogram via a wireless signal to a monitor device similar in form to a personal digital assistant. The monitor can be left in a cradle in the home or carried outside. This device then transmits the data continuously to a monitoring center via a wireless telephone network, or via a wired phone connection, if wireless network access is unavailable. If neither are available, the device has a storage buffer of 48 h of data that is transmitted when either type of telephone connection is established. An alert is triggered when either previously set automatic arrhythmia parameters are met, or when the patient manually marks an event by pressing a button on the device screen. Trained staff at the monitoring center analyze the data, and inform the referring physician of serious arrhythmias. Regular summaries of the gathered data, including detailed information such as atrial fibrillation burden, are sent to the physician.

A study of 100 consecutive patients using MCOT revealed the possible clinical utility of this system [1]. Patients were monitored from 2 to 28 days with a mean of 9.9 days. The indication for monitoring included palpitations, to determine efficacy of drug therapy, dizziness, syncope, and monitoring for ventricular tachycardia (VT). A clinically significant arrhythmia was found in

51 patients, 25 of which were asymptomatic, including 12 with atrial fibrillation, 10 with supraventricular tachycardia, 2 with nonsustained VT, and 1 with atrial flutter. MCOT detected an arrhythmia in 16 of 30 patients in whom previous monitoring with Holter or event recorders did not. Overall, a change in management was undertaken in 34 of the 100 patients with MCOT. These preliminary results, show the successful utilization of this new technology, with its largest advantage being the detection of asymptomatic, infrequent arrhythmias. There has been no evaluation to date of the cost effectiveness of this technology when compared with other standard monitoring systems.

Functional status monitor

The ability to monitor a patient's functional status, activity, and energy expenditure in a noninvasive convenient manner, may have applications in many medical fields. A novel technology has been developed, consisting of a multisensor device affixed to the upper arm with an armband (SenseWear PRO_2, Bodymedia Inc., Pittsburgh, PA) with the ability to transmit data either wirelessly or via a USB cable to personal computer with proprietary software that compiles and analyzes the data. The device is nonintrusive, weighs 2.9 ounces, is powered by two AAA batteries, and can store up to 2 weeks of information. Integrated in the device are five sensors; a two-axis accelerometer, galvanic skin response, heat flux, skin temperature, and near body temperature (Figure 8.1). The data is recorded continuously, and users can timestamp an event by pressing a button on the device. By combining the data from these five sensors, and in conjunction with data, such as age, gender, height, and weight, accurate measures of energy expenditure can be made. Additionally, through constructed data models, physical activity duration, number of steps, duration of recumbency, sleep onset, wake time, and sleep efficiency can be derived. These models have been validated against more standard measures, and have come within 90–97% accuracy. For example, the analyzed data from the armband had a 91.1% (within a 95% confidence interval) accuracy in predicting total energy expenditure, when compared to a VO2 machine (Data on file, Bodymedia, Inc.).

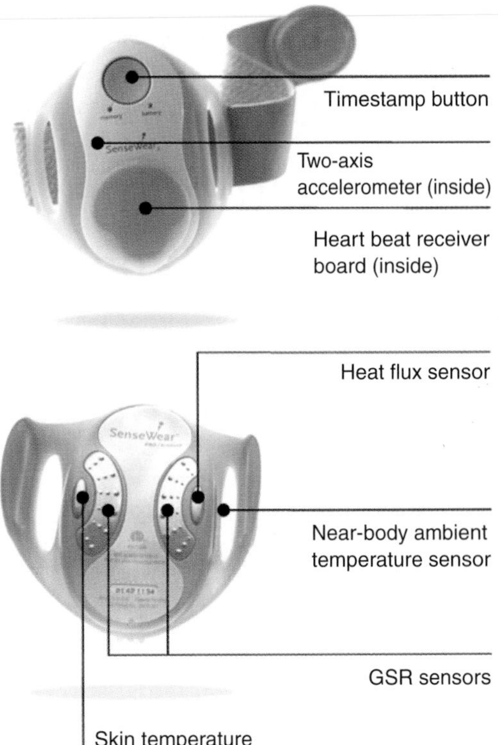

Figure 8.1 Image of the BodyMedia SenseWear Pro_2 Armband device indicating the various embedded sensors. (Reprinted from © BodyMedia Inc. 2004, with permission.)

Contextual data regarding the wearer's activity at any time can also be derived using the data from the sensors.

Currently, applications of this technology are limited to weight management and fitness. However, the addition of external digital data into the armband device, such as weight, blood pressure, and glucometer readings, may extend the usefulness of the device into management of cardiac patients with a wide range of diagnoses. Currently, tests are ongoing for validation of a heart rate sensor integrated in the armband, which could potentially allow for remote electrocardiographic monitoring without traditional leads. This data combined with body position, activity, and other physiologic data, could potentially make this technology a powerful tool in the diagnosis and treatment of patients with arrhythmias, by integrating heart rhythm data with the actual physiologic status of the patient (Figure 8.2).

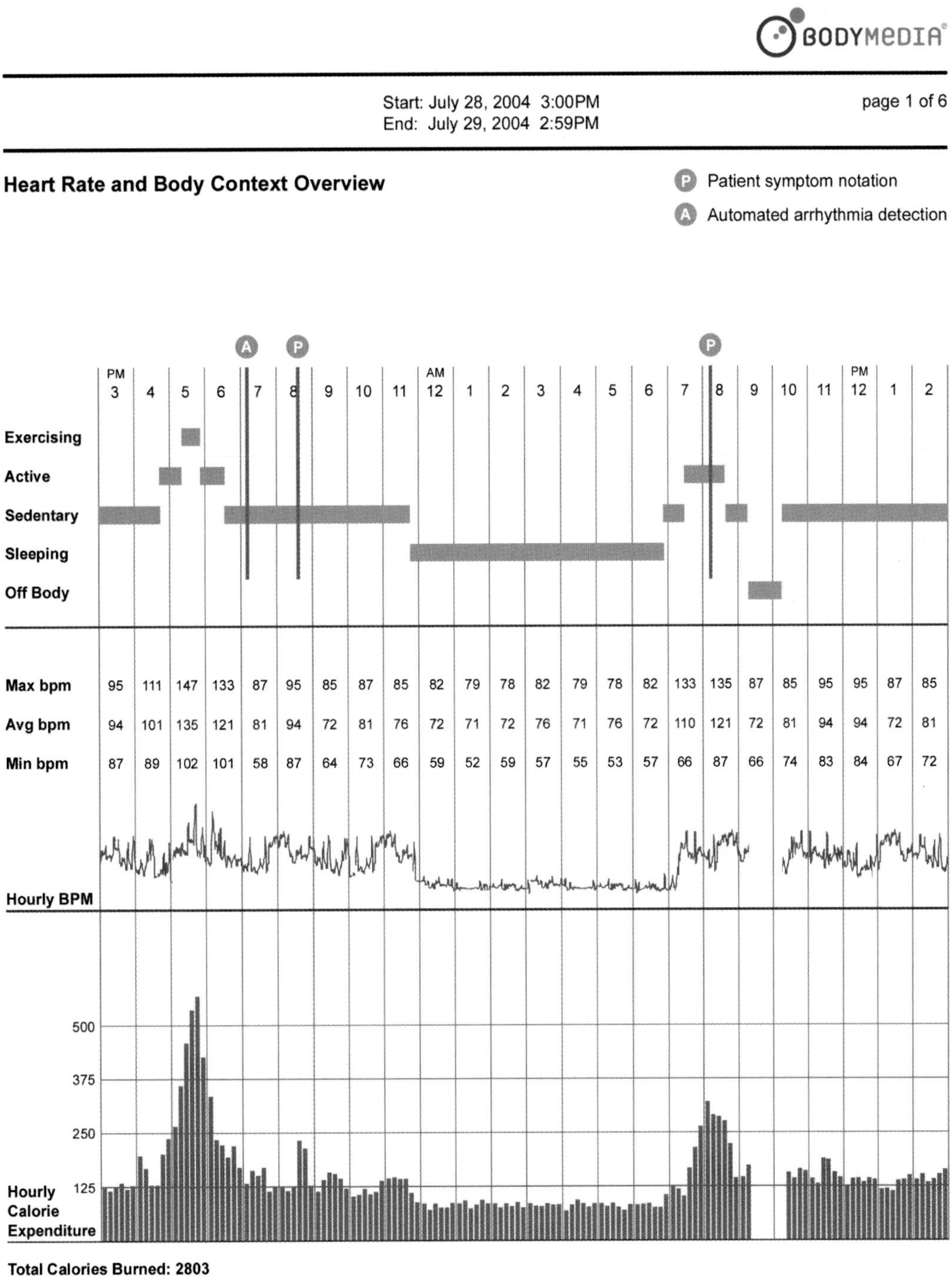

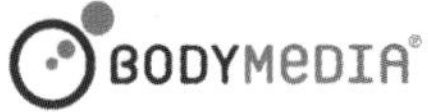

Start: July 28, 2004 3:00PM
End: July 29, 2004 2:59PM

page 1 of 6

Heart Rate and Body Context Overview

P Patient symptom notation
A Automated arrhythmia detection

Exercising
Active
Sedentary
Sleeping
Off Body

	PM 3	4	5	6	7	8	9	10	11	AM 12	1	2	3	4	5	6	7	8	9	10	11	PM 12	1	2
Max bpm	95	111	147	133	87	95	85	87	85	82	79	78	82	79	78	82	133	135	87	85	95	95	87	85
Avg bpm	94	101	135	121	81	94	72	81	76	72	71	72	76	71	76	72	110	121	72	81	94	94	72	81
Min bpm	87	89	102	101	58	87	64	73	66	59	52	59	57	55	53	57	66	87	66	74	83	84	67	72

Hourly BPM

500
375
250
125
Hourly Calorie Expenditure

Total Calories Burned: 2803

Figure 8.2 Simulated report of data from BodyMedia SenseWear Pro$_2$ Armband showing temporal correlation of heart rate, specific activity, along with patient triggered markers, and automated arrhythmia detection markers. (Reprinted from © BodyMedia Inc. 2004, with permission.)

Implantable hemodynamic monitoring

Congestive heart failure (CHF) remains a substantial healthcare challenge with nearly 5 million patients in the United States carrying the diagnosis, and 500 000 patients newly diagnosed cases each year. CHF is the reason for hospital admissions accounting for 6.5 million hospital days per year in the United States [2]. Frequent physical examination and right heart catheterization to assess volume status is costly and impractical. Recently, an implantable hemodynamic monitor (IHM) has been developed, and is being studied clinically [3]. The device is similar to a single chamber permanent pacemaker, and is implanted in a similar transvenous fashion. A passive fixation lead, which houses a pressure sensor at the tip, is placed in the right ventricular outflow tract. The memory device in the pectoral area records right ventricular (RV) systolic and diastolic pressure (Figure 8.3), estimated pulmonary artery diastolic pressure, maximum change in pressure over time (dP/dT), heart rate, activity, and temperature. The accuracy and precision of the measurements were confirmed by comparing the data to simultaneous recordings from a pulmonary artery catheter at 3, 6, and 12 months after implant. The same study showed the data to be accurate regardless of body position or activity level [4].

Numerous studies have shown the IHM to be feasible, safe, and reliable [3–5]. The device is capable of long-term recording of hemodynamic data (Figure 8.4). Only one study has examined the long-term hemodynamic measurements in a series of patients with CHF, with correlation to clinical events [3]. Thirty two patients with CHF had an IHM (Chronicle, Medtronic Inc., Minneapolis, MN) placed. For 9 months, physicans caring for the patients did not have access to the data. For the following 17 months, physicians caring for the patients were given access to the data. A total of 36 volume overload events occurred, during which RV systolic pressures increased by 25 ± 4% ($p < .05$) and heart rate increased by 11 ± 2% ($p < .05$). Twelve of these events required hospitalizations, and in nine of those pressure increases occurred 4 ± 2 days before these heart failure exacerbations. The rate of hospitalizations was significantly less after the physicans were exposed to the IHM data (0.47 per year versus 1.08 per year; $p < .01$). The authors concluded that implantation of an IHM may help to guide daily

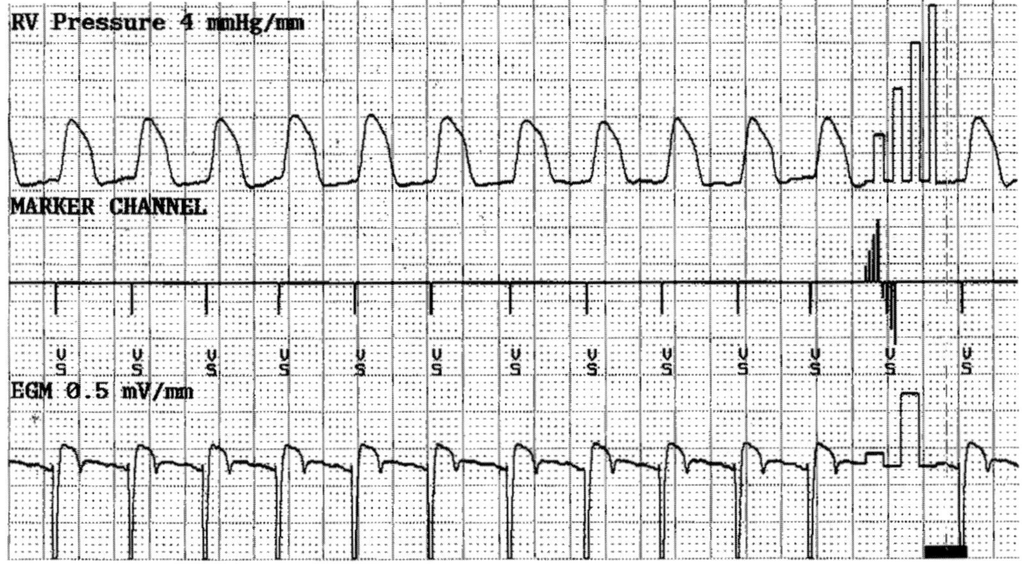

Figure 8.3 Real-time recording output from interrogation of a Medtronic Chronicle Device. The top recording represents RV pressure, middle recording is the marker channel (VS = ventricular sensing), lower recording is the ventricular electrogram (EGM) recorded from the right ventricular lead. (Reproduced with permission from Medtronic Inc., Minneapolis, MN.)

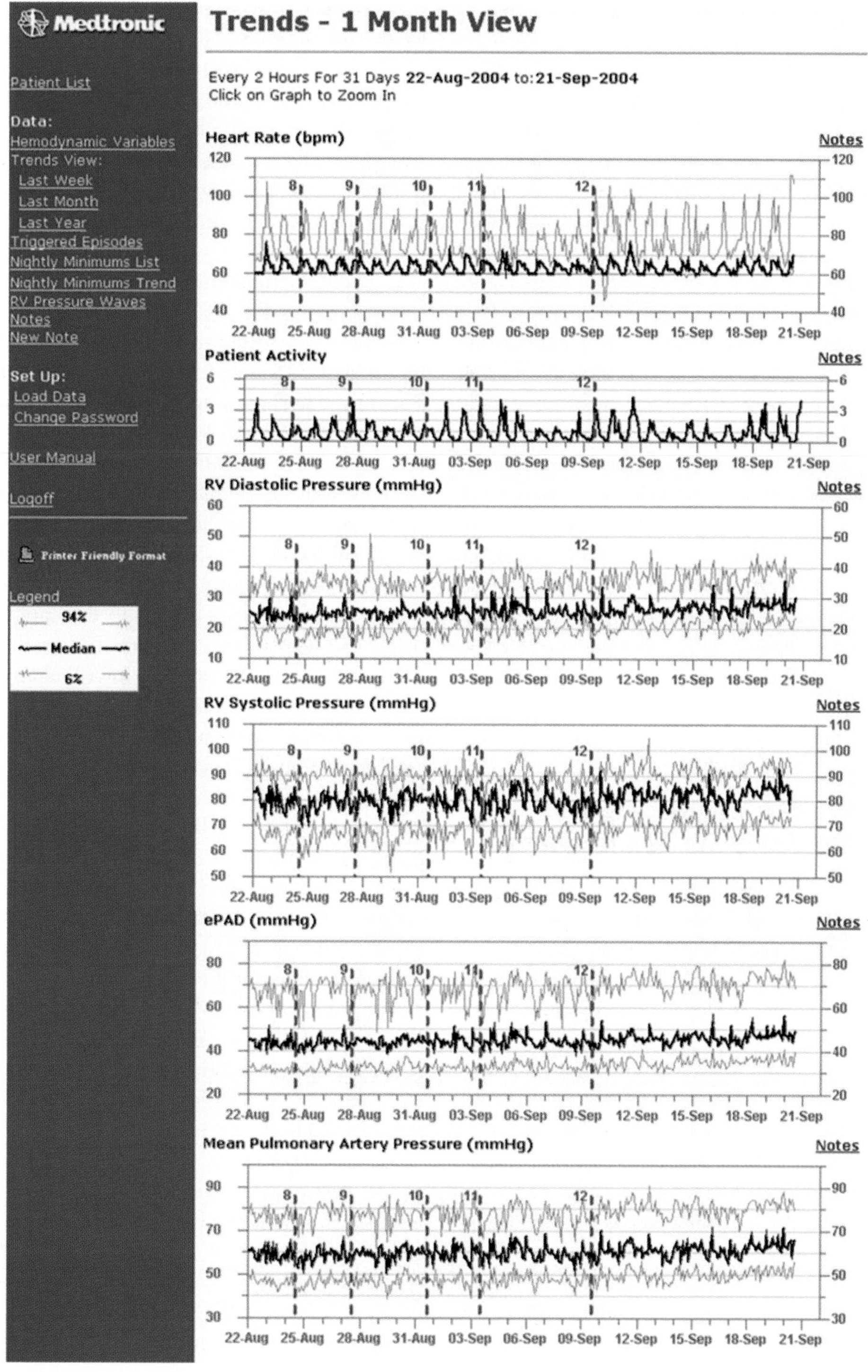

Figure 8.4 One month summary of data recorded from a Medtronic Chronicle device. bpm = beats per minute, RV = right ventricle, ePAD = estimated pulmonary artery diastolic. (Reproduced with permission from Medtronic Inc., Minneapolis, MN.)

care of heart failure patients, and may serve to decrease heart failure hospitalizations.

Currently, the Compass-HF (*C*hronicle *O*ffers *M*anagement to *P*atients with *A*dvanced *S*igns and *S*ymptoms of *H*eart *F*ailure) trial is enrolling patients to examine these issues in a prospective randomized fashion. The study is enrolling patients with NYHA Class III–IV symptoms with a recent emergency visit requiring intravenous therapy, already on standard optimal heart failure therapy. There are a number of exclusion criteria including: expected heart transplant within 6 months, severe COPD, continuous positive ionotropic therapy, mechanical or stenotic right heart valves, or major cardiovascular events in the last 3 months. After meeting inclusion criteria, all patients are to have a chronicle device implanted. Following implant, patients will be randomized for 6 months to a clinician access group, or blocked clinician access group, based on the ablility of the treating physician to view the hemodynamic data. The primary endpoints of the study are safety of the device, and the efficacy of the device measured by the difference in heart failure hospitalizations, and emergent medical visits [6].

Noninvasive electrographic imaging (body surface mapping)

Current technology in the field of electrophysiology is limited to the use of invasive techniques for accurate mapping of cardiac arrhythmias. An emerging technology, noninvasive electrographic imaging (ECGI), has been developed by Rudy and coworkers [7], which promises to accomplish accurate arrhythmia mapping via a noninvasive technique. The human application of this method is derived from published data of animal experiments, in which, for example, an infarcted dog heart was suspended in a human shaped torso tank, and VT was accurately mapped by analysis of measured body surface potentials [8]. The reconstructed maps identified the location of the abnormal substrate for VT (infarction), VT epicardial activation, and epicardial breakthrough sites [8].

The method of ECGI, in humans, combines heart–torso geometry data, acquired from computed tomography images, with data from a 224 channel ECG taken from an electrode vest worn by the patient. This data is reconstructed on the surface of the heart using specialized software and displayed as epicardial potentials, electrograms, and isochrones (Figure 8.5). Recently published data, showed the ability of ECGI to accurately map atrial and ventricular activation and ventricular depolarization in a normal heart, right bundle branch block, and focal activation from right and left ventricular pacing.

In addition the authors were able to noninvasively map typical atrial flutter, which demonstrates the powerful potential applications of this technology [7]. Figure 8.6(a) depicts reconstructed isochrones during sinus rhythm, during which the earliest activation localized to the location of the sinus node. The left atrial appendage was the last to be activated, with atrial activation consistent with normal intratrial activation in humans. Figure 8.6(b) shows isochrones reconstructed during typical atrial flutter at 300 beats per minute. The atrial flutter circuit was mapped noninvasively with ECGI technology. The circuit is confined to the right atrium, propagating in a counterclockwise fashion from the inferior vena cava – tricuspid valve isthmus and up the intraatrial septum, emerging epicardially via bachman's bundle anteriorly. The wavefront then continues down the right atrial free wall and splits in two directions, one through the inferior vena cava – tricuspid valve isthmus, and a second propagating around the IVC, which collides with with a leftward branch of the downward free wall limb of the macro-reeentrant circuit at the crista terminalis. The left atrium was not involved in the macro-reentry circuit and the left atrial appendage was activated latest (Figure 8.6) [7]. This pattern of conduction is consistent with invasive catheter mapping of typical atrial flutter [9, 10].

The developers of ECGI envision such a noninvasive electrophysiologic tool as beneficial in a number of ways: identifying abnormal myocardial substrate as marker for sudden cardiac death risk, specific arrhythmias diagnosis to guide intervention, localization in the heart for specific therapies (ablation, pacing etc.), measuring efficacy of therapy over time, and studying the mechanisms of arrhthymias in humans, where prior study was limited to animals due to the risk of invasive electrophysiologic testing [7].

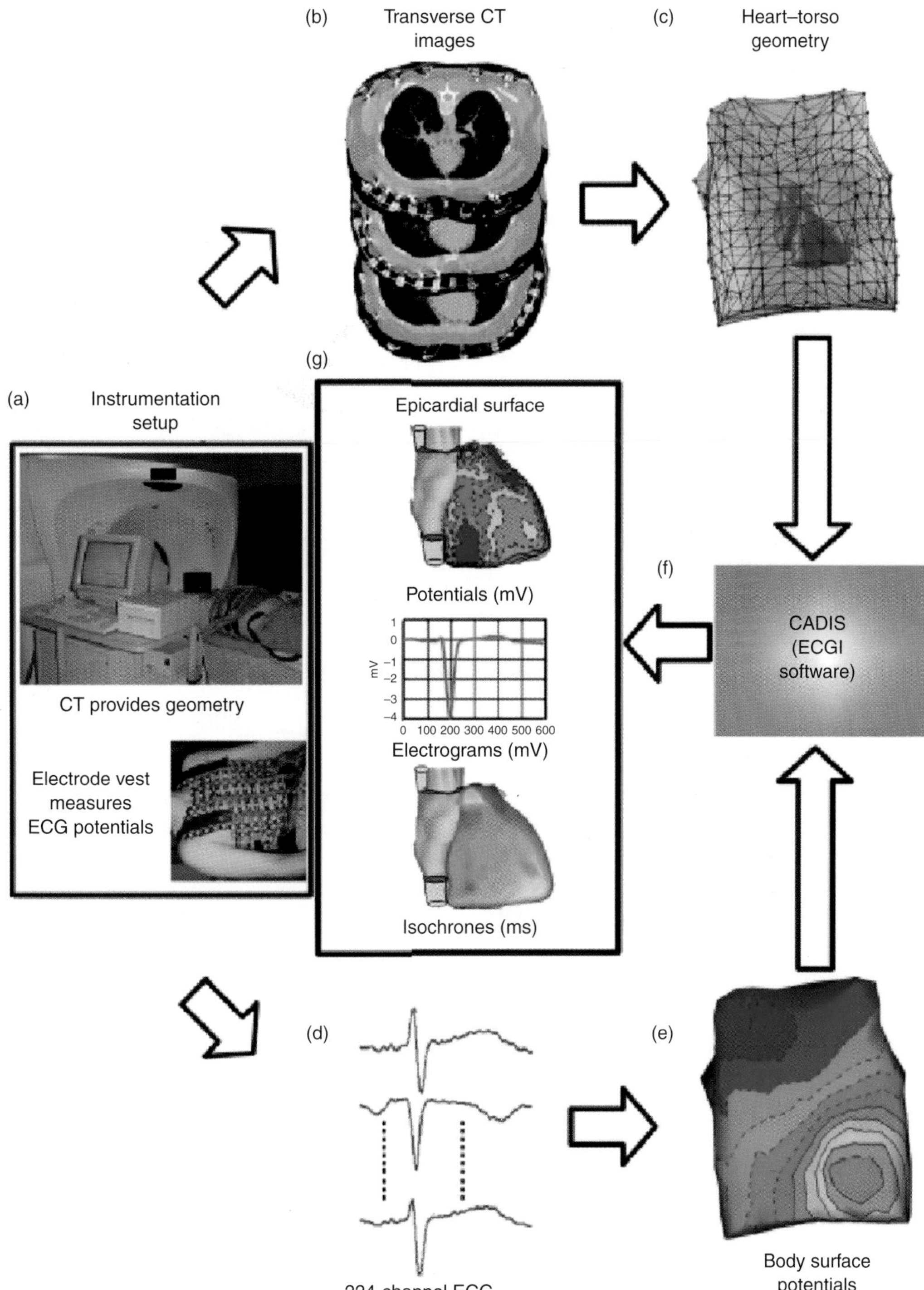

Figure 8.5 Diagram of ECGI technology. (a) Instrument setup. (b) Traverse CT images showing heart contour and position of body surface electrodes. (c) Meshed heart–torso geometry. (d) ECG signals from mapping system. (e) Representation of body surface potentials. (f) ECGI software (CADIS). (g) EGI images, epicardial potentials, electrograms, and isochrones. (Reprinted from *Nature Med* [7], with permission.)

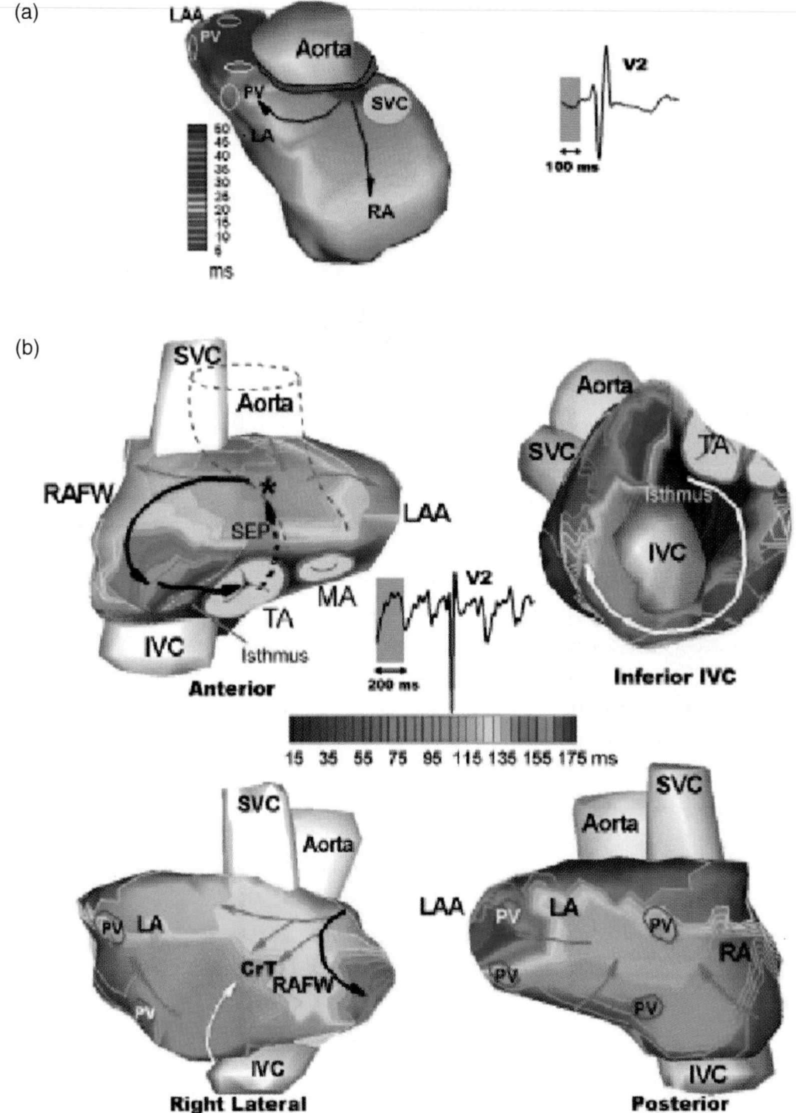

Figure 8.6 ECGI mapping of atrial activation. See text for details. (a) Left superior–posterior view of sinus rhythm. (b) Isochrones from ECGI of typical atrial flutter. ECG of lead V2 with mapped flutter cycle shaded in blue. Black arrows in anterior view indicate propagation of flutter wavefront. Solid arrows show activation of the epicardium and dashed arrows show septal activation. Breakthrough at Bachmann's Bundle indicated by *. White arrows show propagation around inferior vena cava and right anterior free wall. Left atrial activation is shown by white arrows. IVC – inferior vena cava, LA – left atrium, LAA – left atrial appendage, SVC – superior vena cava, TA – tricuspid annulus, MA – mitral annulus, ms – milliseconds, PV – pulmonary vein, RAFW – right atrial free wall, SEP – septum, CrT – crista terminalis. (Reprinted from *Nature Med* [7], with permission.)

Arrhythmia technologies are advancing at a rapid pace. New technologies for arrhythmia monitoring including mobile outpatient cardiac telemetry and a light, user-friendly multisensor armband hold promise in accurately detecting clinical arrhythmias, while providing more detailed information about related patient activity and status. An IHM may, one day, assist in the challenge of heart failure management, and help in keeping patients out of the hospital. Accurate noninvasive mapping of cardiac arrhythmias is an exciting technology that could revolutionize the diagnosis and treatment of patients. Extensive clinical investigation will need to be performed to validate the accuracy, utility, and ultimately cost effectiveness of these emerging technologies.

References

1 Kowey P, Joshi A, Prystowsky E *et al.* First experience with a Mobile Cardiac Outpatient Telemetry (MCOT) system for the diagnosis and management of cardiac arrhythmia. *PACE* 2003; **26**: 1090.

2 Hunt SA, Baker DW, Chin MH *et al.* ACC/AHA guidelines for the evaluation and management of chronic heart failure in the adult: executive summary. A report of the American College of Cardiology/American Heart Association Task Force on Practice Guidelines (Committee to revise the 1995 Guidelines for the Evaluation and Management of Heart Failure). *J Am Coll Cardiol* 2001; **38**(7): 2101–2113.

3 Adamson PB, Magalski A, Braunschweig F *et al.* Ongoing right ventricular hemodynamics in heart failure: clinical value of measurements derived from an implantable monitoring system. *J Am Coll Cardiol* 2003; **41**(4): 565–571.

4 Magalski A, Adamson P, Gadler F *et al.* Continuous ambulatory right heart pressure measurements with an implantable hemodynamic monitor: a multicenter, 12-month follow-up study of patients with chronic heart failure. *J Card Fail* 2002; **8**(2): 63–70.

5 Steinhaus DM, Lemery R, Bresnahan DR, Jr *et al.* Initial experience with an implantable hemodynamic monitor. *Circulation.* 1996; **93**(4): 745–752.

6 Medtronic. *Compass-HF Investigational Plan.* Minneapolis, MN September 2003.

7 Ramanathan C, Ghanem RN, Jia P, Ryu K, Rudy Y. Noninvasive electrocardiographic imaging for cardiac electrophysiology and arrhythmia. *Nat Med* 2004; **10**(4): 422–428.

8 Burnes JE, Taccardi B, Ershler PR, Rudy Y. Noninvasive electrocardiogram imaging of substrate and intramural ventricular tachycardia in infarcted hearts. *J Am Coll Cardiol* 2001; **38**(7): 2071–2078.

9 Rodriguez LM, Timmermans C, Nabar A, Hofstra L, Wellens HJ. Biatrial activation in isthmus-dependent atrial flutter. *Circualtion* 2001; **104**(21): 2545–2550.

10 Daoud EG, Morady F. Pathophysiology of atrial flutter. *Annu Rev Med* 1998; **49**: 77–83.

9

CHAPTER 9

Techniques of prediction of arrhythmia occurrence and stratification for sudden cardiac death

Aseem D. Desai, MD *& Bradley P. Knight,* MD

Background

Sudden cardiac death (SCD), defined as instantaneous death, unwitnessed death, or death occurring within 1 h of the onset of symptoms, is the number one killer in the United States, accounting for approximately 400 000 deaths per year [1–3]. SCD is largely due to ventricular tachyarrhythmias, either ventricular tachycardia (VT) or ventricular fibrillation (VF) [4]. Because the majority of SCD episodes occur outside the hospital where immediate medical attention is unavailable, the survival rate is dismal. Due to this poor survival, there has been an increasing focus on the use of automated external defibrillators (AEDs) by untrained laypersons in public places and the identification of high-risk patients who may benefit from implantable cardioverter defibrillator (ICD) therapy. This chapter will review the past, present, and future methods of risk stratifying patients for the development of VT/VF and SCD.

Prediction of ventricular arrhythmias and SCD

To date, most progress in the prediction of SCD has been in the identification of high-risk patients within a subgroup of cardiac patients, such as survivors of myocardial infarction (MI) or patients with congestive heart failure (CHF). Due to the development of fields such as genetic and molecular cardiology, efforts are now being made in the identification of other subgroups of patients at risk for SCD including patients with long-QT syndrome, Brugada syndrome, arrhythmogenic right ventricular cardiomyopathy, and hypertrophic cardiomyopathy.

Despite these strides, three significant problems remain in the prediction of SCD: (1) the majority of SCD occurs in the general, asymptomatic population where the incidence is low and where current risk stratification methods have not been tested or are impractical [5]; (2) current primary and secondary prevention strategies are directed at patients already known to be at risk based on conventional criteria (prior cardiac arrest or post-MI and ejection fraction (EF) < 30%), who represent a small percentage of the overall population at risk; and (3) etiologies other than VT/VF, including ruptured aortic aneurysm, pulmonary embolism, and acute MI, can cause sudden death. Pratt *et al.* [4] classified 17 of 834 defibrillator recipients as having SCD. After postmortem analysis, only 7 of the 17 had a confirmed arrhythmic cause of death by ICD interrogation.

Nonetheless, the application of defibrillator therapy for primary prevention among patients identified as being high risk has resulted in a significant reduction in total mortality. Examples include patients who are post-MI with a left ventricular EF (LVEF) < 40%, nonsustained VT (NSVT), and inducible VT during electrophysiology testing

(MUSTT and MADIT I) [6, 7], patients who are post-MI with an LVEF < 30% (MADIT II) [8], and patients with CHF and an LVEF < 35% (SCD-HeFT, DEFINITE, COMPANION) [9–11].

The ideal SCD risk stratification test would have the following characteristics: low cost, noninvasive, reproducible, high sensitivity and specificity, and high positive and negative predictive values. Furthermore, one would want specific prediction of arrhythmic death since the primary therapeutic interventions are targeted at termination of VT/VF.

Current risk stratification tests for SCD and VT/VF can be categorized into ones which measure: (1) heart structure and function; (2) coronary ischemia; (3) abnormal electrophysiology; and (4) autonomic imbalance. These will be described below.

Measures of heart structure and function

Measures of heart structure and function include echocardiography, nuclear and magnetic resonance imaging, and contrast ventriculography. These imaging modalities can assess ventricular function and detect structural abnormalities such as aortic stenosis and hypertrophic cardiomyopathy that might be associated with SCD. The relationship between EF and SCD has been studied extensively. The Task Force of Sudden Cardiac Death of the European Society of Cardiology stated that reduced LVEF remains the single most important risk factor for overall mortality and SCD [12].

Three recent ICD trials, MADIT II [8], SCD-HeFT [9], and COMPANION [11], used EF as the primary risk stratifier. The MADIT II study found that patients with a prior MI and an EF < 30% had a 31% reduction in mortality with ICD therapy compared with standard medical therapy [8]. SCD-HeFT found that patients with an ischemic or nonischemic cardiomyopathy, NYHA Class II and III CHF, and an EF < 35% had a 23% reduction in mortality with ICD therapy compared with placebo or amiodarone [9]. Lastly, COMPANION found a significant reduction in the secondary endpoint of all-cause mortality when patients with advanced CHF, an EF < 35%, and a QRS duration > 120 ms were treated with a cardiac resynchronization ICD device (CRT-D) compared with CRT only or optimal drug therapy [11].

In addition to EF, the presence of CHF symptoms is likely additive, and possibly synergistic, in terms SCD risk. Heart failure is associated with many factors that predispose to ventricular arrhythmias, including increased sympathetic tone, electrolyte imbalances, abnormal repolarization, after-depolarizations, and Purkinje system conduction delay. The SCD-HeFT trial found that the presence of CHF identified patients who benefit from defibrillator therapy.

The severity of heart failure, or functional classification, also seems to predict ventricular arrhythmias. The Triggers of Ventricular Arrhythmias (TOVA) study analyzed predictors of appropriate ICD therapy in a large ICD population ($n = 1140$) [13]. The presence of NYHA Class III CHF was the strongest predictor of appropriate ICD therapy for VT/VF (hazard ratio = 2.40), even after adjustment for LVEF. The combination of an LVEF < 20% and NYHA Class III symptoms was associated with a very high risk for appropriate shocks (hazard ratio = 3.90).

Because patients with NYHA Class IV symptoms have not been considered to be appropriate candidates for conventional defibrillator therapy, there is little information regarding the incidence of defibrillator therapy in patients with the most advanced heart failure. However, recent CRT-D trials have provided an opportunity to study these patients. Desai and colleagues identified predictors of appropriate ICD therapy in a CRT-D heart failure study population (VENTAK CHF) [14]. Patients who had either a primary or secondary indication for an ICD were randomized to either therapy with a standard ICD or therapy with an ICD that had CRT capability. After multivariate analysis, two independent predictors of appropriate ICD therapy were identified: NYHA Class IV CHF ($p = .019$) and a history of sustained VT/VF ($p = .002$) [15]. Despite the implications of this study, current guidelines recommend against prophylactic ICD implantation in medically refractory Class IV patients who are not transplantation candidates, since pump failure is a more common mode of death than VT/VF and the short-term mortality of these patients is high and would likely be unaffected by ICD implantation [16–17].

There are several limitations to the use of ventricular function as an optimal risk stratification tool. Limited sensitivity has been demonstrated in several studies. The Maastricht Circulatory Arrest Study of out of hospital cardiac arrest survivors found that 20% of patients had an EF > 50% [18]. Furthermore, the ATRAMI trial demonstrated that 27/49 deaths within 1 month post-MI had an EF > 35% [19]. Moreover, significant reductions in mortality and SCD were seen in the secondary prevention ICD trials CASH, AVID, and CIDS where the mean EF was greater than 30% [20].

Limited specificity is also a problem with using ventricular function as a risk stratifier. Data from the MUSTT study showed there was no difference in the percentage of arrhythmic deaths in patients with an EF < 30% versus those > 30%. In fact, patients with an EF < 30% and no inducible VT had a lower arrhythmic death rate than those with inducible VT and EF > 30%, arguing that factors in addition to EF are important in conferring risk of VT/VF.

Measures of coronary ischemia

It has been known for long that ischemia is associated with the risk of SCD. There exists significant interplay among ischemia, VT/VF, and SCD. Although the mechanisms are not fully understood, ischemia is associated with the development of delayed after-depolarizations, QT prolongation, and abnormal automaticity, all of which can facilitate VT/VF. These arrhythmias can be further maintained by scar-related or functional reentry.

Traditionally, SCD was thought to account for almost 50% of the total mortality in the first year post-MI, with a considerable drop over the subsequent 12–24 months. A recent MADIT II substudy found that mortality rates were higher over time as time from the index MI increased in patients randomized to conventional therapy. Furthermore, ICD therapy had a greater impact among patients with a time since MI ≥ 18 months before ICD implant compared with those <18 months [21].

Abnormal predischarge stress testing in post-MI patients confers an increased mortality, including SCD [22]. Specifically, significant ST segment depression, ventricular ectopy, hypotension, and poor exercise capacity have all been associated with increased events. Markers of the inflammatory response (C-reactive protein), plaque vulnerability (abnormal matrix metalloproteinases), and thrombogenesis (increased D-dimer and apo-B and decreased apo-A1) are currently being investigated as risk factors for sudden death. Coronary vasospasm is also associated with VT/VF and SCD. Genetic variations in systems that control vascular tone, such as the vascular endothelial nitric oxide synthetase (eNOS) system, could predispose to vasospasm. Identification of these genetic variations might be helpful risk assessment tools in the future [23].

Measures of abnormal electrophysiology

Measures of abnormal electrophysiology have intrinsic appeal as predictors of VT/VF and SCD. Various electrophysiologic (EP) tests have been developed to identify abnormal myocardial substrate or potential triggers of SCD.

Spontaneous ventricular ectopy

It has long been recognized that spontaneous ventricular ectopy (SVE) is a risk factor for mortality [24]. Bigger [25] demonstrated that frequent premature ventricular contractions and NSVT identify a high-risk group of post-MI patients, independent of EF. The MADIT trial demonstrated a reduction in mortality with ICD therapy among patients who were required to have spontaneous ectopy. However, studies that have used multivariate analysis of several clinical variables among heart failure patients have shown that ventricular ectopy is not an independent predictor of sudden death. Therefore, when numerous variables are entered into an equation, the presence of NSVT may not add much to a patient's risk of SCD. On the other hand, because ventricular ectopy is a univariate predictor of SCD in patients with heart failure and because ambulatory monitoring is commonly performed in the hospital and as an outpatient, it remains a somewhat useful clinical tool in everyday practice.

Signal-averaged electrocardiogram

Another method to risk stratify patients for SCD is the signal-averaged electrocardiogram (SAECG). The SAECG is used to identify delayed activation of the myocardium, late potentials, using surface electrocardiographic techniques. Patients with an abnormal SAECG have the substrate for sustained

VT due to reentry. Several studies have shown that an abnormal SAECG is a predictor of SCD [11, 20, 26]. In the MUSTT study, a filtered QRS duration >114 ms was associated with the primary endpoint of arrhythmic death or cardiac arrest (28% versus 17%, $p < .001$) [6]. In fact, a QRSf > 114 ms in association with an EF < 30% represented a very high-risk group of patients.

Signal-averaged electrocardiogram has also been felt to have a high negative predictive value. Bailey *et al.* determined that a normal SAECG and normal EF was associated with a <2% incidence of arrhythmic events over 2 years [27]. In contrast, patients with an abnormal SAECG and an EF < 30% had an arrhythmic risk of 38%. The CABG-Patch trial was the only randomized, controlled ICD trial to evaluate the utility of the SAECG as a risk stratifier [28]. This study enrolled 900 patients with CAD, EF ≤ 35%, and an abnormal SAECG prior to CABG. Patients were randomized to ICD or standard therapy. The ICD provided no survival benefit. However, it was felt that the lack of benefit from defibrillator therapy was due to an improvement in the substrate by coronary revascularization. It is, therefore, difficult to judge the ability of the SAECG to risk stratify patients for SCD from the CABG-Patch study. SAECG is limited by the fact that it cannot be performed in patients with a left bundle branch block.

Microvolt T-wave alternans

Microvolt T-wave alternans (MTWA) detects subtle beat-to-beat changes in repolarization. Several publications have been released recently that demonstrate that MTWA testing could be an effective risk stratifier in patients with an ischemic or nonischemic cardiomyopathy [29–30]. Bloomfield *et al.* [31] found that MTWA was better than QRS duration at identifying a high-risk group of MADIT II patients likely to benefit from ICD therapy, and a low-risk group of patients unlikely to benefit. The hazard ratios for 2-year mortality for an abnormal MTWA and a QRS duration >120 ms were 4.8 ($p = .020$) and 1.5 ($p = .367$), respectively. The actuarial mortality rate was significantly lower in patients with a normal MTWA (3.8%, 95% CI = 0.0–9.0) than a QRS duration <120 ms (12.0%, 95% CI = 5.6–18.5). The corresponding false negative rates were 3.5% for MTWA and 10.2% for QRS duration. The ongoing Alternans before Cardioverter Defibrillator (ABCD) trial will compare the positive predictive value of MTWA test with that of an EPS in patients with ischemic heart disease, left ventricular dysfunction with an EF < 40%, and NSVT.

The advantages of using MTWA to risk stratify patients is that it can be performed easily using modifications of currently available exercise equipment, is noninvasive, and is relatively inexpensive. Disadvantages include its requirement that a patient is able to exercise and to be in sinus rhythm. MTWA cannot be performed in patients who have persistent atrial fibrillation or a ventricular paced rhythm.

QT dispersion (QTD), QT variability index (QTVI), and normalized QT variability (QTVN)

Temporal and spatial heterogeneity in repolarization predispose to reentry and ventricular arrhythmias. Several tests have been developed to identify repolarization abnormalities. QTD remains controversial because of its concept, methodology, and conflicting results [32]. In contrast, the QTVI, an index of beat to beat QT duration changes adjusted for heart rate variability (HRV), has been shown to be superior to other risk stratifiers, including VT inducibility and TWA, for arrhythmic events in post-MI patients [33]. Furthermore, QTV may represent a novel method to assess risk of patients who are already in a high-risk group. Haigney *et al.* [34] analyzed the median QTVN in 817 MADIT II patients. In this study, QTV was assessed in 10 min, resting high-resolution electrocardiogram (ECG) recordings using a semiautomated algorithm that measures beat-to-beat QT duration. The authors found that the top quartiles of QTVI and QTVN were independently associated with VT/VF in follow-up (HR 1.8 and 2.18, respectively).

EP testing

Programmed ventricular stimulation is designed to test for the presence of an abnormal myocardial substrate that permits reentry. Inducible monomorphic VT is very uncommon in a patient with a normal heart, but is present in approximately one-third of patients with an EF < 30% following MI. EP testing is useful for risk stratification in patients with prior MI, but is not helpful in patients with a nonischemic cardiomyopathy.

The MADIT I study was the first large-scale, randomized defibrillator trial that enrolled patients who were risk stratified partially based on the presence of inducible VT during EP testing [7]. The MUSTT study, similarly, risk stratified patients based on inducibility during EP testing [6]. In the MUSTT registry study, the outcomes of the 1397 patients that were not inducible were compared with the outcomes of the 353 patients with inducible tachyarrhythmias who received no antiarrhythmic therapy. The primary endpoint of cardiac arrest or death from arrhythmia occurred in 24% of the noninducible group compared with 32% in the inducible group. This contrasts with the 9% mortality in the inducible group treated with an ICD. As the noninducible patients had significantly poorer outcomes than this latter group, there must be a risk factor aside from inducibility to account for the increased mortality, such as low EF or NSVT that were also present in the noninducible group.

Therefore, although EP testing appears to provide additional information regarding the risk of SCD in patients with ventricular dysfunction following MI, the negative predictive value is poor and the absolute risk is sudden death despite a negative EP test being unacceptably high. The test is also limited by its invasive nature and high cost.

Autonomic imbalance

It is becoming increasingly evident that the two components of the autonomic nervous system, sympathetic and parasympathetic, play a significant role in the initiation and modulation of arrhythmias ranging from atrial fibrillation to VT. Abnormal baroreflexes are common following MI and appear to be associated with an increased mortality. Several tests have been developed to identify abnormalities in autonomic function that may be useful in identifying high-risk patients for SCD.

Heart rate variability

Heart rate variability testing is designed to measure the relative activity of the sympathetic and parasympathetic nervous system. Several large studies have shown that patients with a low HRV after an MI have increased mortality compared with those with normal HRV [19, 35–36]. The Defibrillators in Acute Myocardial Infarction Trial (DINAMIT) was a randomized trial that assessed the utility of abnormal HRV to identify patients at risk for SCD after a recent MI (40 days) with an EF $\leq$ 35% [37]. The standard deviation of normal-to-normal R–R intervals was required to be $\leq$70 ms, and patients were randomized to ICD or standard drug therapy. There was no difference in survival, but there was a 50% reduction in arrhythmic death in the ICD group, which was offset by an increase in nonarrhythmic death. Because the negative benefit of ICD therapy in this trial is most likely attributable to an improvement in ventricular function in the immediate post-MI phase, it is difficult to interpret the relative value of HRV from the DINAMIT trial.

Heart rate turbulence (HRT) is a new method for evaluating the response of sinus beats to single ventricular premature beats. The normal response is immediate acceleration with subsequent deceleration of heart rate, whereas a blunted response is considered as a sign of impaired baroreflex sensitivity. Schmidt *et al.* [38] showed that HRT is an independent predictor of total and cardiovascular mortality in two postinfarction populations.

Additional considerations

In addition to the above-discussed tests, there are several other considerations in testing to predict VT/VF and SCD. For example, it has been shown that a combination of tests is more predictive for SCD than each used individually [39]. A nice example of this concept is the MADIT I study that found a 67% probability of an arrhythmic event over 2 years when a low EF, SVE, and positive EP test were all present [7]. Equally important, there is likely a need for repeat testing over time to accurately identify risk. Structural substrates such as a low EF can improve or worsen, thereby affecting risk.

Lastly, over the last several years, there has been an accumulating body of evidence suggesting that there may be molecular and genetic indicators of SCD. The "family clustering" of SCD victims supports this concept. In one study, if there was a history of maternal and paternal SCD events, the relative risk for SCD in offspring was as high as 9.4 [40].

Conclusions

Any clinical predictor of SCD must be easy and reproducible to have widespread applicability. Complicated predictors, even if found to have prognostic power, have limited clinical use. Currently, no single risk stratifying test is adequate to predict a patient's arrhythmic and SCD risk with sufficient positive predictive value. Genomics and proteomics have potential, and will probably guide treatment decisions in the future, but are currently not useful clinically. Furthermore, the interaction between genetics and the environment cannot be overstated.

Ultimately, the identification of a "signature" of clinical, biochemical, and genetic markers of SCD will likely be required. However, a relatively low positive predictive value may continue to limit any test if it is applied to a large population with an overall low risk of SCD. The ultimate value in risk stratification tests will likely be in the identification of a low-risk patient among a conventionally defined high-risk cohort (i.e. prior MI and an EF $< 30\%$). There is emerging data suggesting a benefit of the QTVI and T-wave alternans as helpful tests for the large group of patients with ventricular dysfunction following MI. Further studies are needed to better evaluate these and other techniques, in both the ischemic and nonischemic cardiomyopathies.

References

1 International Statistical Classification of Diseases and Related Health Prloblems, 10th revision, Online version for 2003. Web URL: http://www3.who.int/icd/vol1htm2003/fr-icd.htm.

2 Goldstein S. The necessity of a uniform definition of sudden coronary death: witnessed death within one hour of the onset of acute symptoms. *Am Heart J* 1982; **103**: 156–159.

3 State-specific mortality from sudden cardiac death-United States, 1999. *MMWR Morb Mortal Wkly Rep* 2002; **51**: 123–126.

4 Pratt CM, Greenway PS, Schoenfeld MH *et al.* Exploration of the precision of classifying sudden cardiac death. Implications for the interpretation of clinical trials. *Circulation* 1996; **93**: 519–524.

5 Myerburg RJ, Interian A Jr, Mitrani RM *et al.* Frequency of sudden cardiac death and profiles of risk. *Am J Cardiol* 1997; **80**: 10F–19F.

6 Buxton AE, Lee KL, DiCarlo L *et al.* Electrophysiologic testing to identify patients with coronary artery disease who are at risk for sudden death. Multicenter Unsustained Tachycardia Trial Investigators. *N Engl J Med* 2000; **342**: 1937–1945.

7 Moss AJ, Hall WJ, Cannom DS *et al.* Improved survival with an implanted defibrillator in patients with coronary disease at high risk for ventricular arrhythmia. *N Engl J Med* 1996; **335**: 1933–1940.

8 Moss AJ, Zareba W, Hall WJ *et al.* Prophylactic implantation of a defibrillator in patients with myocardial infarction and reduced ejection fraction. *N Engl J Med* 2002; **346**: 877–883.

9 Bardy GH. SCD-HeFT: the Sudden Cardiac Death in Heart Failure Trial. *American College of Cardiology 2004 Scientific Sessions*. New Orleans, March 7–10, 2004.

10 Kadish A, Dyer A, Daubert JP *et al.* Prophylactic defibrillator implantation in patients with nonischemic dilated cardiomyopathy: Defibrillators in Non-Ischemic Cardiomyopathy Treatment Evaluation (DEFINITE). *N Engl J Med* 2004; **350**: 2151–2158.

11 Bristow MR, Saxon LA, Boehmer J *et al.* Cardiac-resynchronization therapy with or without an implantable defibrillator in advanced chronic heart failure: comparison of medical therapy, pacing, and defibrillation in heart failure (COMPANION). *N Engl J Med.* 2004; **350**: 2140–2150.

12 Priori SG, Aliot E, Blonstrom-Lundqvist C *et al.* Task force on sudden cardiac death of the European Society of Cardiology. *Eur Heart J* 2001; **22**: 16.

13 Whang W, Mittleman MA, Rich DQ *et al.* Heart failure and the risk of shocks in patients with implantable cardioverter defibrillators: results from the Triggers Of Ventricular Arrhythmias study. *Circulation* 2004; **109**: 1386–1391.

14 Higgins SL, Hummel JD, Niazi IK *et al.* Cardiac resynchronization therapy for the treatment of heart failure in patients with intraventricular conduction delay and malignant ventricular tachyarrhythmias *J Am Coll Cardiol* 2003; **42**: 454–459.

15 Desai AD, Burke MC, Hong TE *et al.* Predictors of appropriate defibrillator therapy in patients with an implantable defibrillator that delivers cardiac resynchronization therapy. Unpublished data.

16 MERIT-HF Study Group. Effect of metoprolol CR/XL in chronic heart failure: Metoprolol CR/XL Randomised Intervention Trial in Congestive Heart Failure (MERIT-HF). *Lancet* 1999; **353**: 2001–2007.

17 Gregoratos G, Abrams J, Epstein AE *et al.* ACC/AHA/NASPE 2002 guideline update for implantation of cardiac pacemakers and antiarrhythmia devices: summary article: a report of the American College of Cardiology/American Heart Association Task Force on Practice Guidelines (ACC/AHA/NASPE Committee to

Update the 1998 Pacemaker Guidelines). *Circulation* 2002; **106**: 2145–2161.

18 Gorgels AP, Gijsbers C, de Vreede-Swagemakers J *et al.* Out-of-hospital cardiac arrest – the relevance of heart failure. The Maastricht Circulatory Arrest Registry. *Eur Heart J* 2003; **24**: 1204–1209.

19 La Rovere MT, Bigger JT Jr, Marcus FI *et al.* Baroreflex sensitivity and heart-rate variability in predication of total cardiac mortality after myocardial infarction: ATRAMI (Autonomic Tone and Reflexes After Myocardial Infarction). *Lancet* 1998; **351**: 478–484.

20 Connolly SJ, Hallstrom AP, Cappato R *et al.* Meta-analysis of the implantable cardioverter defibrillator secondary prevention trials: AVID, CASH and CIDS studies (Antiarrhythmics vs Implantable Defibrillator study, Cardiac Arrest Study Hamburg, Canadian Implantable Defibrillator Study). *Eur Heart J* 2000; **21**: 2071–2078.

21 Wilber DJ, Zareba W, Hall WJ *et al.* Time dependence of mortality risk and defibrillator benefit after myocardial infarction. *Circulation* 2004; **109**: 1082–1084.

22 Theroux P, Waters DD, Halphen C *et al.* Prognostic value of exercise testing soon after myocardial infarction. *N Engl J Med* 1979; **301**: 341–345.

23 El-Sherif N, Turitto G *et al.* Risk stratification and management of sudden cardiac death: a new paradigm. *J Cardiovasc Electrophysiol* 2003; **14**: 1113–1119.

24 Cohen JD, Neaton JD, Prineas RJ *et al.* Diuretics, serum, potassium and ventricular arrhythmias in the Multiple Risk Factor Intervention Trial. *Am J Cardiol* 1987; **60**: 548–554.

25 Bigger JT Jr. Relation between left ventricular dysfunction and ventricular arrhythmias after myocardial infarction. *Am J Cardiol* 1986; **57**: 12B.

26 Heart Failure Society of America. Heart Failure Society of America (HFSA) Practice Guidelines: HFSA guidelines for management of patients with heart failure caused by ventricular systolic dysfunction. *J Card Fail* 1999; **5**: 357–382.

27 Bailey JJ, Berson AS, Handelsman H *et al.* Utility of current risk stratification tests for predicting major arrhythmic events after myocardial infarction. *J Am Coll Cardiol* 2001; **38**: 1902.

28 Bigger JT (For the Coronary Artery Bypass Graft (CABG) Trial Investigators). Prophylactic use of implanted cardiac defibrillators in patients at high risk for ventricular arrhythmias after coronary-artery bypass graft surgery: Coronary Artery Bypass Graft (CABG) Patch Trial Investigators. *N Engl J Med* 1997; **337**: 1569–1575.

29 Chow T, Scholss E, Waller T *et al.* Microvolt T-wave alternans identifies MADIT II type patients at low risk of ventricular tachyarrhythmic events. *Circulation* 2003; **108**: IV-323.

30 Hohnloser SH, Ikeda T, Bloomfield DM *et al.* T-wave alternans negative coronary patients with low ejection fraction do not benefit from defibrillator implantation. *Lancet* 2003; **362**: 125–126.

31 Bloomfield DM, Steinman RC, Namerow PB *et al.* Microvolt T-wave alternans distinguishes between patients likely and patients not likely to benefit from implanted cardiac defibrillator therapy: A solution to the Multicenter Automatic Defibrillator Implantation Trial (MADIT) II condundrum. *Circulation* 2004; **110**: 1885–1889.

32 Zareba W. Dispersion of repolarization: time to move beyond QT dispersion. *Ann Noninvasive Electrocardiol* 2000; **5**: 373.

33 Atiga WL, Calkins H, Lawrence JH *et al.* Beat-to-beat repolarization lability identifies patients at risk for sudden cardiac death. *J Cardiovasc Electrophysiol* 1998; **9**: 899.

34 Haigney MC, Zareba W, Gentlesk PJ *et al.* QT Interval variability and spontaneous ventricular tachycardia or fibrillation in the Multicenter Automatic Defibrillator Implantation Trial (MADIT) II patients. *J Am Coll Cardiol* 2004; **44**:1481–1487.

35 Odemuyiwa O, Malik M, Farrel T *et al.* Comparison of the predictive characteristics of heart rate variability index and left ventricular ejection fraction for all-cause mortality, arrhythmic events and sudden death after acute myocardial infarction. *Am J Cardiol* 1991; **68**: 434–439.

36 Kleiger RE. Heart rate variability and mortality and sudden death post infarction. *J Cardiovasc Electrophysiol* 1995; **6**: 365–367.

37 Hohnloser S. Defibrillators in Acute Myocardial Infarction Trial (DINAMIT). *American College of Cardiology 2004 Scientific Sessions*. New Orleans, March 7–10, 2004.

38 Schmidt G, Malik M, Barthel *et al.* Heart-rate turbulence after ventricular premature beats as a predictor of mortality after acute myocardial infarction. *Lancet* 1999; **353**: 1390.

39 Ikeda T, Sakata T, Takami M *et al.* Combined assessment of T-wave alternans and late potentials used to predict arrhythmic events after myocardial infarction: a prospective study. *J Am Coll Cardiol* 2000; **35**: 722.

40 Jouven X, Desnos M, Guerot C *et al.* Predicting sudden death in the population: the prospective Paris study I. *Circulation* 1999; **99**: 1978–1983.

10

CHAPTER 10

Beta-blocker efficacy in long-QT syndrome patients with mutations in the pore and nonpore regions of the hERG potassium-channel gene

Arthur J. Moss, MD, *Derick R. Peterson,* PhD, *Wojciech Zareba,* MD, PhD, *Rahul Seth,* BS, *Scott A. McNitt,* MS, *Mark L. Andrews,* BBS, *Ming Qi,* PhD, *Michael J. Ackerman,* MD, PhD, *Jesaia Benhorin,* MD, *Elizabeth S. Kaufman,* MD, *Jennifer L. Robinson,* MS, *Jeffrey A. Towbin,* MD, *G. Michael Vincent,* MD, *&* *Li Zhang,* MD

The human ether-a-go-go (hERG) gene is one of the seven long-QT syndrome (LQTS)-related genes involved in the hereditary disorder consisting of QT prolongation, arrhythmia-related syncope, and sudden death [1–3]. Mutations involving the hERG gene are associated with a reduction in the rapid component of the delayed rectifier repolarizing current (I_{Kr}) and are responsible for the LQT2 form of LQTS [4]. Our group has shown that untreated patients with mutations in the pore region of the hERG gene are at an increased risk of experiencing arrhythmia-related cardiac events compared with similar untreated patients with nonpore mutations [5]. The objective of this study is to examine the efficacy of beta-blocker therapy on cardiac events in LQT2 patients with mutations in the pore and nonpore regions of the hERG gene after adjustment for relevant covariates.

Methods

Study population

The study population consisted of 275 subjects with genetically confirmed hERG mutations derived from 59 LQT2 families enrolled in the International Long-QT Registry (v. 11a of the database). The hERG mutations were identified in each subject using standard genetic tests. All subjects or their guardians provided informed consent for the genetic and clinical studies. Phenotype characterization of enrollment status in terms of proband (first family member identified with LQTS) and affected family member (individual with LQTS identified during family evaluation of the proband) and QTc measurement is as previously reported [5].

Genotype characterization

The pore region of the hERG channel was defined as the area extending from S5 to the midportion of S6 involving amino acid residues 550 through 650 [1].

Cardiac events

LQTS-related cardiac events were defined as syncope, aborted cardiac arrest, or unexpected sudden death without a known cause. The date and patient age when cardiac events occurred and when beta-blocker therapy was initiated were recorded as part of the Registry database.

Statistical analysis

We performed time to event analyses using Andersen's extension of the Cox proportional-hazards regression model for time-dependent covariates [6]. Separate models were developed for time origins at birth and, conditional on survival, at ages 13 and 21 years. In the past, we used birth as the only time origin, but in the present analyses we include time origins at ages 13 and 21 since these ages span the high-risk adolescent period and allow us to evaluate both beta-blocker therapy and prior event history, neither of which is possible when analyzing time to first event since birth. An indicator of any events prior to the time origin was included since decisions to initiate beta-blocker therapy are often a function of this information. Beta-blocker therapy was added to each regression model as a time-dependent main-effect variable to evaluate the effectiveness of this therapy in reducing the probability of cardiac events. Mutation location and its interaction with beta blockers were evaluated to determine if beta blockers had a different effect in those with pore versus nonpore mutations. The endpoint was the time until the first cardiac event after each time origin. Risk probabilities were quantified by the hazard ratio – the relative risk of experiencing a first cardiac event per unit time after the time origin for patients with the factor present as compared with that among patients not having the factor. QTc was modeled in a time-dependent fashion, using the mean of each patient's prior QTc measurements at any given time, with missing QTc measurements, for example, at birth, imputed by the first available ECG measurement after the specified time origin. Time-dependent enrollment status (proband, affected family member, or not yet known) was included in the analyses. Sex was adjusted for in all models. Grouped jackknife estimates of standard errors were used to adjust *p*-values and confidence intervals for potential within-family dependence not directly modeled by the Cox models.

Results

The clinical characteristics of the patient population with pore and nonpore mutations at each of the three time origins are presented in Table 10.1. Patients

Table 10.1 Clinical characteristics by mutation location and analytic time origin.

Clinical variables	*Nonpore*	*Pore*	*p-value*
Birth as time origin	(n = 229)	(n = 46)	
Female (%)	55	54	.89
Patients with cardiac events before time origin (%)	0	0	—
On beta blockers at time origin (%)	0	0	—
Baseline QTc (s)	0.48 ± 0.05	0.51 ± 0.05	.004
Age 13 as time origin	(n = 165)	(n = 38)	
Female (%)	66	58	.45
Patients with cardiac events before time origin (%)	13	50	<.001
On beta blockers at time origin (%)	8	29	<.001
Mean QTc (s) prior to time origin	0.48 ± 0.05	0.52 ± 0.05	<.001
Age 21 as time origin	(n = 139)	(n = 30)	
Female (%)	68	57	.31
Patients with cardiac events before time origin (%)	27	67	<.001
On beta blockers at time origin (%)	17	40	.006
Mean QTc (s) prior to time origin	0.49 ± 0.05	0.52 ± 0.05	.013

with pore mutations had longer QTc intervals at all three time origins, and at age origins 13 and 21 years, were more likely to have previously experienced cardiac events and to have been placed on beta blockers than patients with nonpore mutations.

The risk factors associated with LQTS-related cardiac events are presented in Table 10.2 for each time origin. The pore mutations were associated with a significantly increased risk for cardiac events only from birth when cardiac events had not yet occurred; pore mutations did not make a significant contribution to the risk models at age 13 or 21 years when cardiac events prior to these ages were included in the risk models. The elevated risk for females was significant at all three time origins, with the risk progressively increasing with age. The risk of prolonged QTc decreased with age, and it was no longer a significant risk factor by age 21. Time-dependent beta-blocker therapy showed a protective effect at all three time origins, with significant protection at the two later time origins. There was no significant interaction of beta-blocker therapy with mutation location (pore versus nonpore) on outcome at any of the time origins. Enrollment status (proband versus affected family member) did not make a significant contribution to any of the models.

Table 10.2 Hazard ratios for LQTS-related cardiac events at different time origins.

Variable	*Hazard ratio*[a]	*95% CI*	*p-value*
Birth as time origin			
Pore	3.61	2.14, 6.09	<.001
Female	1.80	1.16, 2.79	.008
QTc[b]	1.07	1.04, 1.10	<.001
Beta blockers[c]	0.49	0.14, 1.70	.26
Age 13 as time origin			
Pore	1.12	0.53, 2.36	.77
Female	2.18	1.25, 3.81	.006
QTc[b]	1.06	1.01, 1.11	.016
Prior events	2.96	1.75, 5.01	<.001
Beta blockers[c]	0.37	0.14, 0.94	.038
Age 21 as time origin			
Pore	0.69	0.29, 1.64	.40
Female	3.60	1.67, 7.77	.001
QTc[b]	1.03	1.00, 1.06	.069
Prior events	3.84	2.14, 6.89	<.001
Beta blockers[c]	0.35	0.13, 0.91	.032

[a] Risk of experiencing a first cardiac event per unit time after the time origin for patients with the factor present as compared with that among patients not having the factor.
[b] Increase or decrease in the hazard ratio per 10 ms change in the time-dependent mean QTc above or below 500 ms, respectively.
[c] Time-dependent beta-blocker therapy. There was no significant interaction of beta-blocker therapy with mutation location (pore versus nonpore) on outcome at any of the time origins.

Discussion

In LQTS patients with hERG mutations, pore mutations identify patients at significantly increased risk for cardiac events only when using birth as the time origin. The pore effect no longer contributes significant risk when prior cardiac events are included in the later time-origin risk models. Beta blockers provide significant protection with increasing age, but there is no interaction of beta blockers with mutation location, that is, beta blockers did not show greater protection with pore than nonpore mutations. Females have a greater risk at all three time origins.

These findings amplify our previous report on the increased risk with hERG pore mutations in LQT2. In the prior report [5], the hazard ratio for pore mutations using birth as the time origin was 2.5 among probands and 10.7 among affected family members. In the current study, proband and affected family member status was not a significant factor when modeled in a time-dependent fashion. At birth, the hazard ratio for pore mutations was 3.6, a value between 2.5 for probands and 10.7 for affected family members in the prior publication. These findings reveal a more modest but still highly significant hazard ratio for pore mutations when using birth as the time origin, probably related to a larger sample size and more events than in the prior publication [5].

The current analyses provide insight into the reason for the diminishing risk of pore mutations with age. Pore mutations are associated with a significant risk for cardiac events when using birth as the time origin. Those who experience a subsequent cardiac event, say between birth and age 13 or 21 years, are typically at a higher risk for additional events. When we include prior event history as a covariate in the time-origin analyses after birth, the prior event history captures the predictive power of the pore mutation, and pore mutations become an insignificant factor. These findings emphasize the prognostic importance of a history of prior cardiac events when following patients with LQT2 mutations.

In a prior study, we compared cardiac event rates before and after starting beta blockers [7]. We found that beta blockers were protective, but that approach was potentially biased since beta blockers were usually initiated following a prior cardiac event. Such analyses can overestimate the benefit of beta blockers. We tried to reduce this bias by selecting time origins based on age, that is, age 13 and 21 years, rather than the start of beta blockers. The current analyses substantiate the protective effect of beta blockers, especially when evaluating time origins not directly associated with beta blocker initiation or events. The only valid way of estimating the true effect of beta blockers is with a randomized trial, but such a trial does not appear feasible.

Acknowledgment

This work was supported in part by research grants HL-33843 and HL-51618 from the National Institutes of Health, Bethesda, MD.

References

1 Splawski I, Shen J, Timothy KW *et al.* Spectrum of mutations in long-QT syndrome genes. KVLQT1, HERG, SCN5A, KCNE1, and KCNE2. *Circulation* 2000; **102**: 1178–1185.

2 Plaster NM, Tawil R, Tristani-Firouzi M *et al.* Mutations in Kir2.1 cause the developmental and episodic electrical phenotypes of Andersen's syndrome. *Cell* 2001; **105**: 511–519.

3 Mohler PJ, Schott JJ, Gramolini AO *et al.* Ankyrin B mutation causes type 4 long-QT cardiac arrhythmia and sudden cardiac death. *Nature* 2003; **421**: 634–639.

4 Keating MT, Sanguinetti MC. Molecular and cellular mechanisms of cardiac arrhythmias. *Cell* 2001; **104**: 569–580.

5 Moss AJ, Zareba W, Kaufman ES *et al.* Increased risk of arrhythmic events in long-QT syndrome with mutations in the pore region of the human ether-a-go-go-related gene potassium channel. *Circulation* 2002; **105**: 794–799.

6 Andersen PK, Gill RD. Cox's regression for counting processes: a large sample study. *Ann Statistics* 1982; **10**: 1100–1120.

7 Moss AJ, Zareba W, Hall WJ *et al.* Effectiveness and limitations of beta-blocker therapy in congenital long-QT syndrome. *Circulation* 2000; **101**: 616–623.

11

CHAPTER 11

New developments in out-of-hospital cardiac defibrillation: evaluation of AED strategies

Robert J. Myerburg, MD, *Shauntelle Elliott,* RN, *Donald G. Rosenberg,* MD, *Alberto Interian Jr.,* MD, *&* *Agustin Castellanos,* MD

Background and definition of the problem

Estimates of the incidence of sudden cardiac death (SCD) in the United States range from less than 200 000 to more than 450 000 per year. The actual number remains uncertain because of variations in data sources and techniques for estimating event rates [1], but it is likely to be in the range of 300 000–350 000 per year [2]. Thus, SCD is a persisting public health problem. It is generally accepted that out-of-hospital cardiac arrest accounts for 1–2 deaths per 1000 population per year for the middle-aged and older adult populations, this figure representing ~50% of all cardiovascular deaths [3]. For adolescents and young adults, the incidence is ~1 per 100 000 per year [3]. Within the population aged 35 years and older, coronary heart disease accounts for ~80% of all SCDs, with the cardiomyopathies accounting for an additional 10–15%.

In attacking the problem of SCD, it is unrealistic to assume that either primary prevention of disease states, clinical interventions of established diseases, or community response systems will have a major impact as a single approach. Each strategy has a role, in part because large numbers of events occur unexpectedly in the out-of-hospital environment and are not predicted with great accuracy by risk profiling in most clinical circumstances [4]. For example, when coronary heart disease-related SCDs are analyzed according to clinical status at the time of the event, more than two-thirds of the deaths occur as the first clinical event or in a patient defined at relatively low risk for mortality based upon clinical status (Figure 11.1). Conversely, less than 25% of SCDs, and perhaps as few as 10–15% occur among patients who have high-risk markers for arrhythmic death as defined in implantable cardioverter defibrillator (ICD) trials or a hemodynamic status that predicts high risk of an impending mortality [4]. Since strategies intended to identify risk of SCD among the clinically silent or relatively low-risk populations lack sufficient power to guide the use of interventions such as ICDs for primary prevention, strategies that complement advanced interventional therapies are necessary to respond to unexpected cardiac arrests.

Since a large proportion of SCDs are initiated by the mechanism of ventricular fibrillation (VF) or hemodynamically compromising ventricular tachycardias (VTs), community-based defibrillation strategies have emerged as an important approach to the SCD problem. They began first as an extension of the "coronary care unit" concept, expanding subsequently to community-based paramedical

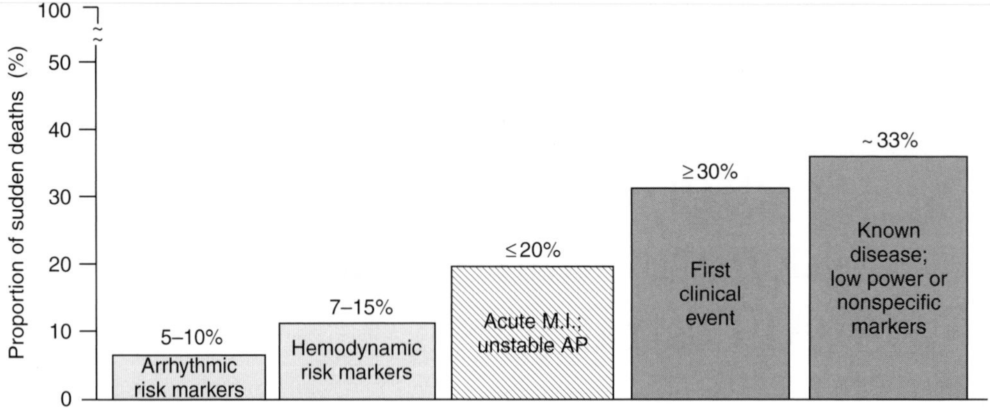

Figure 11.1 Distribution of SCDs among different clinical subgroups in ischemic heart disease. Arrhythmic markers of risk for SCD, which have been used in many of the ICD trials, identify subgroups at high risk for SCD, but account for no more than 5–10% of all events. Based upon estimates from heart failure trials and other observation data, hemodynamic markers have the potential to identify another 7–15% of all events. At the other extreme, more than 30% of all SCDs occur as the first clinical expression of the underlying disease, and another 33% occur in patients with low-risk markers for mortality. These statistics underscore the need for more powerful individual risk profiling for SCD among the general population. (Modified from *J Cardiovasc Electrophysiol* [4], with permission.)

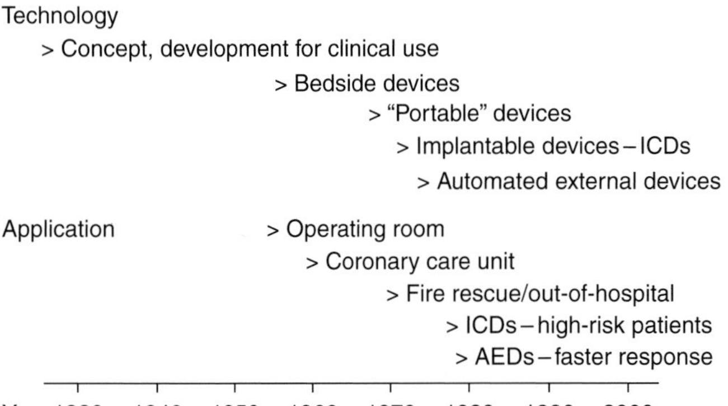

Figure 11.2 Evolution and application of defibrillator technologies. Beginning in the late 1920s and continuing to the present, there has been a transition from concept to application of evolving defibrillator technologies. The initial concept required more than 20 years to evolve, but the evolution of advanced technologies has been more rapid, with their applications following developments. (Reproduced from *J Cardiovasc Electrophysiol* [40], with permission.)

programs, and finally to the placement of automated external defibrillators (AEDs) in the hands of nonconventional responders with training targeted to emergency responses that include CPR and early defibrillation [5, 6] (Figure 11.2).

History of out-of-hospital cardiac arrest survival

Prior to the initial development of community-based emergency rescue systems in Miami [7] and Seattle [8], out-of-hospital cardiac arrests were almost always fatal. The studies carried out between the late 1960s and 1974 in these cities, and published in 1974, yielded 14% and 11% survival rates to hospital discharge. Encouraged by these results, both cities continued to improve their emergency rescue systems. The Seattle system moved effectively into the dual concepts of public education for bystander CPR [9] and a first-responder tier of emergency medical technicians to perform early defibrillation at the scene of a cardiac arrest [10]. Their data reflected benefits of both strategies. By the late 1970s and into the mid-1980s, survival rate from ventricular fibrillation in the Seattle community peaked at a range of 30–35% [11] (Table 11.1) and the Miami data peaked at a 23% survival rate [12]. At the same time, data began to emerge from other sources. For example, a

Table 11.1 History of survival from out-of-hospital cardiac arrest based upon community interventions.

Year	*Community interventions*	*% of survival*
1971–4	Initial Miami/Seattle outcomes	14, 11
1978–85	Peak Miami/Seattle outcomes	25–35
1984	Rural outcomes	
	Standard basic life support	3
	Ambulance-based expanded access	19
1991	Estimated cumulative US survival	1–3
1992–4	Major metropolitan population centers	≤2
1996	Dade-County, FL, current outcomes	9
1996–8	Current US EMS outcomes, cumulative	<5
1999	"Optimized" systems {OPALS}	5

Notes: After the initial studies of emergency rescue responses to out-of-hospital cardiac arrest that provided modestly encouraging results, continued focus on improved systems was accompanied by better outcomes in selected centers. However, cumulative outcomes have been disappointing, with overall US survival currently estimated at <5%. These experiences do not include public access programs with nonconventional responders.

Source: Modified from *J Cardiovasc Electrophysiol* [4], with permission.

study in rural communities in Iowa, having populations of less than 10 000, yielded a disappointing 3% survival rate using standard basic life support and emergency vehicle summons. However, when they added ambulance-based response systems that included capacity for early defibrillation, the survival rate improved to 19% [13]. This was the first data-driven suggestion that nonconventional responders with defibrillators might improve outcomes.

The experience in selected communities, such as Miami and Seattle, was not representative of the cumulative statistics in the United States (Table 11.1). As recently as 1991, the cumulative US survival from out-of-hospital cardiac arrest was estimated to be in the range of only 1–3% [14], and two studies in large population centers, New York [15] and Chicago [16], yielded survival outcomes of 2% or less. In 1996, the survival rates in metropolitan Miami-Dade county were reevaluated, and it was observed that survival from witnessed-onset cardiac arrest due to VF was only 9%, compared with 14% for the City of Miami Fire Rescue System as far back as 1974. Despite enhancements to systems at various locations across the country, estimates for US survival are still under 5%, and an optimized system in Ontario, Canada resulted in an increase in survival from less than 4% to 5%, a significant increase in a relative sense, but still far below desirable survival rates [17]. With this experience spanning 25 years, attention to new strategies for out-of-hospital cardiac arrest responses began to emerge during the 1990s [18] and continues in the present decade [19].

Technical evolution of AEDs

The concepts of the ICD and the AED both emerged during the 1970s (Figure 11.2). AEDs were originally intended for use by high-risk patients in the home, but technical limitations of the early devices interfered with that application. It would have been short-lived anyway, because the ICDs emerged beginning in the early 1980s [20], and the original target population for AEDs soon became ICD candidates. After a quiescent period of uncertainty about the proper role for AEDs, they underwent further technical refinement and were developed for a target population of unexpected cardiac arrest victims in the community, with the notion that they could be operated by nonconventional and less highly trained responders [5]. Their role in this realm is now being expanded [6].

Technological advance in AEDs, combined with the disappointing statistics for out-of-hospital cardiac arrest survival related likely to response times, encouraged a number of deployment strategies, which are undergoing continuous evaluation. Strategic deployment can be classified into four categories: (1) emergency vehicles, (2) public access sites, (3) multifamily dwellings, and (4) single family dwellings. Table 11.2 provides examples and the type of rescuers that can be used in each category. The fundamental principle driving each of these strategies is that minimally trained personnel or lay individuals can learn the operation of AEDs and apply them in the setting of a cardiac emergency. Examples of nonconventional cardiac arrest response by emergency vehicle personnel, beyond the scope of conventional emergency rescue system responders, including standard fire engines, police patrol cars, and ambulances. The rescuers for these strategies have a higher level of training than for some of the other public access strategies that include AED placement in public buildings, stadiums and malls, airports and airliners, and other sites at which people congregate.

Table 11.2 Strategies for AED deployment.

Deployment	*Examples*	*Rescuers*	*Advantages*	*Limitations*
Emergency vehicles	Police patrol cars Fire engines Ambulances	Trained emergency personnel	Experienced users Broad deployment Objectivity	Deployment time Arrival delays Community variations
Public access sites	Public buildings Stadiums and malls Airports and airliners	Security personnel Designated rescuers Random lay persons	Population density Shorter delays Lay and emergency personnel access	Low event rates Inexperienced users Panic and confusion
Multifamily dwellings	Apartment buildings Condominiums Hotels	Security personnel Designated rescuers Family members	Familiar locations Defined personnel Shorter delays	Infrequent use Low event rates Geographic factors
Single family dwellings	Private homes Apartments	Family members	Immediate access Familiar setting	Acceptance; victim alone One-time user; panic

Notes: Examples of deployment strategies, type of rescuers, and the advantages and limitations of each strategy, are provided (see text for details).

Source: From *J Cardiovasc Electrophysiol* [4], with permission.

The responder personnel can include the security guards at various locations, designated rescuers, and even random laypersons with minimal or no prior training. Multifamily dwellings include apartment buildings, condominiums, and hotels, and once again responders may include security personnel, designated rescuers, or family members. The single family dwelling focuses on private homes, with the responder usually being a trained family member. The latter strategy has the disadvantage of rare utilization of devices by the rescuers and the possibility of panic at the time of a suspected cardiac arrest in a family member. Its advantage resides in the fact that a large percentage of cardiac arrest occurs in the home [21]. An alternative suggestion for this general strategy is the concept of neighborhood-designated responders [22] who would require training and coordination that would have to be individualized to each neighborhood. The anticipated effect of the patterns of deployment is to expand the density of availability of AEDs so that the probability of rapid access to defibrillation would be statistically greater during a medical emergency.

Police as cardiac arrest responders

A number of communities, worldwide, have implemented and/or tested the feasibility of placing AEDs in police patrol cars in order to improve response times to cardiac arrest [23–29]. In contrast to fire-department-based or ambulance-based emergency rescue responders, the police offer the potential to be closer (both physically and in time) to the sites of cardiac events, because patrol cars are on the road at all times. Therefore, it is reasonable to expect the police to respond more quickly.

Among the communities that carried out early studies on this concept, Rochester, MN, has provided important data [24]. Their data on 246 cardiac arrests, of which 131 (53%) had shockable rhythms, demonstrate a cumulative survival of 22%, even though police response times were only ~50 s less than standard paramedic response times. The nature of the community, with a low population and traffic density, does not make it surprising that there was not a great difference between response times of police and paramedics, but highlights the fact that the response times for both was less than what is seen in major metropolitan areas (see below). Their outcome data revealed that spontaneous return of circulation by shock only was equivalent for both police responders and the paramedic responders (~20–30%), with the remainder requiring ACLS, which was provided only by paramedics. One of their important observations was that survival to hospital discharge was nearly 100% in the subgroup in whom shock only was sufficient to result in return of circulation. This outcome was equivalent for both police and paramedic responders.

The Amsterdam Resuscitation Study, which provided data on police and emergency medical service (EMS) response times in one section of that city, demonstrated a significantly improved response time by police. Fifty percent of the police responses occurred in 6 min or less, compared with approximately 11 min for EMS [25]. Less encouraging statistics emerged from rural Indiana, where placement of AEDs in police cars in sparsely populated areas did not provide a significant benefit, with police arriving first at the scene of cardiac arrest in only 6% of the instances [27].

The Miami-Dade county, Florida, police-AED project

Because of the disappointing reduction in survival rates from out-of-hospital cardiac arrest in metropolitan Miami-Dade county, Florida, a decision was made to place AEDs in all metropolitan Miami-Dade county police vehicles. The program was setup to include a data acquisition system in order to allow for the accumulation of data to determine whether there was benefit from this strategy in a large, densely populated, complex metropolitan area [29].

Automated external defibrillators were deployed in all Miami-Dade county, Florida, police vehicles, beginning on February 1, 1999. Distribution to all officers was completed on July 1, 1999. The startup process included a training program for all police officers prior to deployment, using a modified version of the American Heart Association's "Heart Saver Program." The 4-h training session included hands-on instruction on the use of AEDs. The educational program employed a "train-the-trainer strategy," in which selected police officers with a special interest in the project were trained to be educators, and participated in training other groups of officers. The training program and deployment were carried out sequentially in the nine Miami-Dade county police districts; 1900 officers were trained during the 5-month implementation period. The cumulative area of Miami-Dade county, excluding incorporated municipalities having independent law enforcement programs, is 1792 square miles, divided into nine police districts ranging from 15 to 722 square miles (median = 37 square miles), and district population densities ranging from 261 to 6647 inhabitants/square mile (median = 635 inhabitants per square mile). Thus, the mean density of AED deployment in the county was 0.94 AED/square mile. The total population of the county is 1 181 612 (based on the 2000 census), with a mean population density of 660 persons/square mile.

911 communications system

The Metropolitan Miami-Dade county Emergency Communications System (911) was modified for the police-AED project as a dual-dispatch program. Prior to implementation, 911 calls coming into central emergency telecommunications consoles were deployed to EMS if they were medical emergencies and to police for conventional police incidents. In order to implement the police-AED program, selected codes for medical emergencies were simultaneously relayed to both police and fire rescue, and the telecommunication consoles for the two services dispatched the appropriate vehicles. The codes initially selected were: code 6-D – breathing problems; code 9 – cardiac-respiratory arrest; code 10-D – chest pain; code 12-D – seizures/convulsions; code 14-D – drowning and diving; 15-D – electrocution; codes 19-C and 19-D – heart problems; code 23-D – overdose/ingestion; code 25-D – suicide attempt; 31-D – unconsciousness/fainting (nontraumatic); and code 32 – unknown (man down). Most of the actual cardiac arrest responses were classified under codes 6, 9, 10, and 31. A few were classified as codes 12, 19, and 32.

Response strategies

The AED-equipped police and fire rescue vehicles (standard EMS vehicles), were simultaneously deployed as a strategy intended to achieve diagnosis, AED availability, and defibrillation as quickly as possible if VT or VF is observed by the first responder at the scene. If the EMS vehicle arrived first, police were diverted and relieved of further responsibility to the call. If police arrived first, they deployed their AEDs and carried out defibrillation and/or CPR, based on the initial rhythm diagnosed and subsequent responses. When EMS arrived at the scene, police were relieved of further responsibility. Police responsibilities are limited to basic life support and defibrillation, whereas EMS personnel have the added responsibility of providing advanced life support. Transportation to the nearest appropriate medical facility was carried out by EMS personnel in all cases. Police retain the AEDs in their vehicles when off duty. The intent was to maintain availability of the devices in the community for *ad hoc* use by officers in their neighborhoods when not on duty.

In order to estimate effectiveness of the program, the study design of a case series with historical controls was used to evaluate the effect of police-AED deployment on response times and survival. Police-AED runs were compared to simultaneously deployed EMS runs in the dual dispatch system; and both were compared to recent (1997–9) historical EMS controls. As soon as AEDs were deployed in each police district, the data were analyzed for the dual deployment program, based on individual response times and first responder times. The historical control comparison is based upon EMS response time data and survival outcomes from September 1, 1997 until AED deployment was completed on or before July 1, 1999. For the period February 1–July 1, 1999, each district was counted among the historical controls until it received its AEDs.

Inclusion criteria, data acquisition and analysis

For inclusion in the cardiac arrest response analysis, the protocol required a witnessed or unwitnessed loss of consciousness, not anticipated by prior hemodynamic status, in the absence of trauma or other exogenous influences as a definable precipitating event. Nonetheless, for inclusion as a medical emergency triggering police dispatch, a broader range of deployment codes was used. These included codes for witnessed and unwitnessed unexpected loss of consciousness, symptoms of impending loss of consciousness or other cardiac events, and a broad array of codes indicating a possible or existing medical emergency (see above). Because initial experience yielded a large number of dispatches that were inappropriate for the intent of the police-AED program, codes that yield no cardiac arrests are continuously evaluated for discontinuation from the list of police dispatches.

Special police forms were developed for the program, and the data from these forms were validated and supplemented by information from standard EMS forms generated during the simultaneous EMS runs. All such data were entered into a dedicated computer database, developed for the purpose of these observations. The available information provides time intervals measured from 911 call to police dispatch, arrival at scene, arrival at patient's side, deployment of the AED, defibrillation and arrival at hospital emergency departments. Survival to hospital discharge was the primary endpoint in the analysis.

In order to achieve accurate and comparable time points for multiple timed elements of the program, the internal clocks in the AEDs and the clocks in the county emergency communications center, telecommunication consoles, and computer-assisted dispatch (CAD) systems are all synchronized to atomic clock time. When a 911 call is received, the CAD system assigns an automatic time stamp, and the time of dispatch of both police and EMS vehicles are linked to that atomic clock standard. The time of arrival at the scene must be called in by both police and EMS and logged into the CAD, generating a time stamp linked to the 911 incoming call standard. However, the time from arrival at scene to arrival at patient's side is not uniformly called in to the CAD operator, and therefore not linked to atomic clock time. Since the AED internal clocks are also linked to the atomic clock, standard time references are available for power-up and delivery of shocks. Because of this, the primary definition of response time, for the purpose of comparing police-AED and EMS, was based on the interval from 911 call to arrival at scene, since these time points were uniformly linked to the atomic clock, therefore providing true comparisons. Finally, time estimates from onset of cardiac arrest to 911 call was called for on the police forms, but were approximations not uniformly available and not linked to a standard time.

Data on response time and survival benefits

From February 1, 1999 to April 30, 2001, 911 calls were assigned as dual police-AED and standard EMS dispatches to possible or definite medical emergencies, and averaged 2086 per month (70 per day county-wide, or 8 per district). Based on the number of shifts and cars, this accounts for 1.1 dispatches per AED/month.

Among the police medical emergency runs, 0.75% ($n = 420$) were determined to be actual cardiac arrests. During the historical control period from September 1, 1997 until complete implementation of the police-AED program, the standard EMS system deployed 318 sole responders to actual cardiac arrests. Since initiation of the police-AED program, police were the first responders to 237 of the 420 dual dispatches to actual cardiac arrests (56%). EMS arrived before police in 138 instances (33%), and police and EMS arrived simultaneously in 45 (11%).

The mean age of the 420 cardiac arrest victims responded to in the police-AED program was 67.8 ∀ 16.3 years (mean ∀ SD), and 257 (61%) were males. Among the 318 historical EMS controls, the mean age was 69.5 ∀ 15.1 years, and 186 of the 318 (59%) were males. The initial rhythm recorded at the scene of cardiac arrest was a shockable VT/VF in 163 (39%) of the police-AED responses and 122 (38%) of the standard EMS responses. The corresponding nonshockable initial rhythms were 257 (61%) and 196 (62%).

Police-AED response times from 911 call to arrival at the scene of cardiac arrest, and from call to patients' side, was shorter than corresponding EMS response times. Among the 420 responses for cardiac arrest after implementation of the police-AED program, the mean (∀ SD) time from the 911 call to arrival of police at the scene of a cardiac arrest was 6.16 ∀ 4.27 min (median = 6 min). During the same period, the mean police response time from 911 call to the scene of nonmedical police emergencies was 4.15 ∀ 1.40 min ($p < .0001$) (Figure 11.3).

The response time to the scene of cardiac arrest by simultaneously dispatched EMS vehicles after implementation of the police-AED program was 7.56 ∀ 3.60 min (median = 7 min; $p < .001$ compared to police). Since EMS was the actual first responder in 33% of the paired police-AED/EMS runs, the time for the first rescuer to arrive at the scene was analyzed separately. In this analysis, the arrival time of the first responder during the police-AED program was reduced to 4.88 ∀ 2.88 min, with a median of 5 min ($p < .001$, compared to EMS controls) (Figure 11.3). The historical control response time for standard EMS during the 17 months before implementation of the police-AED program, plus the proportional 5 month phase-in period, was available for 315 of the 318 runs (99%). The response time was 7.64 ∀ 3.66 min (median = 7 min), not different from the actual EMS response time of 7.56 ∀ 3.60 min during the paired observation period after police-AED deployment.

Analyses of the distribution of response times among police-AED responders, paired EMS responders, and historical EMS responders demonstrate that the proportion of response times less than 5 min from 911 activation is significantly higher for the police-AED responses than for either of the EMS analyses. Of the police responses, 34% were achieved in less than 5 min, compared with 14% for concurrent EMS ($p < .001$), and 11% for historical EMS deployments prior to the police program ($p < .001$) (Figure 11.4). Moreover, the first responder time to the scene of cardiac arrest during the police-AED

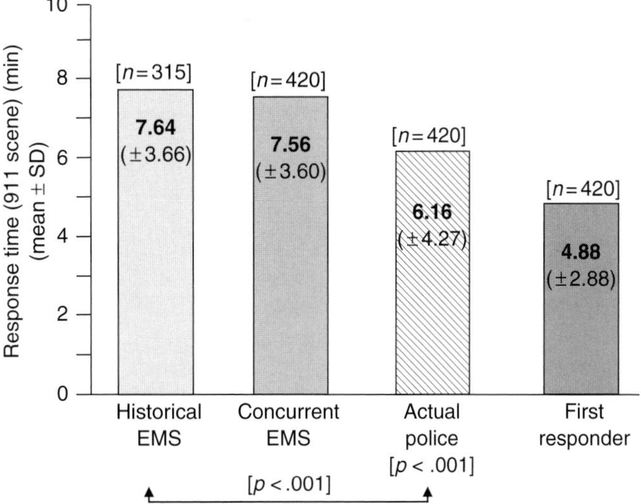

Figure 11.3 Cardiac arrest response times in metropolitan Miami-Dade county, Fl. The vertical bars demonstrate the mean (∀ SD) response time for the historical EMS controls (n = 315), compared with EMS responses concurrent with actual police responses (n = 420). The time of arrival of the first service at the scene of a cardiac arrest (first responder) was significantly improved by the dual-response system. (Reproduced from *Circulation* [29], with permission of the American Heart Association.)

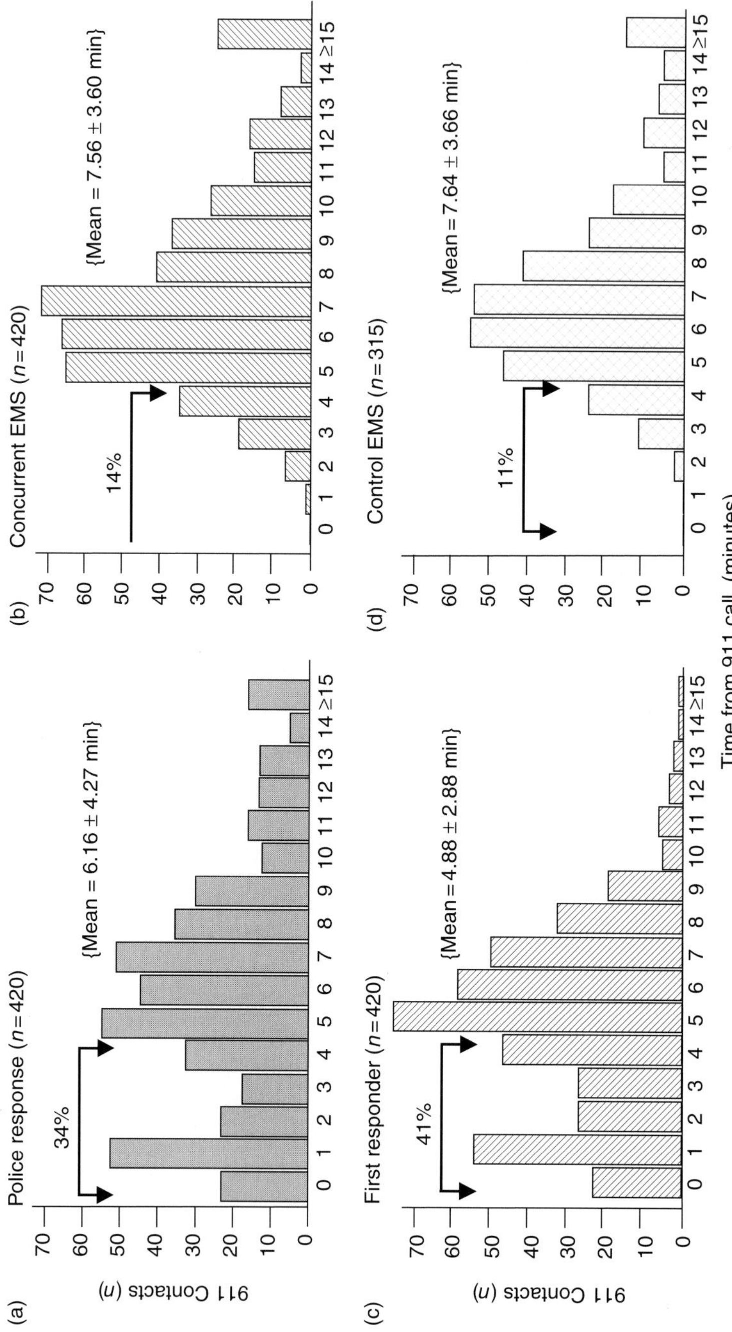

Figure 11.4 Distribution of responses to individual cardiac arrest calls. (a) Police responders, (b) concurrent EMS, (c) arrival of the first service at the scene (first responder), and (d) the historical control EMS responders are compared. See text for details. (Reproduced from *Circulation* [29], with permission of the American Heart Association.)

program was less than 5 min in 41% of the runs ($p < .001$, compared with historical EMS controls). Thus, despite the relatively small difference in mean response time between police and EMS, the skewed response times demonstrate that a dual dispatch police/EMS system offers a response-time advantage to a substantial segment of the population at risk. After the anthrax panic in 2001, police response times deteriorated for ~6 months. Police were inundated with calls about possible anthrax exposures and the cardiac arrest calls were delayed or handled by standard EMS. Response times improved after the anthrax scare abated.

Among the 163 victims in shockable rhythms responded to during the police-AED program, 28 (17.2%) survived to hospital discharge, compared with 11 of 122 (9.0%) in the standard EMS program ($p = .047$) (Figure 11.5). In contrast, the survival rate for victims in nonshockable rhythms was very low, and was not benefitted by the police-AED program. Thus, while the VT/VF subgroup benefitted significantly from the police-AED program, cumulative survival data to hospital discharge revealed only a small survival benefit from the police-AED program (32 police-AED survivors (7.6%) versus 19 standard EMS survivors (6.0%), odds ratio = 1.3; $p = NS$).

The survival benefit of the police-AED deployment strategy for victims in shockable rhythms was slightly higher for those victims with shockable rhythm in whom the onset of cardiac arrest was witnessed. Witnessed onset yielded a 24.0% (23 of 96) survival rate for police-AED and 10.5% (6 of 57) for standard (historical) EMS, and a similar proportional benefit for police-AED compared to standard EMS (odds ratio = 2.7 (95% CI = 1.0–7.0); $p < .05$).

Public access AEDs

Interest in public access AEDs has emerged rapidly in recent years, in part as a consequence of a series of studies on the effectiveness of these devices. The initial reports focused on those sites where people congregate or are at a distance from conventional medical response systems. Several models have been tested [6]. A large study on general public access in shopping malls and other public areas has recently

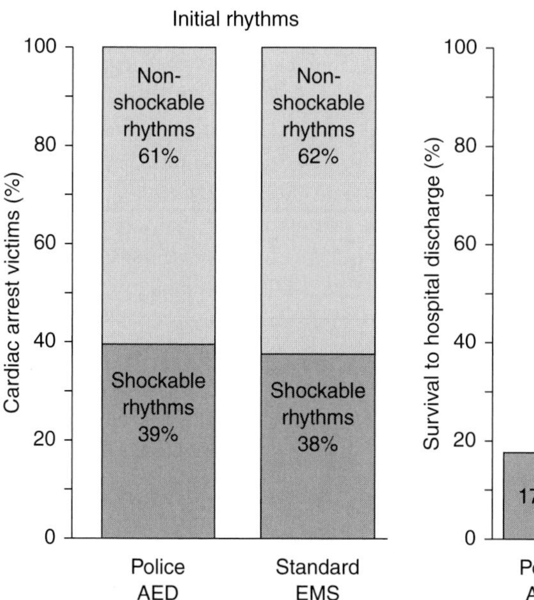

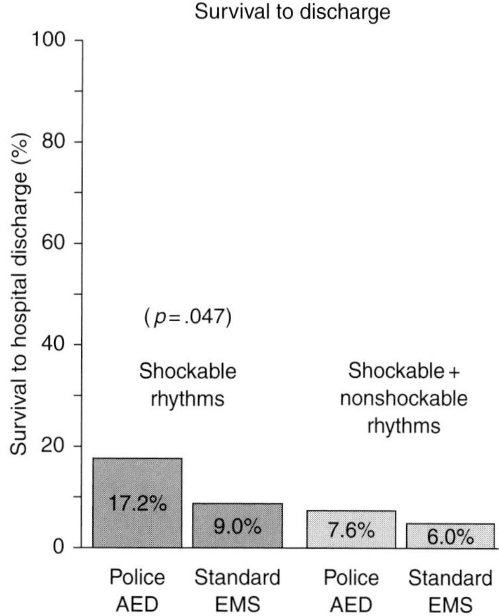

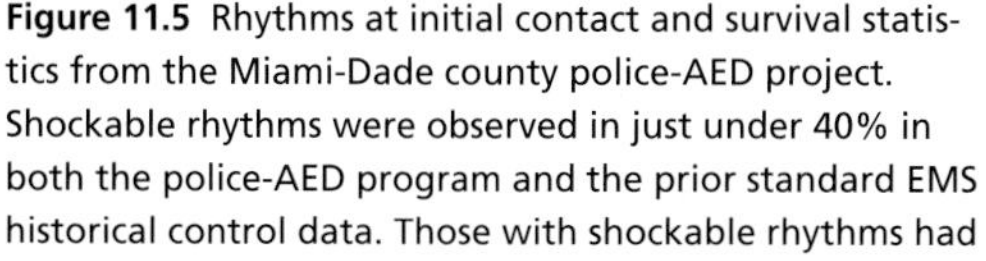

Figure 11.5 Rhythms at initial contact and survival statistics from the Miami-Dade county police-AED project. Shockable rhythms were observed in just under 40% in both the police-AED program and the prior standard EMS historical control data. Those with shockable rhythms had an improved survival to hospital discharge with only a small improvement when both shockable and nonshockable rhythms were included in the analyzed data. (Modified and reproduced from *Circulation* [29], with permission of the American Heart Association.)

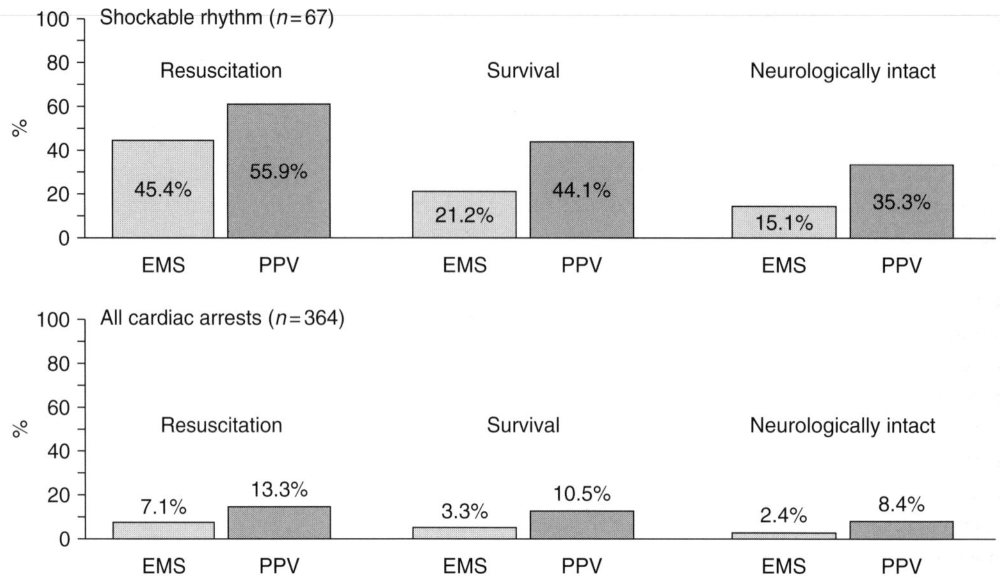

Figure 11.6 Public access defibrillation. A study of public access defibrillation, blended with conventional response systems, was carried out in Piacenza, Italy. Rapid defibrillation by strategically deployed AEDs resulted in improved outcomes from cardiac arrest due to shockable rhythms, including both initial survival and survival to hospital discharge without neurological impairment. The population impact of this observation is limited by the observation that the majority of responses were to patients who were in nonshockable rhythms at the time of initial contact by the responder. Nonetheless, the significant improvement in outcome for patients with shockable rhythms encourages this strategy. (Reproduced from *Circulation* [31], with permission.)

been reported [30]. The data suggested a relatively small benefit in absolute terms, but survival was twice as high with AED availability compared with CPR alone. In addition, the Piancenza, Italy, experience has demonstrated a benefit of public access AEDs in the community for victims of cardiac arrest due to VF [31], but impact was limited by the high proportion of responses in which nonshockable rhythms were identified at first contact (Figure 11.6). In addition, from the perspective of currently available data, there are two additional strategies that are particularly instructive, namely the airport and airline data and casino data.

AEDs in airports and on passenger airliners

The first substantive body of information that was released on the potential benefit of AEDs for in-flight cardiac arrest came from Qantas Airlines, but the data were disappointing [32]. The initial published data from the Qantas experience, in which airports and trans-Pacific airliners were equipped with AEDs in the early 1990s, suggested effectiveness in airports, but limited benefit in flight. The ground-based responses in major airports in Australia demonstrated that 79% of the cardiac arrests were due to shockable rhythms (VT/VF), and the cumulative survival rate among those victims was 21% (24% among the VT/VF subgroup). In contrast, the in-flight data from the Qantas program demonstrated that only 6 of 27 events were due to recognized shockable rhythms (22%), although 2 of those 6 did survive. The remaining 21 of the 27 victims (78%) had bradyarrhythmias or asystole. Among these, about one-half were thought to have been sleeping when they were actually in cardiac arrest, and were found to be asystolic when their status was finally recognized. The other one-half appeared to have had primary bradyarrhythmic events, still an excess compared with ground-based experience. Subsequent data from American Airlines also demonstrated that the majority of cardiac arrests in the air were due to nonshockable rhythms, although the proportion of nonshockable rhythms was lower [33]. More optimistically, however, the victims who had shockable rhythms had a 40% survival rate, yielding an overall survival rate of ~17%.

The AED experience in casinos

The Las Vegas casino AED project provides data on the efficacy of public access defibrillation in a setting that is particularly well suited to rapid responses. The system used security personnel in casinos to respond to cardiac arrest with AEDs in the casinos themselves. Since the gambling tables in casinos are under constant video surveillance, the recognition of onset of loss of consciousness was relatively easily achieved. The study demonstrated that CPR was begun 2.9 ∀ 2.8 min after recognized onset of cardiac arrest, and time to the first AED shock was 4.4 ∀ 2.9 min [34] (Figure 11.7). This resulted in an overall success rate of 38% for all cardiac arrests with documented VT/VF and 59% with the subgroup of witnessed onset of cardiac arrest due to VT/VF. As anticipated, survival was significantly better when the time from collapse to shock was 3 min or less compared with >3 min. While this is a unique environment, it provides a model for testing the efficacy of rapid access defibrillation, and the data clearly show importance of time, particularly within the first 3 min. Thus, while this particular model is of limited relevance to the community at large, it does provide a goal to be achieved in other settings for improved outcomes.

Other community-based AED strategies

Automated external defibrillator deployment strategies are being considered and evaluated in settings beyond those described above. The four categories of strategies each have advantages and limitations, as listed in Table 11.2. The most rational approach for determining the validity of AED deployment strategies will derive from scientific support for their efficacy and incremental benefit over conventional systems. This is best done by

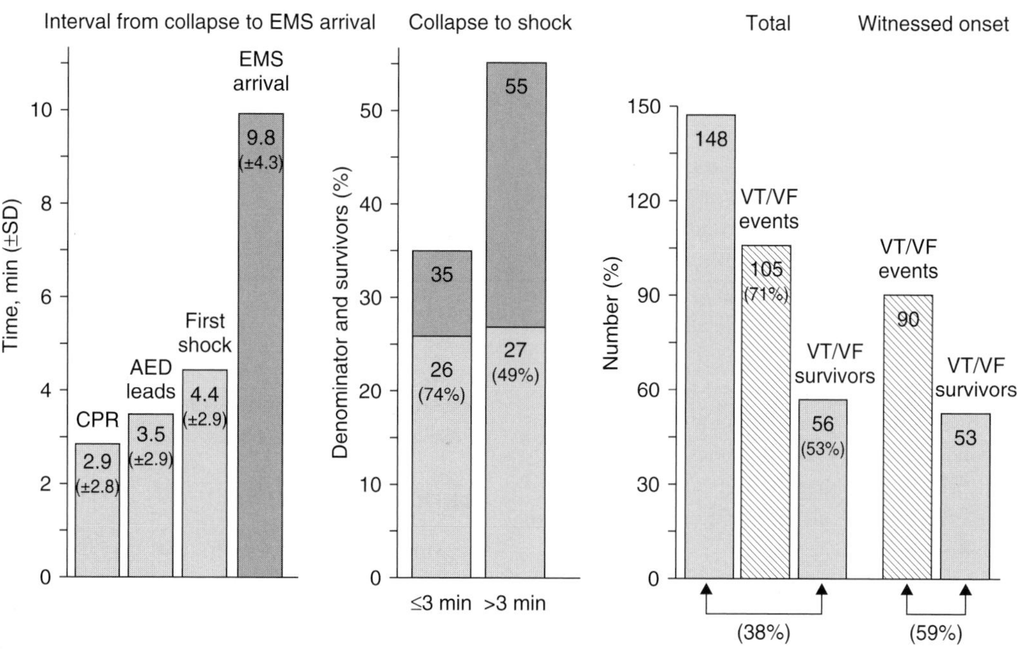

Figure 11.7 Las Vegas casino AED data. AED deployment in a controlled environment in which onset of cardiac arrest frequently can be witnessed, demonstrated short intervals from onset of collapse to CPR and AED shocks. Response times were reduced by more than 50% compared with standard EMS. For those found in VT/VF, survival was better than expected from other community-based systems and approached 60% for witnessed onset VT/VF. When response time was <3 min, survival for VT/VF was more than 70%. (Reproduced from *N Eng J Med* [34], with permission. See text for details)

observations of well-controlled emergency systems initially, such as police and ambulance-based deployments, and simultaneously by extension into other public access sites in which a broader array of personnel is trained to use the devices [12, 13]. These might include security personnel in public buildings, stadiums, airports, and shopping malls. Data from the Chicago airport is encouraging. Among 18 cardiac arrests in which VF was observed at initial contact, 11 (61%) victims survived to hospital discharge [35]. Six of the survivors had been responded to by persons with no prior use or training in AED deployment. Additional studies are underway to determine the impact of deployments in other public venues. Beyond that, AED deployment in multifamily dwellings, best controlled by defined users such as security personnel, in which device use is more sporadic, should be scrutinized with carefully designed registry studies.

Interaction between CPR, ACLS, defibrillation, and survival

Two recent studies have suggested the potential for improving outcomes with out-of-hospital defibrillation by a period of CPR prior to an attempted defibrillation. The studies suggest that if defibrillation can be carried out in <5 min after the onset of cardiac arrest CPR does not add benefit in regard to outcome [36]. However, in the time frame from 5 to 10 min between the onset of cardiac arrest and defibrillation a brief period (60–90 s) of CPR prior to defibrillation appears to improve outcome (Table 11.3). This appears to be based on oxygenation of myocardial tissue prior to defibrillation after maximal oxygen extraction has occurred creating a metabolic deficit. It is unlikely that delays longer than 10 min would be benefited by CPR, given the dismal outcome observed with or without CPR [37].

In another study, the question of added benefit of advanced life-support responses in the setting of an optimized response system for rapid defibrillation was evaluated [38]. There was no incremental improvement, further supporting the notion that broader application of immediate access to defibrillation is the key to further improving survival.

Table 11.3 CPR prior to defibrillation.

	CPR first (n = 104)	*Standard (n = 96)*	*Odds ratio (95% CI)*	*p*
≤5 min				
Hospital discharge (1°)	9 (23%)	12 (29%)	0.70 (0.26–1.91)	.61
ROSC	21 (52%)	23 (56%)	0.87 (0.36–2.08)	.82
1-year survival	8 (20%)	12 (29%)	0.60 (0.22–1.69)	.44
>5 min				
Hospital discharge (1°)	14 (22%)	2 (4%)	7.42 (1.61–34.3)	.006
ROSC	37 (58%)	21 (38%)	2.22 (1.06–4.63)	.04
1-Year survival	13 (20%)	2 (4%)	6.76 (1.42–31.4)	.01

Notes: For victims of cardiac arrest, a brief period of CPR prior to defibrillation improves survival for those with an interval between onset and shock of >5 min. For those to whom a shock is delivered within <5 min, there is no added benefit of an initial period of CPR.

Source: [37]. See text for details.

Conclusion

A rational and comprehensive approach to the problem of SCD must include better understanding of the basic science underpinnings of the pathophysiology of potentially fatal arrhythmias [1], more accurate profiling of individual risk among the large population segments who have a relatively low excess risk [1–3, 39], and effective strategies for community-based responses to impending or actual cardiac arrests [1, 4, 6, 29]. In respect to the latter, broadening our approaches to include strategies that respond from multiple points of attack is anticipated to lead to higher survival rates.

Acknowledgments

Dr. Myerburg is funded in part by the Louis Lemberg Chair in Cardiology and the American Heart Association Chair in Cardiovascular Research at the University of Miami, Miami, Florida. Portions of the work cited were supported by grants and contracts from the Miami Heart Research Institute (University of Miami/Miami Heart Research Institute Cardiovascular Genetics Program), and the Public Health Trust, Miami, Florida.

References

1 Myerburg RJ. Scientific gaps in the prediction and prevention of sudden cardiac death. *J Cardiovasc Electrophysiol* 2002; **13**: 709–723.

2 Myerburg RJ, Kessler KM, Castellanos A. Sudden cardiac death: epidemiology, transient risk, and intervention assessment. *Ann Intern Med* 1993; **119**: 1187–1197.

3 Myerburg RJ, Castellanos A. Cardiac arrest and sudden cardiac death. In: Braunwald E, ed. *Heart Disease: A Textbook of Cardiovascular Medicine*. 6th edn. WB Saunders Company, Philadelphia, PA, 2001: 890–931.

4 Myerburg RJ. Sudden cardiac death: exploring the limits of our knowledge. *J Cardiovasc Electrophysiol* 2001; **12**: 369–381.

5 Nichol G, Hallstrom AP, Kerber R *et al.* American Heart Association report on the second public access defibrillation conference, April 17–19, 1997. *Circulation* 1998; **97**: 1309–1314.

6 Marenco JP, Wang PJ, Link MS, Homoud MK, Estes NAM, II. Improving survival from sudden cardiac arrest: the role of the automated external defibrillator. *JAMA* 2001; **285**: 1193–1200.

7 Liberthson RR, Nagel EL, Hirschman JC, Nussenfeld SR. Prehospital ventricular fibrillation. Prognosis and follow-up course. *N Engl J Med* 1974; **291**: 317–321.

8 Baum RS, Alvarez H, Cobb LA. Survival after resuscitation from out-of-hospital ventricular fibrillation. *Circulation* 1974; **50**: 1231–1235.

9 Thompson RG, Hallstrom AP, Cobb LA. Bystander-initiated cardiopulmonary resuscitation in the management of ventricular fibrillation. *Ann Intern Med* 1979; **90**: 737–740.

10 Eisenberg MS, Copass MK, Hallstrom AP *et al.* Treatment of out-of-hospital cardiac arrests with rapid defibrillation by emergency medical technicians. *N Engl J Med* 1980; **302**: 1379–1383.

11 Cobb LA, Weaver WD, Fahrenbruch CE, Hallstrom AP, Copass MK. Community-based interventions for sudden cardiac death. Impact, limitations, and changes. *Circulation* 1992; **85**(Suppl. I): I98–I102.

12 Myerburg RJ, Conde CA, Sung RJ *et al.* Clinical, electrophysiologic and hemodynamic profile of patients resuscitated from prehospital cardiac arrest. *Am J Med* 1980; **68**: 568–576.

13 Stults KR, Brown DD, Schug VL, Bean JA. Prehospital defibrillation performed by emergency medical technicians in rural communities. *N Engl J Med* 1984; **310**: 219–223.

14 Cummins RO, Ornato JP, Thies WH, Pepe PE. Improving survival from sudden cardiac arrest: the chain of survival concept. *Circulation* 1991; **83**: 1832–1847.

15 Lombardi G, Gallagher J, Gennis P. Outcome of out-of-hospital cardiac arrest in New York City. the pre-hospital arrest survival evaluation study. *JAMA* 1994; **271**: 678–683.

16 Becker LB, Ostrander MP, Barrett J, Kondos GT. Outcome of CPR in a large metropolitan area – where are the survivors? *Ann Emerg Med* 1991; **20**: 355–361.

17 Stiell IG, Wells GA, Field BJ *et al.* Improved out-of-hospital cardiac arrest survival through the inexpensive optimization of an existing defibrillation program: OPALS study phase II. Ontario Prehospital Advanced Life Support. *JAMA* 1999; **281**: 1175–1181.

18 Smith SC, Hamburg RS. Automated external defibrillators: time for federal and state advocacy and broader utilization. *Circulation* 1998; 97: 1321–1324.

19 Becker L, Eisenberg M, Fahrenbruch C, Cobb L. Public locations of cardiac arrest: implications for public access defibrillation. *Circulation* 1998; **97**: 2106–2109.

20 Mirowski M, Reid PR, Winkle RA *et al.* Mortality in patients with implanted automatic defibrillators. *Ann Intern Med* 1983; **98**: 585–588.

21 de Vreede-Swagemakers JJ, Gorgels AP, Dubois-Arbouw WI *et al.* Circumstances and causes of out-of-hospital cardiac arrest in sudden death survivors. *Heart* 1998; **79**: 356–361.

22 Zipes DP. The neighborhood heart watch program: save a victim everywhere (SAVE). *J Am Coll Cardiol* 2001; **37**: 2004–2005.

23 Mosseso VN Jr, Davis EA, Auble TE, Paris PM, Yealy DM. Use of automated external defibrillators by police officers for treatment of out-of-hospital cardiac arrest. *Ann Emerg Med* 1998; **32**: 200–207.

24 White RD, Hankins DG, Bugliosi TF. Seven years' experience with early defibrillation by police and paramedics in an emergency medical services system. *Resuscitation* 1998; **39**: 145–151.

25 Waalewijn RA, de Vos R, Koster RW. Out-of-hospital cardiac arrests in Amsterdam and its surrounding areas: results from the Amsterdam resuscitation study (ARREST) in "Utstein" style. *Resuscitation* 1998; **38**: 157–167.

26 Kette F, Sbrojavacca R, Rellini G *et al.* Epidemiology and survival rate of out-of-hospital cardiac arrest in northeast Italy: the F.A.C.S. study. Friuli Venezia Giulia Cardiac Arrest Cooperative Study. *Resuscitation* 1998; **36**: 153–159.

27 Groh WJ, Newman MM, Beal PE, Fineberg NS, Zipes DP. Limited response to cardiac arrest by police equipped with automated external defibrillators: lack of survival benefit in suburban and rural Indiana – the police as responder automated defibrillation evaluation (PARADE). *Acad Emerg Med* 2001; **8**: 324–330.

28 Newman MM, Mosesso VN Jr, Ornato JP *et al.* Law enforcement agency defibrillation (LEA-D). Position statement and best practices recommendations from the National Center for Early Defibrillation. *Prehosp Emerg Care* 2002; **6**: 346–347.

29 Myerburg RJ, Fenster J, Velez M *et al.* Impact of community-wide police car deployment of automated external defibrillators on out-of-hospital cardiac arrest. *Circulation* 2002; **106**: 1058–1064.

30 The Public Access Defibrillation Trial Investigators. Public access defibrillation and survival after out-of-hospital cardiac arrest. *N Eng J Med* 2004; **351**: 637–646.

31 Capucci A, Aschieri D, Piepoli MF, Bardy GH, Iconomu E, Arvedi M. Tripling survival from sudden cardiac arrest via early defibrillation without traditional education in cardiopulmonary resuscitation. *Circulation* 2002; **106**: 1065–1070.

32 O'Rourke MF, Donaldson E, Geddes JS. An airline cardiac arrest program. *Circulation* 1997; **96**: 2849–2853.

33 Page RL, Joglar JA, Kowal RC *et al.* Use of automated external defibrillators by a U.S. airline. *N Engl J Med* 2000; **343**: 1210–1216.

34 Valenzuela TD, Roe DJ, Nichol G, Clark LL, Spaite DW, Hardman RG. Outcomes of rapid defibrillation by security officers after cardiac arrest in casinos. *N Engl J Med* 2000; **343**: 1206–1209.

35 Caffrey SL, Willoughby PJ, Pepe PE, Becker LB. Public use of automated external defibrillators. *N Engl J Med* 2002; **347**: 1242–1247.

36 Cobb LA, Fahrenbruch CE, Walsh TR *et al.* Influence of cardiopulmonary resuscitation prior to defibrillation in patients with out-of-hospital ventricular fibrillation. *JAMA* 1999; **281**: 1182–1188.

37 Wik L, Hansen TB, Fylling F *et al.* Delaying defibrillation to give basic cardiopulmonary resuscitation to patients with out-of-hospital ventricular fibrillation: a randomized trial. *JAMA* 2003; **289**: 1389.

38 Stiell IG, Wells GA, Field B *et al.* (for the Ontario Prehospital Advanced Life Support Study Group) Advanced cardiac life support in out-of-hospital cardiac arrest. *N Engl J Med* 2004; **351**: 647–656.

39 Huikuri HV, Castellanos A, Myerburg RJ. Sudden death due to cardiac arrhythmias. *N Eng J Med* 2001; **345**: 1473–1482.

40 Myerburg RJ, Veiez M, Rosenberg DG, Fenster J, Castellanos A. Automative external defibrillators for prevention of out-of-hospital sudden death: effectiveness of the automative external defibrillator. *J Cardiovasc Electrophysiol* 2003; **14**: S108–S116.

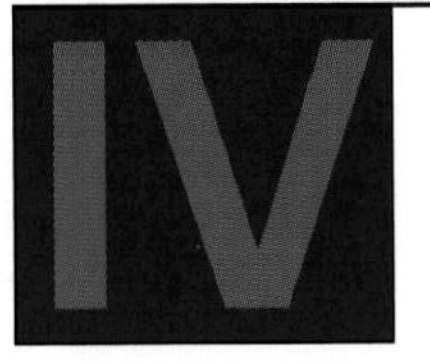

PART IV
Advances in pacing

12

CHAPTER 12

Sensor and sensor integration

Robert F. Rea, MD

Four sensors dominate the rate-adaptive pacemaker market at the present time: those that sense low-frequency vibration resulting from bodily movement, those that sense bodily acceleration in a specific vector, those that sense minute ventilation (MV) as reflected by changes in transthoracic impedance, and those that sense the QT interval. To overcome the limitations of any single sensor, dual-sensor pacemakers were developed to allow more faithful mimicking of the normal sinus node response to exertion. This chapter will focus on the mechanisms by which these sensors work, their clinical effects, and finally the algorithms by which dual-sensor pacemakers process sensor input to modulate the paced heart rate. Following this there will be a brief review of novel although less widely used sensor systems.

Vibration sensor

The key component in the vibration sensor is a piezoelectric crystal that is bonded to the pulse generator canister as shown in Figure 12.1. In response to mechanical deformation, a piezoelectric crystal generates a weak electrical current. With body movement, low-frequency vibrations are transmitted through the bones and muscles to the region of the pulse generator. These vibrations deform the piezoelectric crystal slightly and the resultant weak electric current is used to change the pacing rate.

Given the nature of this sensor, interindividual differences in overall body mass, height, posture, gait, and position of the pulse generator in the chest among others will affect the way in which body motion is detected by the sensor. However, within a given patient, provided no significant change occurs in body habitus, after maturation of the pacemaker pocket, the relation between body activity and output of the sensor is reasonably constant.

The electrical output from the crystal is sensed by counting the number of times of a voltage threshold. To tailor the pacemaker rate response to an individual patient the voltage threshold for spike counting can be programmed as shown in Figure 12.2.

Accelerometer

Accelerometers sense changes of body motion in a specific direction in contrast to vibration sensors which nonspecifically respond to pressure waves resulting from activity. As such, the accelerometer sensor may be more specific in rejecting nonexertional noise. The design of the accelerometer, illustrated in Figure 12.3, allows one to appreciate this. Piezoelements are bonded to a cantilever beam that functions as a seismic mass. This beam is anchored

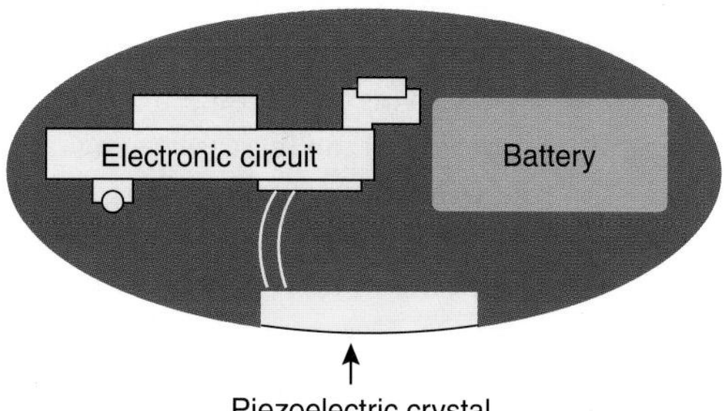

Figure 12.1 In a vibration-sensing pacemaker pulse generator, the piezoelectric crystal is bonded to the canister. Placement of the pulse generator against the chest wall allows low-frequency signals generated by exertion to deform the crystal and thereby increase heart rate.

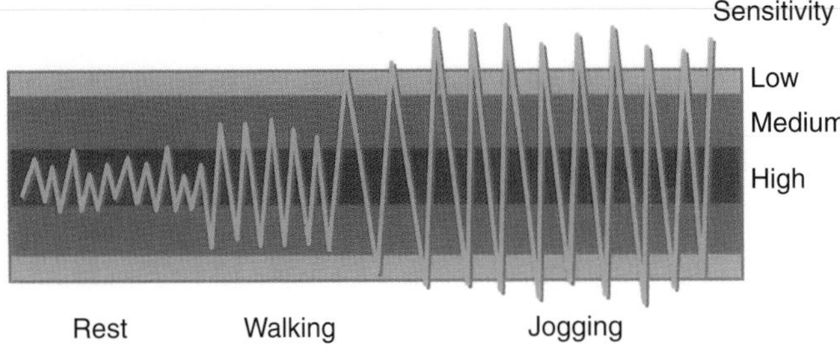

Figure 12.2 Outputs from the piezoelectric crystal shown here as spike oscillations are counted as they cross a programmable threshold level. With a programmed low sensitivity, only high-amplitude spikes are counted. Conversely with a programmed high sensitivity even some signal spike are counted at rest.

to a base (in a pacemaker the hybrid circuit board is used). Movement perpendicular to the beam exerts a force on the mass. Inertial resistance of the mass causes bending and deformation of the piezoelements, like a diver on a board, that generates an electrical signal (piezoelectric), change in resistance (piezoresistive), or change in capacitance (piezocapacitive) [1]. Unlike a vibration sensor equipped pacemaker, however, the altered electrical signal undergoes integration rather than threshold dependent spike counting as shown in Figure 12.4. This may be important as greater degrees of acceleration that produce a single deformation of the seismic mass are translated into higher-amplitude electrical transients that are more proportionally represented by integration than by simple threshold dependent spike counting.

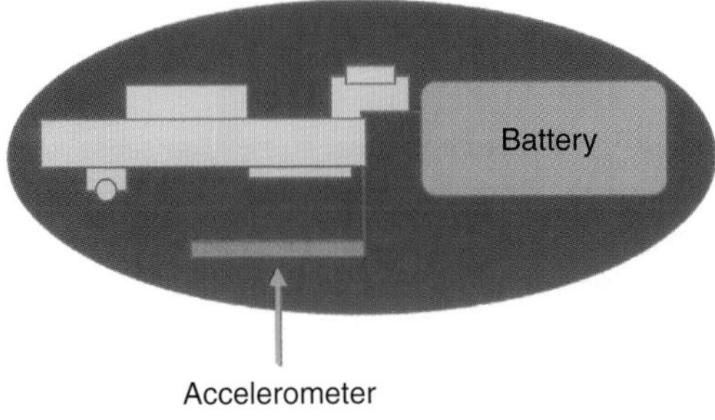

Figure 12.3 In an accelerometer-based pacemaker the piezoelement is suspended by a cantilever beam from the hybrid circuitry in the pulse generator. With movement perpendicular to the plane of the piezoelement, electrical signals are generated that increase heart rate.

Differences between vibration and acceleration sensor pacemakers

Potentially, clinically important differences between these sensors derives from differences in the mechanisms by which they work. Since vibration sensors are nondirectional, body movement in the up and down direction (as might result from riding in a car on a bumpy road) can increase pacing rate. In addition, the frequency response range of the vibration sensor is up to as high as 40 Hz well out of the range of pressure waves generated by typical exercise (1–8 Hz) [2]. In contrast, accelerometers respond more to movement in the forward–backward direction and upper limit of their frequency response is about 10 Hz, much more in line with the expected frequency range of body motion. Finally, since the accelerometer mechanism is not bonded to the pacemaker canister, deformation of

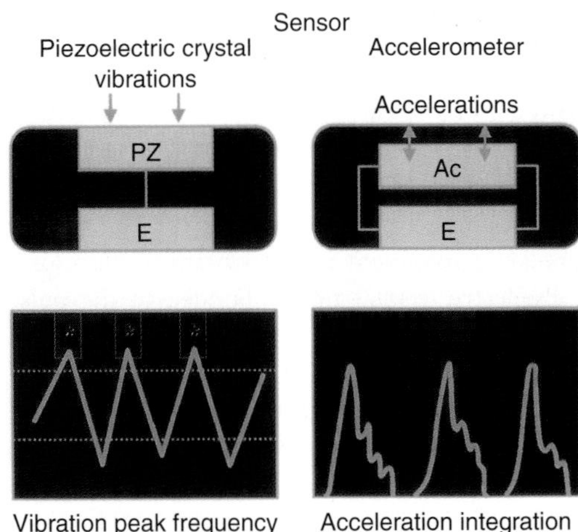

Figure 12.4 This shows how signals are processed differently in piezoelectric (PZ) vibration and accelerometer (Ac) rate-adaptive pacemakers. E denotes the electronic circuit board in the pulse generator. As shown in Figure 12.2, the vibration sensor device counts any signals above a given voltage threshold. In contrast, the accelerometer sensor device integrates the voltage from the piezoelement. By differentially weighting large amplitude deflections of the piezoelement, a more proportional response to exertion is achieved.

the canister with direct local pressure will not increase heart rate.

Advantages and disadvantages of accelerometer and vibration sensor pacemakers

The chief advantage of both of these sensors is the rapidity with which they respond to changes in the level of activity. Since the time from onset of change in body movement to change in generated pressure waves is virtually instantaneous, and since the piezoelement response is similarly rapid, pacemakers with these sensors are capable of extraordinarily rapid (and sometimes inappropriate) rate shifts. Indeed, one chief function of the modulating circuitry in the pacemaker is to temper the rate response both with respect to heart rate acceleration and deceleration.

Vibration sensors, however, are hampered by poor proportionality between the sensor driven paced rate and workload. For example, during descending of stairs at a step rate equivalent to ascending stairs, the sensor driven heart rate was higher, exactly the opposite response of normal volunteers [3]. In addition, relatively nonjarring activities, such as cycling, may not activate the vibration sensor sufficiently to accelerate heart rate to the required degree. Accelerometer responses, however, may be more proportional owing to their lack of dependence on sensed vibration. Thus, ambulating on a soft or hard surface would produce equivalent antero-posterior acceleration but quite different low-frequency vibrations [4].

Both sensors are limited by a lack of response to nonexertional stimuli, such as emotional arousal, static exercise, fever, and hypotension. For this reason, other sensors were developed as reviewed below.

MV sensor

Minute ventilation (MV), the product of respiratory rate and tidal volume, is a faithful marker for oxygen uptake (VO_2), the most accurate measure of human energy expenditure [5]. Below about 70% of $VO_{2\ max}$, the relation between MV and heart rate is roughly linear. As the anaerobic threshold is approached with high workloads, however, MV increases more briskly as a result of accelerated CO_2 production with anaerobic glycolysis [6]. This nonlinearity must be accounted for in pacemaker design to prevent overpacing at high workloads.

Minute ventilation sensors rely on measurements of transthoracic impedance to derive the MV signal. As shown in Figure 12.5 current (I) is injected between the pacemaker canister and the ring electrode. Voltage (V) is measured from the canister to the tip electrode. The amount of battery drain from this current injection is quite small and is limited by the narrow pulse width (7–30 μs) and output (1 mA) at 20 Hz [7]. By solving Ohm's law (resistance = voltage/current), transthoracic impedance (or resistance) is calculated. With inspiration, increased transthoracic volumes increase resistance, and vice versa.

Limitations of MV sensors

While MV sensors track a more physiological signal than vibration or acceleration sensors, they are limited clinically by a sluggish response at the start of exercise related in part to the method by which rest and exercise MV values are compared. And, as noted above, at high workloads near the anaerobic threshold ventilation increases more than heart rate. While MV sensors avoid many of the inappropriate changes in heart rate seen with vibration sensors, nonexercise-related stimuli, such as upper extremity movement, phonation, cough, and pathological breathing patterns, may affect the pacing rate [8]. Low-pass filtering of the MV signal at ~60 Hz is done in some pacemakers to limit the

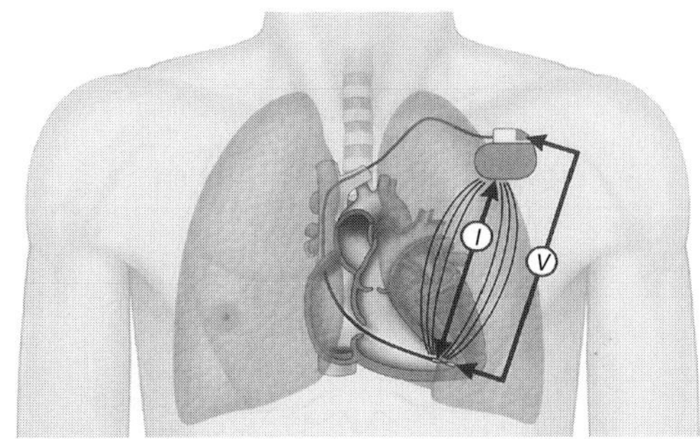

Figure 12.5 Diagram of an MV sensor showing that current (I) is injected between the ring electrode and the pacemaker pulse generator and voltage (V) is measured between the pulse generator and tip electrode. Resistance (or impedance) (R) is calculated by using Ohm's law ($R = V/I$).

influence of such stimuli but this may also limit responsiveness to breathing rates above 60/min as may be encountered in children [9]. Finally, nonexertional stimuli, such as emotional excitement, fever, or hypotension, that do not result in changes in ventilation will not result in changes in paced heart rate.

QT interval sensor

In general, changes in the QT interval reflect changes in sympathetic drive to the heart. This concept is the underpinning for the use of QT interval as an activity sensor since exercise is associated with increases in sympathetic outflow. In one study, peripheral venous plasma levels of norepinephrine correlated with the QT sensor-driven heart rate during and after exercise [10]. It is important to appreciate, however, that the first autonomic change occurring with exercise is withdrawal of parasympathetic drive to the heart. Accordingly, the QT sensor may be sluggish in altering heat rate early in exercise, an effect that has been observed clinically. Recent improvements include steeper rate response slopes at the onset of exercise that partially overcome this limitation.

Since the unpaced T-wave may be difficult to discern from an intracardiac electrode, and since paced and spontaneous QT intvervals may differ, currently available pacemakers utilize the unipolar paced QT interval for detection. Even with this technique the true end of the T-wave may be difficult to discern. Hence a surrogate, the peak negative slope of the T-wave, is used as shown in Figure 12.6.

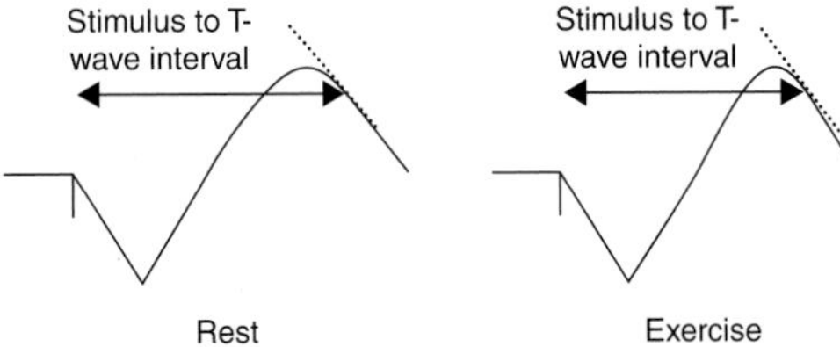

Figure 12.6 This schematically illustrates measurement of the stimulus-T interval in a QT-sensing pacemaker. The maximal rate of T-wave downslope change is assessed mathematically (dotted line) and the interval from the pacing spike is measured. Sympathetic excitation with exercise shortens the stimulus-T interval and triggers an increase in heart rate.

An advantage of the QT sensor is its responsiveness to nonexertional stimuli, such as emotional excitement, pain, or hypotension, each of which is associated with augmentation of sympathetic outflow. In addition, diurnal variation in QT interval, with lengthening during sleep, has been suggested as a mechanism by which pacing rates might be lowered with somnolence [11].

Limitations of QT sensor

Despite the attractiveness of a sensor that monitors a key determinant of cardioacceleration with exercise, several limitations attend QT sensor driven pacemakers. First, an increase in heart rate itself shortens the QT interval leading to the possibility of a positive feedback loop wherein rate-related QT interval shortening stimulates yet higher paced rates. Some of this is overcome in current devices that automatically adjust the rate responsiveness with a self-learning algorithm. Second, drugs and myocardial disease may affect the QT interval and the relation between sympathetic drive and the paced QT interval. Third, programming of steep initial rate response slopes may be required to overcome sluggishness at the onset of exercise. This can lead to overly rapid heart rates later in exercise and oscillation between lower and upper pacing rates with small changes in QT interval [8].

Dual-sensor pacemakers

Rate-adaptive sensors differ with respect to the speed with which they respond, the proportionality of their response with respect to exertion, and their specificity and sensitivity to stimuli that should alter heart rates. No one sensor is perfect. This has led to the development of pacemakers that utilize more than one sensor and integrate their outputs to provide better rate control.

Combination sensors currently in wide use include activity (vibration) and QT interval, and MV and activity (accelerometer or vibration). There are a few algorithms by which the outputs of these sensors may be combined. In a "faster win" algorithm, illustrated in Figure 12.7(a), the sensor suggesting the higher rate is given control of heart rate. In a "blending" algorithm shown in Figure 12.7(b), the inputs are combined, often with different degrees of sensor dominance dependent on prevailing heart rate. Also the presence of a second sensor allows for sensors to crosscheck one another to improve the specificity of heart rate response and avoid pacing in response to nonexertional stimuli. This is illustrated in Figure 12.7(c).

For example, in a Guidant MV + accelerometer pacemaker a "faster win" algorithm is employed. When the accelerometer suggests a heart rate higher than the MV sensor, as is common early in exercise, it controls the magnitude of the response. This is illustrated in Figure 12.8. If, however, the accelerometer suggested rate is still higher than MV at the maximum sensor rate, the MV sensor assumes control. This is an example of sensor

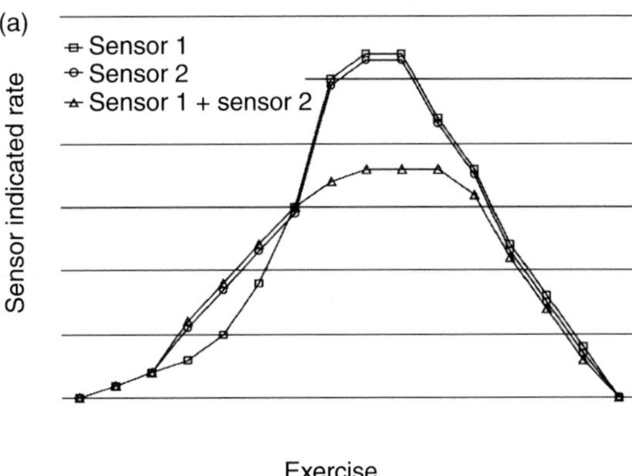

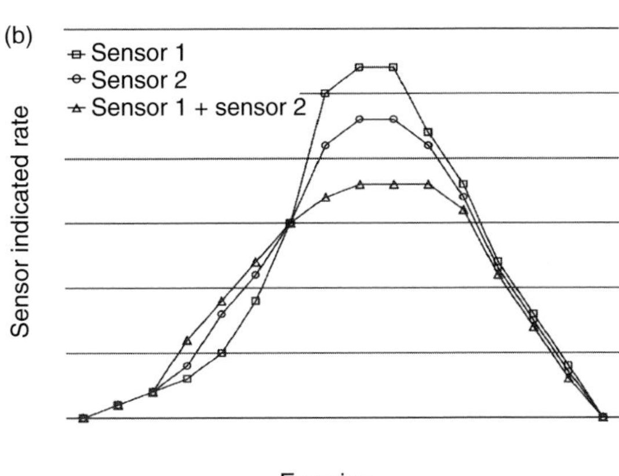

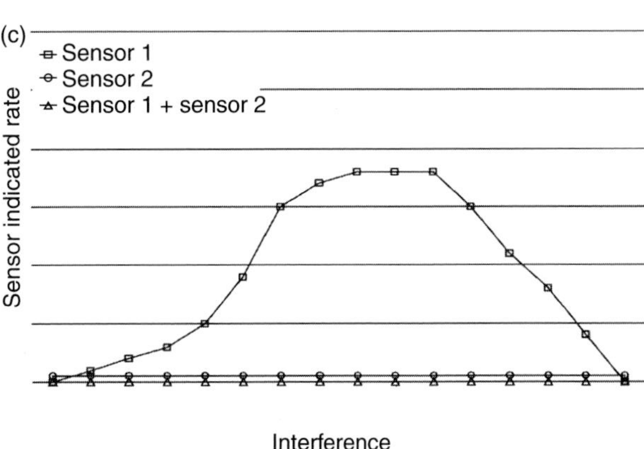

Figure 12.7 (a) Schematic of how two sensors interact in the "faster win" algorithm in a dual-sensor pacemaker. Early in exercise sensor 2 (open triangles) dictates the paced rate. Later sensor 1 assumes control as the output from sensor 2 lags. In recovery the decline in rate again follows the sensor indicating the higher rate. (b) Schematic of blending of sensor inputs in a dual-sensor pacemaker. The paced rate is between that indicated by sensor 1 and sensor 2. (c) Schematic of sensor crosschecking. Sensor 1 responds to a nonexercise stimulus labeled interference. Since sensor 2 detects no exercise signal, the circuitry assumes a noise input to sensor 1 and does not increase heart rate. (Adapted and reprinted from *Cardiol Clin* [8], with permission from Elsevier.)

crosschecking [4]. But when the MV sensor suggested rate is higher, as typically occurs at steady state or during recovery from exercise, it assumes control. As noted above, however, since MV may increase dramatically as the anaerobic threshold is reached, control of heart rate by the MV sensor may be limited by a specified "high-rate break point."

In a Medtronic dual-sensor device a form of sensor blending is employed. At heart rates up to a programmable set point called the Activities of Daily Living (ADL) Rate the dominant sensor driving heart rate is an accelerometer as shown in Figure 12.9. Above this rate the MV sensor assumes control. This permits rapid acceleration of rate with short-lived bouts of exercise as encountered in routine activities but a more proportional heart rate response to sustained exertion as afforded by the MV sensor.

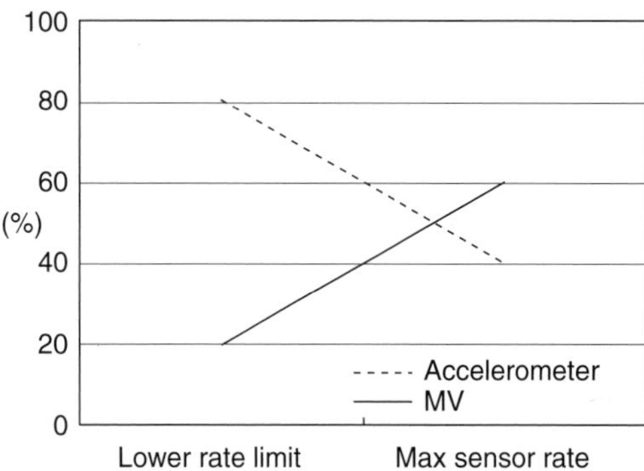

Figure 12.8 Illustration of the relative inputs from the accelerometer and MV sensor in a Guidant pacemaker. There is a gradual shift from accelerometer to MV sensor dominance as heart rate increases. (Adapted and reprinted from *Am J Cardiol* [12], with permission from Elsevier.)

The activity + QT sensor pacemaker by Vitatron incorporates both sensor blending and crosschecking. The relative sensor contribution is programmable as "activity < QT" (30 : 70 ratio), "activity = QT" (50 : 50 ratio), and "activity > QT" (70 : 30 ratio). Since this is a piezoelectric crystal activity sensor that may increase heart rate inappropriately with nonexercise stimuli, only a brief period of purely activity-driven rate response is allowed unless confirmed by similar directional changes from the QT sensor. This is an example of crosschecking at low heart rates. Studies have demonstrated a more gradual rate response with the activity + QT mode than with activity alone [13].

Other rate-adaptive sensors

Several other interesting physiological sensors have been developed but have not gained widespread use in the United States.

Temperature-sensing pacemakers require a special lead capable of monitoring the temperature of the intracardiac blood pool. At the onset of exercise, central blood temperature initially declines as cooler peripheral blood is pumped back to the heart. With continued exercise, however, core body

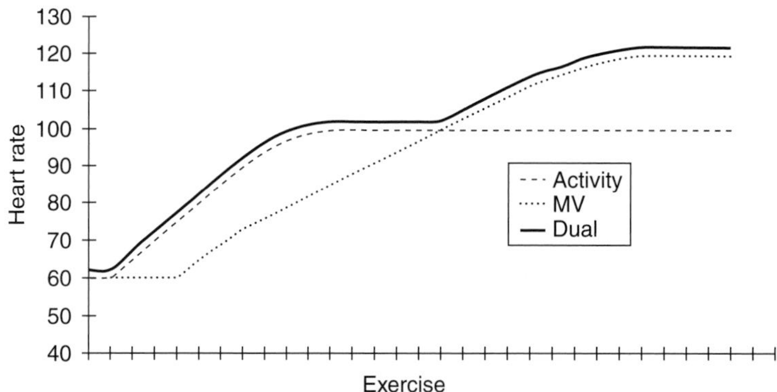

Figure 12.9 Illustration of the relative inputs from activity and MV sensors in a Medtronic pacemaker. Up to a programmable heart rate referred to as the ADL rate, the activity sensor dominates. Thereafter, the MV sensor assumes control. (Reproduced with permission from Medtronic.)

temperature increases as a result of the increased metabolic rate. About three-fourth of the energy consumed with exertion generates heat, while only about one-fourth generates mechanical energy [14]. A limitation of pacemakers incorporating this sensor is the slow onset of change in core blood temperature and relatively inadequate response to low workloads [15].

Impedance measurements made with a special lead in the right ventricle can estimate cardiac chamber volumes and thereby stroke volume. With exercise and normal heart rate responsiveness, stroke volume tends to remain constant. During exercise at a fixed heart rate, stroke volume will increase in an attempt to maintain adequate cardiac output. This upward drift in stroke volume can be used to trigger increase in pacing rate that bring stroke volume back toward baseline. The impedance catheter may also be used to measure preejection interval, that is, the time from the pacing spike to the onset of ventricular contraction. This interval normally shortens with exercise and this may be used as a signal to increase heart rate.

Right ventricular pressure monitoring with a special sensing/pacing lead allows determination of d*p*/d*t* increases, which correlate well with exercise levels. An offshoot of this technology is a purely monitoring device for patients with heart failure or pulmonary hypertension. Clinical decompensation is often preceded by increases in intracardiac pressures or declines in d*p*/d*t*. Since these parameters may be measured at home and transmitted by modem/Internet, it is hoped that preemptive intervention based on these measurements may forestall the development of worsening symptoms and prevent hospitalizations [16].

Other hemodynamic-based sensors include those that measure peak-endocardial acceleration (PEA) with the use of a microaccelerometer sealed in the tip of a special lead. PEA correlates with right ventricular d*p*/d*t* and increases with exercise and sympathetic excitation. Local myocardial contractility can be estimated with impedance measurements from a unipolar electrode embedded in the right ventricle. Injection of current into this lead, with the pacemaker canister as the indifferent electrode, allows estimates of local changes in volume as the right ventricle contracts about the lead tip. As with other similar sensors, increases in contractility accompany increases in sympathetic drive.

Finally a novel sensor that measures the ventricular depolarization gradient (VDG) has been developed. This sensor measures the vector integral of the paced QRS complex. This parameter normally stays fairly constant since cardioacceleration increases and sympathetic excitation decreases VDG. In the presence of chronotropic insufficiency, VDG decreases a signal that can be used to trigger hear rate increases.

References

1 Ousdigian KT. Rate-adaptation by motion. In: Webster JG, ed. *Design of Cardiac Pacemakers*. IEEE Press, Piscataway, NJ, 1995: 305–334.

2 Alt E, Matula M, Theres H, Heinz M, Baker R. The basis for activity controlled rate variable cardiac pacemakers: an analysis of mechanical forces on the human body induced by exercise and environment. *PACE* 1989; **12**(10): 1667–1680.

3 Alt E, Combs W, Willhaus R *et al*. A comparative study of activity and dual sensor: activity and minute ventilation pacing responses to ascending and descending stairs. *PACE* 1998; **21**(10): 1862–1868.

4 Strobel JS, Kay GN. Programming of sensor driven pacemakers. *Cardiol Clin* 2000; **18**(1): 157–176, ix.

5 Mond HG. Respiration. In: Alt, EBSS, & Stangl, K, eds. *Rate Adaptive Cardiac Pacing* Springer-Verlag, Berlin, 1993: 98–110.

6 Lewalter T, Jung W, MacCarter D *et al*. Heart rate during exercise: what is the optimal goal of rate adaptive pacemaker therapy? *Am Heart J* 1994; **127**(4 Pt 2): 1026–1030.

7 Webster JG. Rate adaptation by minute ventilation. In: Webster JG, ed. *Design of Cardiac Pacemakers* IEEE Press, Piscataway, NJ, 1995: 397–404.

8 Leung SK, Lau CP. Developments in sensor-driven pacing. *Cardiol Clin* 2000; **18**(1): 113–155, ix.

9 Kay GN. Basic concepts of pacing. In: Ellenbogen KA, Wood MA, eds. *Cardiac Pacing and ICDs*, 3rd edn. Blackwell Science, Malden, 2002: 48–128.

10 Jordaens L, Backers J, Moerman E, Clement DL. Catecholamine levels and pacing behavior of QT-driven pacemakers during exercise. *PACE* 1990; **13**(5): 603–607.

11 Bexton RS, Vallin HO, Camm AJ. Diurnal variation of the QT interval – influence of the autonomic nervous system. *Br Heart J* 1986; **55**(3): 253–258.

12 Clementy J, Barold SS, Garrigue S *et al*. Clinical significance of multiple sensor options: rate response

optimization, sensor blending, and trending. *Am J Cardiol* 1999; **83**(5B): 166D–171D.

13 Connelly DT. Initial experience with a new single chamber, dual sensor rate responsive pacemaker. The Topaz Study Group. *PACE* 1993; **16**(9): 1833–1841.

14 Mayotte MJ. Rate adaptation by temperature. In: Webster JG, ed. *Design of Cardiac Pacemakers*. IEEE Press, Piscataway, NJ, 1995: 335–368.

15 Hayes DL. Rate-adaptive pacing. In: Hayes DL, ed. *Cardiac Pacing and Defibrillation: A Practical Approach*. Futura, Armonk, 2000: 325–346.

16 Magalski A, Adamson P, Gadler F *et al.* Continuous ambulatory right heart pressure measurements with an implantable hemodynamic monitor: a multicenter, 12-month follow-up study of patients with chronic heart failure. *J Card Fail* 2002; **8**(2): 63–70.

13

CHAPTER 13

New electrode and lead designs for pacemakers

Charles J. Love, MD, FACC

Basic pacemaker lead design has not changed since the first transvenous lead was implanted nearly 50 years ago. The lead is a device consisting of an electrical connector at one end for attachment to the pulse generator. At the other end are one or more surfaces to contact and deliver the electrical stimulus to the myocardium. These two ends of the lead are connected by one or more conductor coils. Each conductor is covered with at least one layer of insulating material. While these four basic components themselves have not changed, the technology within each of them has changed significantly.

Connectors have gone from being proprietary, large, and bulky, to the widely accepted International Standard-1 (IS-1) configuration. IS-1 leads have truly become the standard, and have eliminated the need for using adapters in nearly all situations as leads from different manufacturers are mixed and matched with different pacemakers and ICDs. In addition, the trend toward smaller pacemakers has resulted in the connector block taking up an increasingly large percentage of the device volume. The smaller 3.2 mm IS-1 connector has allowed the size of the connector block on the pacemaker to be downsized significantly, compared with the 5 and 6 mm connectors that it replaced. IS-1 has also made virtually all modern pacemakers and lead systems compatible, replacing what had been at least a half dozen different and incompatible designs. The IS-1 standard has served the industry and implanters well, and should continue to remain a widely used connector for the foreseeable future. However, new challenges have created new connector designs.

Over the past several years, there have been a growing number of devices placed for the purpose of cardiac resynchronization. The transvenous approach using a pacing wire placed into a descending cardiac vein is the most widely used method to pace the left ventricle. Placement of the lead into a cardiac vein nearly always involves cannulation of the coronary sinus with a sheath system through which the pacing lead is inserted and guided to the target vein. Guidant has recently introduced a telescoping sheath system that allows the operator to subselect the target vessel with an inner sheath, through which the pacing lead can be placed. This smaller sheath system, as well as even the "standard" sheath systems, will not allow an IS-1 connector to pass through it as the sheath is removed from the patient. The approach taken by Guidant was the development of the "LV-1" connector. This is very low profile connector that is not compatible with the IS-1 connector in pacemakers and implantable defibrillators. The LV-1 connector will pass through the sheath systems used to place them without the need to slit or peel away the introducer sheath. This connector has provided relief to those not comfortable with the latter two techniques. The only disadvantage of the LV-1 is the lack of compatibility with existing connectors without the use of an adapter.

Another connector design is now being introduced to the pacing world; International Standard-4 (IS-4) as shown in Figure 13.1. The major innovation of this design is allowing for up to four electrical connections to be placed on a 3.2 mm diameter connector, thus eliminating the need for a "yoke"

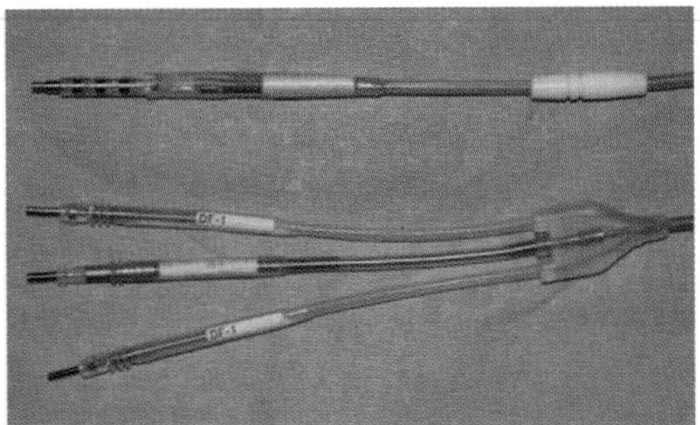

Figure 13.1 IS-4 connector (top) and standard quadrapolar lead with yoke. The IS-4 connector consists of a distal pin and three ring electrodes to allow a total of four electrical contacts on a single connector. Compare this to the much more bulky and complex "standard" set of connectors.

with multiple connectors to insert into the pacemaker. The yoke is the confluence of connections on a multipolar lead. This tends to be large, but more importantly it can be a weak point of the lead as well. Finally, it adds length to the lead which cannot be used for intravascular positioning or slack. By reducing the number of terminal pins, the pacemaker can be made smaller as the device needs fewer connector ports. An additional benefit is the reduced chance of placing one of the many connectors into the wrong pacemaker port. Though the IS-4 connector is initially being used for implantable defibrillator leads, the design is also being applied to cardiac vein leads with up to four pacing electrodes. This will allow selectivity of pacing at one or more sites without having to reposition the lead. By programming the polarity over a wider array of electrodes, the need to reposition a lead due to diaphragm stimulation or exit block may be reduced. Another application of the IS-4 connector will be on lead that incorporates additional components, such as a right ventricular pressure sensor. By placing the auxiliary sensor and traditional pacing/ sensing functions together, the lead connections can be made more simple and reliable.

The electrodes that interface with the myocardium were initially a polished metal alloy. Though functional, they had a large surface area with resulting low charge density and thus high current requirements. They were also prone to exit block. Many tip designs have evolved over the years, using many types of metals and surfaces. Without question, the addition of a steroid elution device to the electrode as introduced by Medtronic in the 1980s has made the greatest impact in terms of low chronic pacing thresholds. It has also virtually eliminated the transient threshold rise seen during the acute maturation of the lead to myocardium interface. It is now very uncommon to see exit block on endocardial leads. While steroid reduced the threshold rise, pacing surface area was being reduced to boost the impedance of the lead and to increase the charge density. Properly designed higher impedance leads use less current at a given voltage, resulting in greater device longevity. More recently, steroid has also been applied to epicardial leads. However, this has been limited to the sew-on leads at this time. There are studies underway to evaluate the effect of steroid on screw-in epicardial leads at this time, as these are very popular, but very prone to developing high thresholds or exit block.

An interesting innovation with regard to electrodes has been developed to deal with the problem of far-field sensing. This problem occurs not uncommonly when the atrial lead not only allows sensing the local atrial electrogram, but also allows sensing of the ventricular electrogram. In such a situation, the device will double count the heart rate. This can have a significant impact on mode switch algorithms, atrial tachyarrhythmia detection and treatment algorithms, atrial arrhythmia suppression algorithms, and even ventricular tachyarrhythmia detection schemes that look at the relationship of the atrial rate to ventricular rate. By designing the atrial lead that is engineered to minimize this far-field sensing, additional acceptable sites for pacing in the atrium are available. Proper design and interelectrode spacing may prevent the problems that can be caused by the oversensing, and allow these to be prevented by the lead instead of needing to be resolved by an algorithmic approach in the device, or even by being simply covered up by a blanking period.

Between the connector and the "working end" of the lead are the conductor coil and insulation. Many different types of conductor designs have been used. The multifilar coil has been the predominate coil design used for many years. The current versions have been proven to be reliable with proper implant technique. Mulifilar coils have been used as a single coil in unipolar applications, or in side by side, coaxial and triaxial arrangement for bipolar or tripolar leads. The most recent variation on the multifilar coil is the coradial design. In this iteration, each individual filament within the wire is insulated, with positive and negative filaments being wound together into a single coil structure (Figure 13.2). This allows for a very small lead body while providing a multipolar lead. The conductor coil has traditionally not only functioned to pass the electrical current to the lead tip, but also to pass a positioning stylet through the center of the coil. However, as the diameter of the lead body gets smaller, a coil conductor is no longer practical, and the use of a cable design is necessary. Cable conductors do not have a lumen through which to pass a stylet, thus a different method to position the lead becomes necessary.

In order to accommodate newer "lumenless" lead designs, new delivery systems are required. These systems are evolving, but the current concepts revolve around steerable and deflecting tip catheters that are placed at the target site (Figure 13.3). A lead with an exposed and fixed helix is then introduced through the sheath and fixed into place by rotating the lead, attaching it to the myocardium. In addition, as there continues to be a growing interest in placing leads at nontraditional sites, these tools will become even more important. There is a growing body of evidence that suggests that pacing the right ventricular apex (with the attendant dyskinesis) is hemodynamically a suboptimal site at which to pace the ventricles. Placement of the lead on the interventricular septum or in right ventricular outflow tract is made more rapid and accurate with this type of implant system. Pacing the Bundle of His can be successfully performed by mapping to that site and fixing a lead into position. By allowing placement of leads as small as 2 French in diameter, multiple site pacing is made more acceptable, as opposed to having multiple larger and more bulky leads in the veins and heart. In the atrium, multisite pacing is felt by some to reduce the incidence of atrial fibrillation. There has been interest in pacing the interatrial septum, Bachman's Bundle, and areas around the coronary sinus in the Triangle of Koch. Again, implant systems that allow one to precisely pace a lead to an anatomic target are becoming more important. The traditional bent stylet techniques that have been used for many decades are too slow and imprecise to allow for fast, accurate, and reproducible lead placement. There are newer stylet technologies that allow one to steer and deflect the placement stylet, such as the Locator™ from St. Jude Medical, allowing more control during the implant process.

Covering the conductor coils requires placing one or more layers of an insulating material to separate the conductors from the body tissues, and to prevent multiple conductors from touching each other. Silicone rubber was used from the early days of pacing, and is still a popular insulator. It has the advantage of being a stable compound in the body, and has a proven track record. It is, however, rather soft and sticky, and is prone to damage via nicks, abrasion, tension, and compression. Polyurethanes

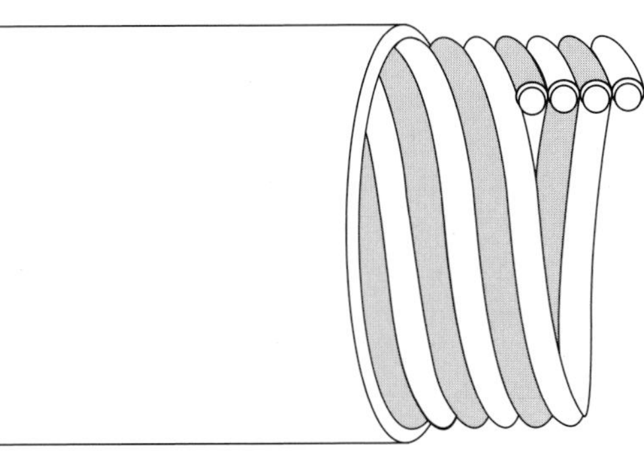

Figure 13.2 Coradial conductor coil design. Each individual filament of the lead is insulated. The filaments are wound together to make a single coil, however, this is actually multipolar and not unipolar.

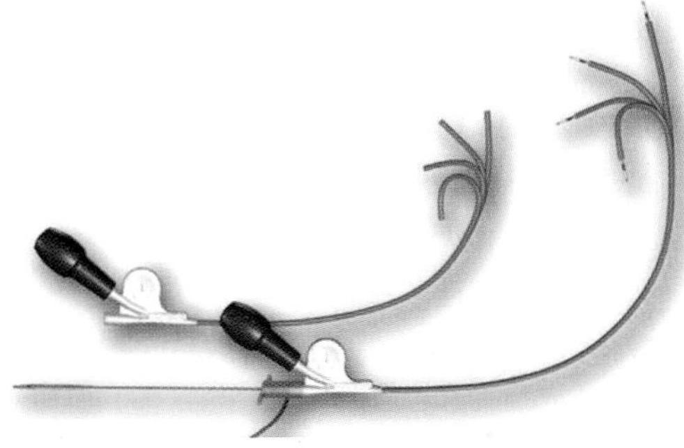

Figure 13.3 Deflecting tip introducer sheath. This sheath is able to be deflected and can be steered to the desired implantation site. A small lead is passed through the sheath and fixed into place after which the sheath is withdrawn.

became popular in that they are much stronger and resistant to the challenges just noted. Due to their strength, thinner insulators were made possible. However, the softer urethanes such as Pellathane-80A were found to have severe issues that could affect the stability of the insulation during the manufacturing processes, as well as being prone to metal ion oxidation (MIO) and environmental stress cracking (ESC). These were problems that could (and in many cases did) destroy the integrity of the insulator over time. The resultant problems created massive alerts and recalls for several manufacturers of pacing leads. New insulators are very difficult to bring to market due to the extensive testing for biocompatibility and reliability that are required. Improvements to silicone over time have resulted in so-called high performance compounds that are tougher than previous compounds. Newer copolymers that are a combination of silicone and urethane have also been developed and are undergoing testing at this time.

Another innovation that is being used is that of engineering the lead body to have different handling characteristics in different sections. For example, a lead designed to be stiffer near the connector end may be more reliable and allow more control while pushing or applying torque to the lead. It may also allow for more stability in the vessel and even more durability in the device pocket. By using a different coil winding or insulation closer to the electrode, the lead may be made more flexible to prevent perforation, or in the case of over-the-wire leads, more likely to track easily over the guidewire. Some insulators, such as polyurethane, have less friction, or insulators may be coated with a biocompatible lubricant to facilitate movement in and out of the point of insertion. These designs also help to reduce the chance of moving an adjacent lead when a single stick/retained guidewire technique is utilized.

Pacing from the cardiac venous system has become not only a routine procedure, but is critically important to improve cardiac performance in patients with abnormal ventricular contraction patterns. There are several challenges to placement of these leads: accessing the coronary sinus, placing the lead into the target vessel, finding and maintaining a stable position, finding a site with adequate pacing parameters, and avoiding extra-cardiac stimulation. There have been many tools developed to access the coronary sinus, and though critical for cardiac vein lead placement, it is not the subject of this chapter. Maintaining a stable position is frequently a challenge. Some leads utilize tines at the pacing tip that are effective when wedged into the target vessel or one of its branches. However, if the vessel is not of the right caliber or if it does not have a branch at the right location, this method of stabilization may not work well. This is especially true of larger-size vessels when the optimal pacing site is more basilar on the ventricle. For sites such as this, leads that have a preformed curve seem to be more stable. Another shape that has been developed is that of a spiral (Figure 13.4). For all of the preshaped leads, once the lead is positioned by a stylet or over a guide wire or simply pushed into position, the shape maintains the position in the vessel. Some leads of this design are a bit more stiff and/or larger in diameter. These will have more difficulty navigating smaller or more tortuous veins. By far, the most important innovation to allow rapid placement of leads in the cardiac veins has been the "over-the-wire" leads. These leads have a small hole in the electrode tip that allows a guidewire to pass through it. By positioning a guidewire in the target vessel, the pacing lead can slide over the wire to the desired spot. This

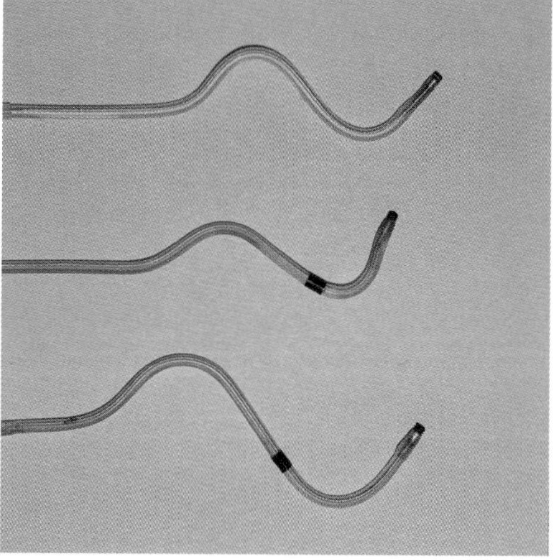

Figure 13.4 One of the new lead cardiac vein lead designs that consists of a spiral shape to hold the lead in position. These are available in different sizes and with one or more pacing electrodes.

technique allows the implanter to have access to the wide array of guidewires that have been at the disposal of the interventional cardiologist for many years. In my own lab, use of this system with proper lead selection has reduced the average complete implant time for these systems to well under 60 min for the entire operation.

Epicardial leads were the first type of lead system to be used in permanent pacing back in 1958. However, once transvenous systems came into widespread use, the need for epicardial leads was greatly limited to special applications and situations such as use in patients after corrective congenital heart surgery and patients with endocarditis. Improvements in conductor design occurred over time to make them less prone to fracture. Fixation with sew-on, stab-in, and screw-in electrodes is available. The addition of steroid eluting technololgy has been applied to epicardial leads, but is limited to the sew-on design only at this time. There is an increasing interest in epicardial leads once again due to the rising popularity of cardiac resynchronization therapy. In some cases, placement of a transvenous left ventricular lead via the cardiac venous system may not be possible. The latter may be due to failure to access the coronary sinus, lack of adequate target veins, high capture thresholds at the target sites, or extra-cardiac stimulation at the target sites. Placement of an epicardial lead using a minimally invasive approach allows one to have a successful implant when the transvenous approach fails.

Sensors are being added to lead systems for the purpose of enhancing our ability to monitor the physiologic status of our patients. The most common sensor currently is the right ventricular pressure monitor (Figure 13.5). This is a piezoelectric device that is integrated into the lead body of a ventricular pacing lead. By its location in the right ventricle, an estimated pulmonary artery pressure can be obtained, and this can be used to follow the volume status of patients with congestive heart failure. The addition of special sensors creates significant issues in terms of lead size, positioning, and reliability. The current sensor requires an 11 French introducer that is quite large compared with the 7 French size that has become the standard. Lead positioning is a challenge due to the fact that the stylet does not go beyond the sensor, leaving several centimeters of "floppy" lead and the electrode tip without direction and support. As this design continues to evolve, we will expect that the latter issues will be resolved.

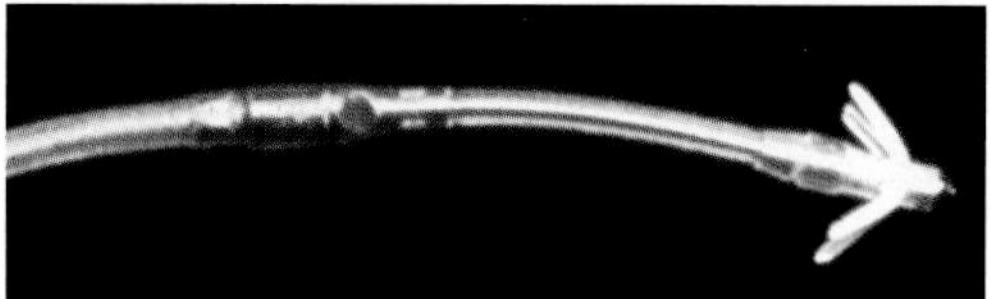

Figure 13.5 Pacing lead with integrated right ventricular pressure sensor.

Yet another lead with an imbedded sensor to measure pressure is in the early stage of development. This is a product from Savacor, Inc. that is designed to be placed in the interatrial septum. A transseptal puncture is made and the lead is advanced into the left atrium. The distal fixation tines are exposed by pulling the introducer sheath back and the lead is pulled against the left side of the septum. The sheath is pulled back further and the proximal tines are deployed on the right side of the septum, fixing it into place. The exposed pressure sensing tip becomes covered with fibrous tissue within 3 months, and does not pose a threat for thrombus formation after that time. A microchip is imbedded into the lead tip to directly record left atrial pressure. These data are transmitted over a standard coaxial bipolar pacing lead to a transmitting device implanted subcutaneously. By recording left atrial pressure directly, this lead allows an accurate assessment of left ventricular filling pressure.

Though basic lead components have not changed very much over the past five decades, the technology within each part of the lead system has evolved significantly. We will expect to see leads with more electrodes, and leads with specialized sensors. All of this, while they continue to get smaller, yet maintaining a high degree of reliability.

CHAPTER 14

Current concepts in intravascular pacemaker and defibrillator lead extraction

Dhanunjaya R. Lakkireddy, MD, *Atul Verma,* MD, *&*
Bruce L. Wilkoff, MD

Introduction

Implantable cardiac devices, such as permanent pacemakers and defibrillators have become more sophisticated with ever-expanding indications over the last decade. At the present time an ~3.9 million patients have functioning pacemakers and 460 000 patients have working implantable cardioverter defibrillators (ICDs) all over the world. (Ross Meisner, personal communication: World Wide Medtronic Marketing estimates from historical industry implants, patient mortality and device registry database 8/30/2004.) With this sudden explosive increase in device implantation, the rate of complications as well as the need for their extraction has increased proportionately. Lead extraction remains a crucial step in the treatment for many common device and lead-related problems. The potential for life-threatening complications, such as lead breakage, venous or myocardial tear, and tamponade, makes lead extraction the least favorable procedure even to the most experienced implanter.

Percutaneous intravascular lead extraction has evolved from simple traction through weight and pulley system to a more advanced modern day laser and radiofrequency technique. The success of simple uncontrolled traction was limited to only recently implanted leads with a significant risk for unsuccessful lead removal, ventricular invagination, or rupture for chronic leads. A more invasive open-heart surgical technique through a midline sternotomy or a limited atriotomy technique was developed, and continues to be a last resort answer to difficult lead extractions that are not suitable for percutaneous techniques [1, 2]. However, the invasiveness, morbidity, and long recovery time of open-heart surgical removal makes them less desirable if the job could be done through percutaneous means. Fortunately, technology has advanced significantly, providing clinicians with newer and safer methods of lead extraction.

Pathology of lead fibrosis

The point of venous entry, entry curve, and the distal tip of the lead are the most common sites of fibrosis [3]. Foreign body reaction to the lead with fibrosis forms the basis for the complexity of lead extraction and the vessel/myocardial tears associated with it. Immediately after the implantation, thrombus forms at the lead–vessel wall and lead–myocardial interface. Later over the course of weeks to years, the thrombus starts to fibrose and may even calcify, further strengthening the fibrous adhesions [3, 4] (Figure 14.1). The degree of fibrosis is directly proportional to the surface area of the lead in contact with the endocardium or endothelium – thicker older leads and defibrillation leads with coils are prone for significant fibrosis compared with thin newer pacemaker leads. Passive fixation leads appear to elicit more intense reaction than active fixation at the tip due to greater contact and movement between the tip and the endocardium in the earlier. The primary goal of any lead extraction technology is to release these fibrous attachments from the lead surface without causing damage to the structures it is attached to.

Indications

The indications for transvenous lead extraction can be categorized into two groups – patient related and lead related. Patient-related indications are infection, ineffective therapy (high defibrillation threshold), perforation, migration, embolization, induction of arrhythmias, venous thrombosis, unrelenting pain, device interactions, device upgrades, and/or presence of multiple abandoned leads. Lead-related indications include lead recalls, lead failure, and/or lead interactions [5]. The North American Society for Pacing and Electrophysiology (NASPE), now the Heart Rhythm Society (HRS), published a policy statement that outlined accepted indications for lead extraction as summarized in Table 14.1 [6].

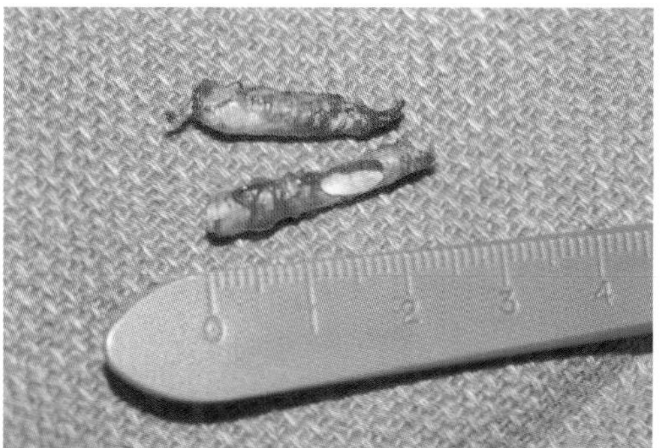

Figure 14.1 Fibrocalcific tissue samples with tubular configuration seen around the leads after extraction.

Principles of extraction

The most important factors that determine the success of lead extraction while minimizing the risk to the patient are:

1 Control of the lead body and tip.
2 Controlled disruption of the fibrous tissue using counterpressure.
3 Bracing the cardiac wall using countertraction.

Table 14.1 NASPE/HRS guideline indications for lead removal.

Class I (general agreement that leads should be removed)	• Sepsis (including endocarditis) as a result of documented infection of any intravascular part of the pacing system, or as a result of a pocket infection when the intravascular portion of the system cannot be aseptically separated from the pocket • Life-threatening arrhythmia secondary to a retained lead fragment • Retained lead or fragment that poses an immediate physical threat • Clinically significant thromboembolic events caused by a retained lead or fragment • Obliteration or occlusion of all useable veins with the need to implant a new pacing system • Lead that interferes with the operation of another implanted device
Class II (leads are often removed, but there is some divergence of opinion)	• Localized pocket infection, erosion, or draining sinus that does not involve the transvenous part of the lead system, when the lead can be cut through a clean incision that is completely separate from the infected area • Occult infection for which no source can be found and for which the pacing system is suspected • Chronic pocket or lead insertion site pain that causes significant discomfort and is not manageable by medical or surgical techniques short of removal • A lead that due to design or failure poses a potential, but not immediate, threat to the patient • A lead that interferes with treatment of a malignancy • Traumatic injury to the lead entry site for which the lead may interfere with reconstruction of the site • Leads preventing access to the venous circulation for newly required implantable devices • Nonfunctional leads in a young patient
Class III (general agreement that removal of leads is unnecessary)	• The risk posed by removal outweighs the benefit of removal • Single, nonfunctional transvenous lead in an older patient • Normally functioning lead that may be reused at the time of pulse generator replacement, provided the lead has a reliable performance history

Control of the lead body includes binding of its elements with application of uniform force on the entire length of the lead, to remove it in one piece with minimal disruption. The locking stylets provide the lead control facilitating complete lead removal and controlled disruption of the fibrous adhesions along the lead. Controlled disruption of the fibrous tissue is achieved through intravascular counterpressure, the pulling force applied on the proximal end and the body of the lead, against the tools dissecting the fibrosis. This force is applied tangentially to the vessel wall and adhering fibrous tissue. Sufficient traction must be applied on the lead, often by using a locking stylet, so that the sheath can follow the lead around the bends in the vein. If too much pressure is applied, or if the lead has insufficient traction, the sheath may tear through the vascular wall, resulting in a life-threatening complication. Operator experience is vital in knowing how much lead tension and counterpressure needs to be applied (Figure 14.2).

Once the sheath is advanced to the lead tip–myocardial interface, countertraction is utilized. Countertraction involves opposing the traction placed on the lead by bracing the myocardium with the overlying blunt sheath. This focuses the traction force perpendicular to the heart wall and limits it to the scar tissue immediately surrounding the lead tip. Therefore, the lead can be torn out of the scar tissue while minimizing the risk of myocardial invagination or a large tear (Figure 14.2).

Instruments

Locking stylets

The development of the locking stylet was a significant advance, enabling sufficient counterpressure during lead extraction with excellent lead control. Locking stylets are designed to lock within the lumen of the lead near the distal electrode tip, so that traction is applied along the entire length of

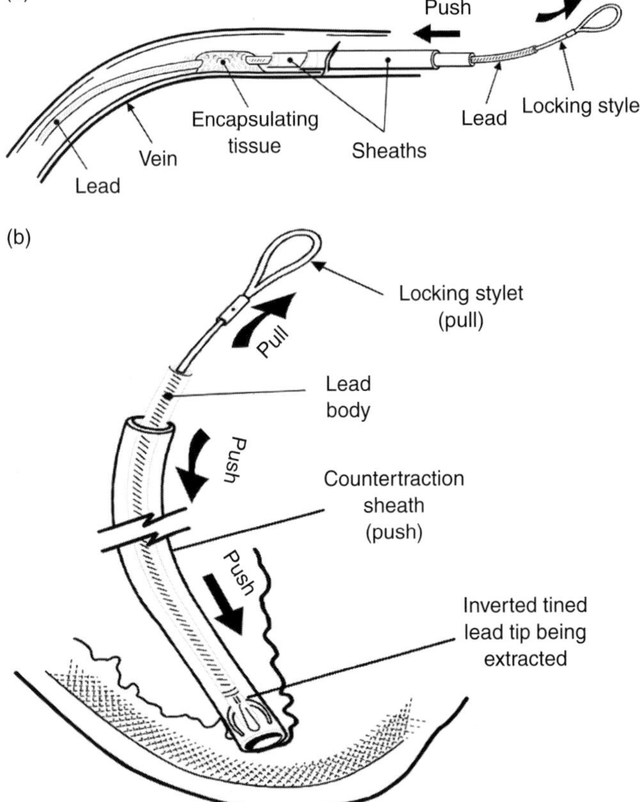

Figure 14.2 Diagrammatic representation of (a) counterpressure and (b) countertraction used during lead extraction.

the lead, and not just the proximal end. This provides stiffness to the lead, minimizes the chance of lead breakage during traction, and promotes intact lead extraction [7]. Currently available locking stylets include (1) Liberator stylet (Cook Vascular Inc, PA) and (2) Spectranetics LLD (Colorodo Springs, CO). While the locking stylet minimizes the chance of lead breakage, it does not eliminate the other complications associated with traction. Tears in the myocardium or vasculature may occur, and the lead may become impacted in fibrous tissue as it is pulled out [8].

Telescoping sheaths

Telescoping sheaths are a vital component of intravascular lead extraction. Their use is based on the two important concepts of *counterpressure* and *countertraction* described earlier [9]. The sheaths are pushed along the lead applying a tangential force shearing off the fibrous tissue from the vessel wall. Telescoping sheaths have an inner guide sheath that fits inside of a larger, more rigid outer sheath [10]. They are available in 11–16 French sizes to accommodate various lead diameters and come in a variety of materials including stainless steel, Teflon™, or other plastics. Steel sheaths are used solely to break through the dense fibrosis, tissue, and sometimes bone that blocks the subclavian venous entry site. Once access into the vein has been obtained, the steel sheaths are changed to flexible plastic sheaths to reduce the risk of vascular damage. The plastic sheaths can easily maneuver around the curves in the vein. Maintaining the angle of the sheath parallel to the lead minimizes the risk of vascular perforation. Fluoroscopic visualization must be used during advancement of any type of sheath to follow its intravascular course. The counterpressure force must be applied judiciously, and if the required force is more than what can easily be applied by the sheath, other extraction devices must be considered. Passage of a sheath down to the heart is most successful in leads that have been implanted for <8 years [10].

Femoral snares

Some leads are not accessible from the venous entry site, such as leads that have been cut or fractured, causing them to retract into the vein or prolapse into the heart. In these cases, the femoral approach for lead extraction may be favored. Femoral extraction requires the use of a large 16 French sheath (Byrd workstation), which is carefully inserted via the femoral vein [11]. The sheath acts as a conduit for the snare as well as acting as the outer telescoping sheath for countertraction. A snare can then be inserted thorough the sheath to grasp the lead, pull it down from the superior veins, and from the heart with countertraction. The most commonly employed snares are the *Dotter basket* – tip deflecting guidewire and the *Needle's Eye snare* (Cook Vascular Inc, PA). The Dotter basket apparatus has a deflecting tip, which can wrap around the lead. The tip is pulled into the basket and the basket may be rotated to entangle the lead within it. The basket is then pulled into the femoral sheath at which point the sheath can be advanced into the heart to provide countertraction [12]. The Needle's Eye works in a similar fashion where the hook of the snare is draped over the lead, the "needle" is advanced through the hook, and the inner sheath is advanced so that the lead is trapped between the hook and needle [13]. The lead can then be pulled out through the sheath.

Techniques of lead extraction

A good history and physical examination, details of the hardware, proper equipment in the operating room, cardiothoracic surgery backup, and operator experience are crucial to successful lead extraction. Most of the leads can be extracted in an electrophysiology lab under local anesthesia with intravenous sedation. General anesthesia may be required for complicated extractions. The accurate location of the leads in the heart is very crucial. The possibility of septal defects, persistent superior vena cava (SVC), migration across the myocardium, and coronary sinus deployment should be borne in mind prior to planning the extraction to minimize complications. The principles described in earlier section apply to any method of lead extraction with minor differences in the type of instruments used – mostly the telescoping sheaths.

Conventional mechanical extraction

This technique involves the use of conventional tools including the blunt Teflon or steel telescoping sheaths with appropriate locking stylets using the principles of counterpressure and countertraction. A linear incision is made to obtain better access to the vein of insertion and the generator is explanted. Dissect the soft tissue as close as possible to the vein and remove the suture sleeves. Identify each lead, its model, course, and its chamber for choosing appropriate equipment. Pay attention to the leads that are not to be removed from being damaged or pulled out while working on the target leads. Cut the terminal pin of each lead leading sufficient length of the proximal end outside the venous insertion. Prepare the cut end by circumferentially incising the insulation. For coaxial bipolar leads the inner insulation should also be incised. Then a standard pacemaker stylet is passed through the electrode to its distal tip to ascertain the distance through which the locking stylet has to travel and to clear the debris. Then assess the size of the electrode using guage pins. Select an appropriate size locking stylet and advance it to the farthest reach of the lead and tie a 0-guage suture around the insulation tightly with a square knot. The long end of the suture is then tied to the looped end of the locking stylet providing for parallel and simultaneous traction on the outer insulation and on the conductor coil. This latter step is applied to all except for Teletronics ACCUFIX "J" lead. And this may not be of much clinical relevance in today's practice and the prophylactic extraction of these leads is not indicated any more.

Straight telescoping stainless steel sheaths greatly facilitate the vessel entry, although this is no longer necessary with the new laser of radiofrequency sheaths. Pass the lead-locking stylet combination through the inner sheath of the two telescoping sheaths securing the loose end with one hand. Assure the triaxial alignment of the sheaths with the course of the lead so that the sheaths slide over the monorail-like lead and rotate while advancing slowly. Once the steel sheaths pass the bend of the lead, they should be exchanged for either Teflon™ or polypropylene sheaths quickly, obstructing the outer sheath to avoid air embolism. It is preferable to use relatively stiffer sheaths as long as there is strong control of the lead. Apply a retraction force on the looped end of the locking stylet equal to which allows advancement of the sheaths while holding the lead away from the outer arc of the insertion vein and into the heart. The sheaths should always be advanced under direct fluoroscopic guidance. These sheaths should not be advanced directly against the vessel wall but rather the leads should be peeled away from the wall of the vessel bringing the lead into the center of the vascular lumen. Failure to advance the sheath after initial progress is likely to be due to damage to their leading edge and requires their replacement.

Once the lead is freed up to the endocardial attachment of its tip slow steady pressure is required. If the locking stylet is still locked with good control, the outer sheath will exert sufficient countertraction to prevent the ventricular wall from invaginating. Sometimes the lead will release from the myocardium but the fibrosis will be too large to enter the sheath. It is therefore helpful to periodically gently retract the lead and sheaths together to see if the job is completed (Figure 14.3(a)–(c)). Occassionally, the large fibrous remnants at the lead tip may not permit the removal of the sheath from the subclavian vein, once the system is withdrawn from the heart into the SVC, additional attempts at retraction of the inner sheath and lead into the outer sheath are usually successful. After removal of the sheaths, bleeding can be contained with simple pressure though at times, a purse string or figure-of-8 suture may be required.

With infected devices, the generator pocket should be completely excised to prevent the microbial reseeding and closed with mattress sutures allowing healing by secondary intention. In noninfected extraction, new hardware can be implanted during the same procedure.

Excimer laser extraction

The steps involved in laser sheath extraction are same as in conventional technique except for the use of the Excimer laser inner telescoping sheaths (Spectranectics Corporation, Colorado Springs, CO) used in conjunction with an outer Teflon™ sheath. A circumferential zone of optic fibers run along the sheath delivering a 308 nm laser beam that ablates the fibrous tissue within 1 mm of the tip, greatly minimizing the amount of counterpressure required.

The laser sheath is one of the most effective extraction tools and has been prospectively studied

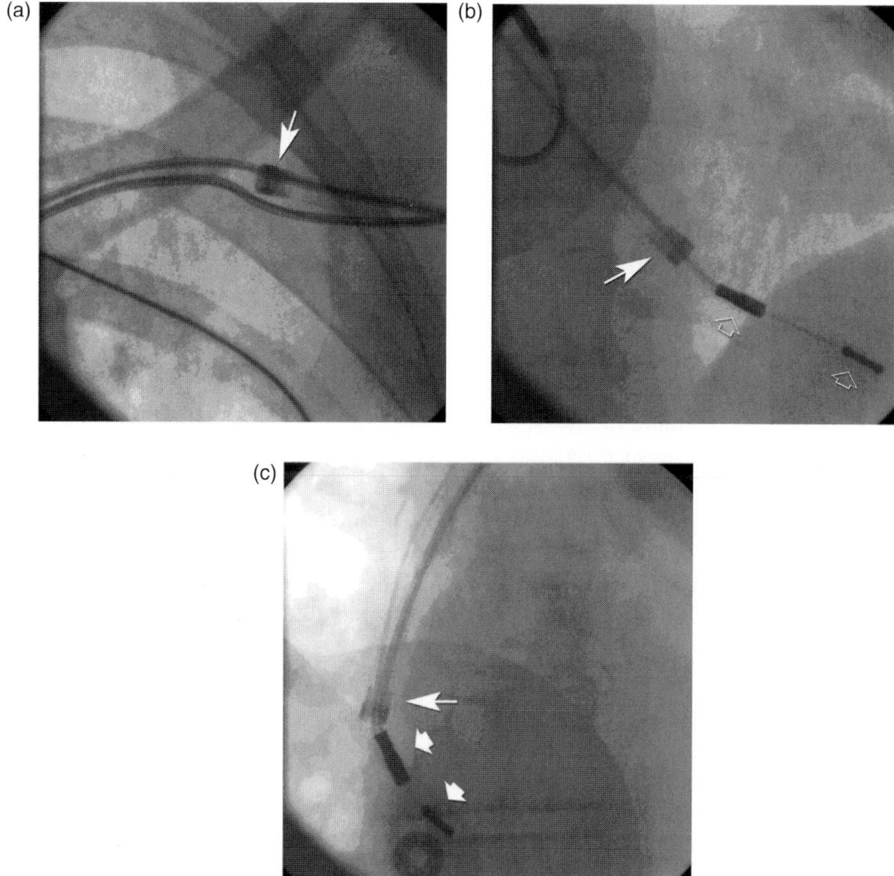

Figure 14.3 (a)–(c) Extraction of the old pacemaker leads within the left brachiocephalic vein using Excimer laser sheath (long arrow). (Atrial lead, short solid arrow; ventricular lead, short open arrow.)

in the randomized PLEXES trial in comparison to traditional extraction with locking stylets and telescoping sheaths [14]. Laser resulted in a higher percentage of complete lead removals (94% versus 64%, $p = .001$) and also reduced the time required for removal (10.1 ± 11.5 min versus 12.9 ± 19.2 min, $p < .04$). Life-threatening complications (including one death) occurred in the laser group, while none occurred in the traditional group, but this difference was not statistically different given the small numbers overall. Whether a true difference exists requires further evaluation, but there is little doubt that the laser has improved the efficacy and speed of lead extraction.

Further trials were performed using the larger diameter 14 and 16 French laser sheaths for larger leads, such as defibrillator leads [15, 16]. The efficacy and complication rates were similar to those reported above, and the extraction time was only 2–4 min longer per lead.

Radiofrequency extraction

This electrosurgical technique is similar to the above mentioned methods except for the use of an electrosurgical sheath, which operates similar to a surgical cautery tool [9]. The electrosurgical sheath has two bipolar tungsten conductors that run along the length of the sheath and terminate exposed electrodes emitting radiofrequency energy disrupting the immediate fibrous tissue. Again, an outer Teflon™ sheath is used to help maneuver the electrosurgical sheath and to provide countertraction once the sheath is advanced to the lead tip.

The electrosurgical sheath provides hypothetical advantages over the laser. First, the sheath is designed to be more supple and therefore may be better able to maneuver around bends in the vein compared with the laser sheath. Second, the radiofrequency energy is supposed to be gentler than the laser, allowing more careful dissection of the tissue and reducing the chance of vascular damage. Finally, the electrosurgical sheath is less expensive [12]. While there are no randomized trials published to date using the electrosurgical sheath, our preliminary experience from the Cleveland Clinic Foundation suggests that this tool compares favorably to the laser sheath. We studied 450 consecutive lead extractions at our institution between November 1998 and November 2001 (Wilkoff BL, personal communication). Of these extractions, laser was used to extract 354 leads and the electrosurgical sheath 96 leads. There were no complications in the electrosurgical group compared to two deaths in the laser group. Furthermore, procedure time was significantly lower in the electrosurgical group versus the laser (130 ± 49 min versus 158 ± 65 min, respectively, $p < .002$). Fluoroscopy time was also reduced (13.3 ± 10.6 min versus 17.1 ± 15.1 min, respectively, $p < .05$). However, there was some selection bias in this series since the lead implant duration was significantly longer in the laser group compared with the electrosurgical group (8.2 ± 5.0 years versus 6.6 ± 4.4 years, $p < .005$). Regardless, it would seem that the electrosurgical sheath has comparable success rates to the laser.

Based on our experience, the electrosurgical sheath may be the tool of first choice for extraction of leads with shorter implant durations in patients who are at higher risk of complications, such as those of advanced age. However, for cases requiring multiple lead extractions and for leads with longer implant durations that have a higher rate of calcification, we have found that the laser is the best option to use.

Defibrillator lead extraction

Defibrillator leads theoretically represent a greater challenge for extraction than pacemaker leads. The leads are generally larger in diameter, requiring larger extraction sheaths, which may increase the risk of vascular injury. The defibrillator coils also tend to stimulate more fibrosis on the vascular wall, so that there are often dense bands that bind the lead to the venous or myocardial surface around the superior vena caval and ventricular coils. However, in experienced hands, extraction of defibrillator leads can be accomplished using the same tools used for pacer leads with similar success rates [17–19]. In a series of 161 patients at the Cleveland Clinic, successful complete extraction of implantable defibrillator leads was achieved without major complication in 96.9% of patients [20]. Failure occurred in only three patients. Two patients had major complications including one death. These compare favorably to data from our pacemaker lead experience, although further data is still required to confirm whether complication risks are higher with defibrillator lead extraction. Procedure time (171.2 min versus 140.8 min, $p < .01$) and fluoroscopy time (11.0 min versus 9.9 min, $p < .01$) were longer for patients undergoing defibrillator lead extraction compared with pacemaker leads, but these times are still quite comparable. Thus, defibrillator lead extraction may have excellent success rates with currently available tools in experienced centers.

Coronary sinus lead extraction

Cardiac resynchronization therapy using biventricular pacing has expanded the implantation of transvenous coronary sinus lead insertion. Though these are typically nonactive fixation, and nontyned thin bodied leads, they are still capable of triggering significant fibrotic responses within the coronary sinus [21]. Extraction of leads from fragile coronary sinus branches, which are highly susceptible to dissection or rupture with excessive instrumentation, can be very challenging. Similar to regular atrial or ventricular leads, coronary sinus leads implanted under 6 months may be extracted with simple traction. There is dearth of data regarding chronic coronary sinus lead extractions. A small report on 14 patients showed 100% successful extraction without major complications and very short procedure and fluoroscopy times (13 min and 1.8 min, respectively) [22]. However, more than one-third of these leads had been implanted for less than 6 months. Currently, a 7 French electrosurgical dissection sheath (EDS) is available for extracting coronary sinus leads. Although, further data regarding the risks and success of coronary sinus lead extraction will be required, especially as the number of these lead implants grows over the next few years. With the use of newer, thicker, bipolar coronary sinus leads, extraction may not be as simple and less traumatic as the thin unipolar leads. The issues surrounding the extraction of these newer leads are yet to be understood.

Extraction in stenosed veins

The mechanical stress associated with pacemaker wires may lead to vessel wall inflammation, fibrosis and thrombus formation, and ultimately to venous stenosis and occlusion anywhere from the site of entry up to the SVC. Patients who need lead revisions with stenosed veins can be successfully treated with a one-step percutaneous approach. This consists of percutaneous retrieval of pacemaker system using the above-described techniques followed by venous revascularization with angioplasty and stenting and installation of new system (Figure 14.4(a)–(c)). There are several small case series that emphasize the role of angioplasty with either metallic of nitinol stents as a safe alternative to this complex problem [23, 24]. The true long-term benefit of this approach requires further observation of large series of patients for several years. Occassionally one may encounter very challenging situations in the form of a stenosed brachiocephalic and SVC, angioplastied and stented with the leads jailed between the stent and the vein wall (Figure 14.5(a) and (b)).

Success and complication rates

In 1999, the US Extraction Database showed a 95% success rate among 4223 leads extracted in 2437 patients [25]. Partial extractions were accomplished

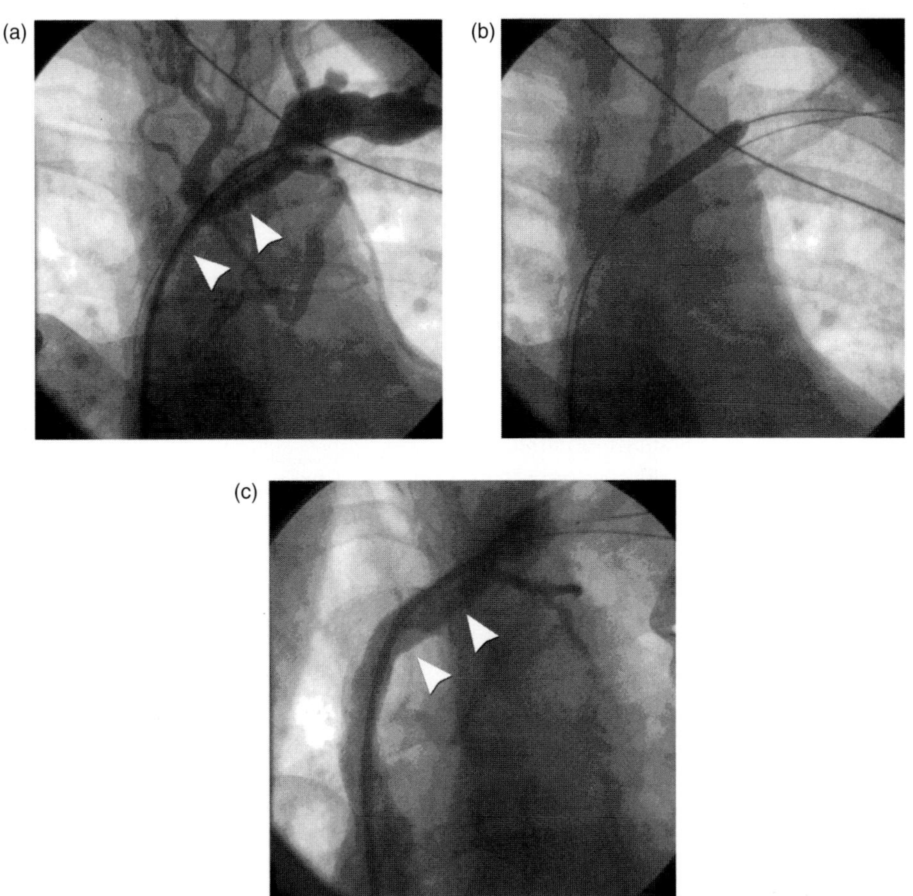

Figure 14.4 (a) Stenosed left brachiocephalic and superior vena cava indicated by two arrow heads. (b) Balloon angioplasty of the stenosed section. (c) Left brachiocephalic and superior vena cava after the deployment of NITINOL stent.

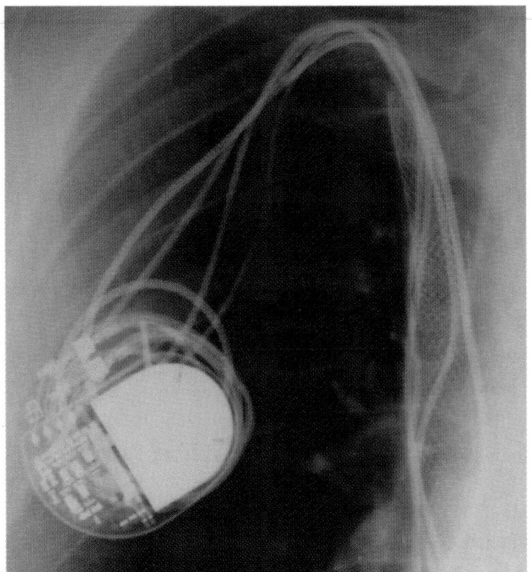

Figure 14.5 Stenosed brachiocephalic and SVC, angioplastied and stented with the leads jailed between the stent and the vein wall.

in 3% of patients, with failure to extract occurring in 2%. Major complications of lead extraction are life threatening and include myocardial avulsion, vascular tear, pneumothorax, pulmonary embolism, arteriovenous fistula, and death. Minor complications are not life threatening, but often require intervention such as pericardial effusion, hematoma, venous thrombosis, and arrhythmia [26, 27]. A report on consecutive patients from the US Extraction Database spanning 1998–1999 showed that major complications occurred in 1.9% of all patients (Wilkoff BL, personal communication). Death occurred in 0.4%, urgent cardiovascular surgery in 0.8%, and pericardial or pleural drainage in 0.5%. Predictors of increased major complication risk included longer implant duration, female gender, multiple leads, and defibrillator leads.

Reimplantation

The need and the timing of reimplantation is dependent on the indication for extraction. If the indications for continued pacemaker or defibrillator therapy no longer exist or patient wishes to discontinue, reimplantation should not be considered. Lead extraction for device infection should be followed by at least 2–4 weeks of intravenous antibiotics with proven negative blood cultures prior to reimplantation. Patients dependent on device therapy can be appropriately treated using bridging therapies, such as temporary transvenous pacing leads or external defibrillator patches in the hospital, and wearable cardioverter defibrillators (LIFECOR Inc., Pittsburgh, PA) in outpatients. For noninfectious indications of lead extraction the new hardware can be simultaneously reimplanted on the same side or on the opposite side. One-step extraction, angioplasty with stenting followed by reimplantation should be considered for patients with symptomatic venous stenosis requiring lead extraction.

Future directions in lead manufacturing and extraction

Intravascular lead extraction is a field that has advanced immensely over the last decade. The array of tools and techniques now available is a far cry from the days of simple traction by a pulley and weight system. The advent of new generation thinner, coated leads will decrease fibrosis and make extraction less complicated. As technology continues to improve, so too will our ability to handle future challenges provided by newer lead technologies.

References

1 del Rio A, Anguera I, Miro JM, Mont L, Fowler VG, Jr, Azqueta M, Mestres CA. Surgical treatment of pacemaker and defibrillator lead endocarditis: the impact of electrode lead extraction on outcome. *Chest* 2003; **124**: 1451–1459.

2 Nouraei SM, Bexton RS, Hasan A. Surgical extraction of infected pacemaker leads after cardiac surgery. *Asian Cardiovasc Thorac Ann* 2003; **11**: 167–168.

3 Love CJ. Current concepts in extraction of transvenous pacing and ICD leads. *Cardiol Clin* 2000; **18**: 193–217.

4 Epstein AE, Kay GN, Plumb VJ, Dailey SM, Anderson PG. Gross and microscopic pathological changes associated with nonthoracotomy implantable defibrillator leads. *Circulation* 1998; **98**: 1517–1524.

5 Brodell GK, Wilkoff BL. A novel approach to determining the cause of pacemaker lead failure. *Cleve Clin J Med* 1992; **59**(1): 91–92.

6 Love CJ, Wilkoff BL, Byrd CL *et al.* Recommendations for extraction of chronically implanted transvenous pacing and defibrillator leads: indications, facilities, training. North American society of pacing and electrophysiology

lead extraction conference faculty. *PACE* 2000; **23**: 544–551.

7 Kennergren C, Schaerf RH, Sellers TD *et al.* Cardiac lead extraction with a novel locking stylet. *J Interv Card Electrophysiol* 2000; **4**: 591–593.

8 Fearnot NE, Smith HJ, Goode LB, Byrd CL, Wilkoff BL, Sellers TD. Intravascular lead extraction using locking stylets, sheaths, and other techniques. *PACE* 1990; **13**: 1864–1870.

9 Byrd CL, Wilkoff BL. Techniques and devices for extraction of pacemaker and implantable cardioverter-defibrillator lead. In: Wilkoff BL, ed. *Clinical cardiac pacing and defibrillation.* WB Saunders, Philadelphia, PA 2000: 669–706.

10 Gilligan DM, Dan D. Excimer laser for pacemaker and defibrillator lead extraction: techniques and clinical results. *Lasers Med Sci* 2001; **16**: 113–121.

11 Byrd CL. Advances in device lead extraction. *Curr Cardiol Rep* 2001; **3**: 324.

12 Espinosa RE, Hayes DL, Vlietstra RE, Osborn MJ, McGoon MD. The Dotter retriever and pigtail catheter: efficacy in extraction of chronic transvenous pacemaker leads. *PACE* 1993; **16**: 2337–2342.

13 Klug D, Jarwe M, Messaoudene SA *et al.* Pacemaker lead extraction with the needle's eye snare for countertraction via a femoral approach. *PACE* 2002; **25**: 1023–1028.

14 Wilkoff BL, Byrd CL, Love CJ *et al.* Pacemaker lead extraction with the laser sheath: results of the pacing lead extraction with the excimer sheath (PLEXES) trial. *J Am Coll Cardiol* 1999; **33**: 1671–1676.

15 Epstein LM, Byrd CL, Wilkoff BL *et al.* Initial experience with larger laser sheaths for the removal of transvenous pacemaker and implantable defibrillator leads. *Circulation* 1999; **100**: 516–525.

16 Kennergren C. Excimer laser assisted extraction of permanent pacemaker and ICD leads: present experiences of a European multi-centre study. *Eur J Cardiothorac Surg* 1999; **15**: 856–860.

17 Cooper JM, Stephenson EA, Berul CI, Walsh EP, Epstein LM. Implantable cardioverter defibrillator lead complications and laser extraction in children and young adults with congenital heart disease: implications for implantation and management. *J Cardiovasc Electrophysiol* 2003; **14**: 344–349.

18 Kantharia BK, Padder FA, Pennington JC III *et al.* Feasibility, safety, and determinants of extraction time of percutaneous extraction of endocardial implantable cardioverter defibrillator leads by intravascular countertraction method. *Am J Cardiol* 2000; **85**: 593–597.

19 Le Franc P, Klug D, Jarwe M *et al.* Extraction of endocardial implantable cardioverter-defibrillator leads. *Am J Cardiol* 1999; **84**: 187–191.

20 Saad EB, Saliba WI, Schweikert RA *et al.* Nonthoracotomy implantable defibrillator lead extraction: results and comparison with extraction of pacemaker leads. *PACE* 2003; **26**: 1944–1950.

21 Tacker WA, Vanvleet JF, Schoenlein WE, Janas W, Ayers GM, Byrd CL. Post-mortem changes after lead extraction from the ovine coronary sinus and great cardiac vein. *PACE* 1998; **21**: 296–298.

22 Tyers GF, Clark J, Wang Y, Mills P, Bashir J. Coronary sinus lead extraction. *PACE* 2003; **26**: 524–526.

23 Chan AW, Bhatt DL, Wilkoff BL. Percutaneous treatment for pacemaker-associated superior vena cava syndrome. *PACE* 2002; **25**(11): 1628–1633.

24 Teo N, Sabharwal T, Rowland E. Treatment of superior vena cava obstruction secondary to pacemaker wires with balloon venoplasty and insertion of metallic stents. *Eur Heart J* 2002; **23**: 1465–1470.

25 Smith HJ, Fearnot NE, Byrd CL, Wilkoff BL, Love CJ, Sellers TD. Five-years experience with intravascular lead extraction. U.S. Lead Extraction Database. *PACE* 1994; **17**: 2016–2020.

26 Alt E, Neuzner J, Binner L *et al.* Three-year experience with a stylet for lead extraction: a multicenter study. *PACE* 1996; **19**: 18–25.

27 Byrd CL, Wilkoff BL, Love CJ *et al.* Intravascular extraction of problematic or infected permanent pacemaker leads: 1994–1996. U.S. Extraction Database, MED Institute. *PACE* 1999; **22**: 1348–1357.

15

CHAPTER 15

Left ventricular epicardial lead implantation: Anatomy, techniques, and tools

Jennifer Cummings, MD, *William Belden*, MD, & *Bruce L. Wilkoff*, MD

Introduction

The technical obstacles to the implementation of cardiac resynchronization therapy (CRT) are largely related to implantation and have been only partially ameliorated by the accumulated experience. The tools and techniques used to meet these challenges are continually evolving. However, with these rapid changes, it has become critical that physicians performing these procedures become well versed in the broad armamentarium available in order to ensure successful and effective left ventricular (LV) lead placement. Crucial to the successful implementation of these tools and techniques is a thorough understanding of the right atrial (RA) and cardiac venous anatomy. This chapter will briefly review a compilation of the tools, techniques, and the anatomical and conceptual basis behind tool selection and utilization.

Though the tools available in CRT change faster than most publications can keep up with, the general steps to implantation have remained the same. First, it is necessary to obtain venous access. Second is placement of all pacing leads (RA, right ventricular (RV), and coronary sinus (CS)). Placement of the CS lead involves several steps: (1) engaging the CS, (2) identifying and selecting a target vessel, (3) placing the LV lead into the targeted vessel, and (4) removing the implantation tools.

Definitions

Sheath/introducer

For the purposes of this discussion, sheath and introducer are used synonymously. In the context of a telescoping system, the sheath serves as a stable conduit between pectoral area and the CS for the *guide catheter*. In this role, the sheath becomes the CS *platform* or workstation for the telescoping system. When referring to the size of a sheath/introducer it is important to remember that the French size refers to the internal diameter while the French size of guides and catheters refer to the external diameter. Guides and catheters are designed to be placed in the body through a sheath or introducer. For example, a 7 French catheter/guide fits through a 7 French introducer/sheath.

Directional device (guide/catheter)

The directional guide/catheter fits within the sheath. The internal diameter of the directional device distinguishes a *directional catheter* or *directional guide*. When the internal diameter of the directional device is large enough to deliver only the angioplasty wire, it is referred to as the *"directional catheter."* As part of a telescoping system, the *directional catheter* is placed in the CS through the *sheath/introducer*. It provides direction, support, and a low-friction environment for an angioplasty wire. Various shaped directional catheters are used depending on the venous anatomy. Recall that the French size of a catheter refers to the outer diameter (OD). The internal diameter of all 6 French (OD) and smaller catheters are too small for the available pacing leads. In contrast, when the internal diameter of the directional device is large enough to deliver the pacing lead, it is referred to as the *"directional guide."* As part of a telescoping system, the directional guide is placed in the CS through a sheath. It provides direction, support, and a low-friction environment for a pacing lead or an angioplasty wire. Various shaped directional guides are used depending on the venous anatomy. Recall that the French size of a guide refers to the OD. The internal diameter of most 7 French (OD) interventional guides are large enough to deliver the most LV leads directly.

Venous Access

Generally, techniques in obtaining access for CRT placement have not dramatically changed from that of standard pacing devices. Both right and left subclavian access can be used, with both approaches having unique advantages and disadvantages. Approach through the right subclavian provides the implanting physician the ability of using the left anterior oblique (LAO) view of fluoroscopy without having the imaging equipment interfering with the surgical field and thus decreases operator radiation exposure. However, this approach presents a challenge when attempting to engage the CS OS in that the catheter needs to make two opposite right-angle turns to first enter the heart then to enter the CS itself. Though specific catheters have been designed for this approach, some argue that stability of the catheter placed from the right remains challenging [1]. In contrast, the left subclavian provides gentler curves that allow catheters to enter the heart and then the CS. Though this allows for deeper seating of the catheter and thus improved stability, the operator is often working around the image intensifier above the surgical field. The left approach is by far the more common approach, especially in the United States, but most operators should not only be comfortable with both approaches but also be able to select optimal tools to maximize success from either side.

Preferred methods of obtaining venous access vary between institutions and operators. No one technique has proven to be ideal, but general concepts appear to make the procedure easier. The primary concerns in obtaining access include the risk of pneumothorax, hemothorax, and damage to the vein itself. Use of cephalic vein cutdown for pacemaker lead access is considered ideal by many physicians in that it provides good hemostatic control and virtually no risk of pneumothorax. Though this is sufficient for the RA and RV leads, there is not sufficient room for the sheath required for CS lead placement. Thus, even when a cephalic vein is used for the RV and RA leads, a separate sheath, placed in the subclavian or axillary vein, is necessary.

Another approach to the subclavian is direct access through either a proximal puncture near the medial curve of the clavicle or a distal puncture where the subclavian becomes the axillary vein as it courses over the first rib. However, even using this type of access requires a separate puncture and sheath for the placement of the CS lead. Having a separate site greatly facilitates the additional manipulation of the sheaths, catheters, and leads necessary for ideal placement.

With an increase in the number of patients with previous devices presenting to the EP lab for "upgrade" to a biventricular device, it is important to take into consideration patency of the subclavian vein currently being used by their device leads as well as the integrity and function of the leads in place. Though some physicians favor venography in all implants both old and new, visualization of the subclavian vein is important in this patient population. Thrombosis from chronic or multiple leads as well as tortuous anatomy associated with scarring from previous leads may make addition of a CS lead at the same site difficult or even impossible. Angiography either by manual peripheral injection in the EP lab immediately prior to the procedure or by interventional radiology can provide information as to the course, size, and patency of the venous system. Also, attention to the condition, age, and thresholds of the current leads is imperative. Though lead assessment is typically done during the procedure, the need for an RV or RA lead in addition to the CS or even extraction may alter location of the device or allocation of lab resources.

The CS: engaging the ostium

The first step in placing the LV lead is engaging the CS OS in a manner that allows advancement of the guide catheter. Located just superior the tricuspid valve on the posterior wall of the right atria, the CS OS is protected on its superior–posterior aspect by the Thebesian valve as well as the Eustachian ridge (Figure 15.1(a)). These structures make a direct (anterograde) approach along the inferior–posterior wall of the right atrium to the CS OS difficult (Figure 15.1(b)). However, these structures actually

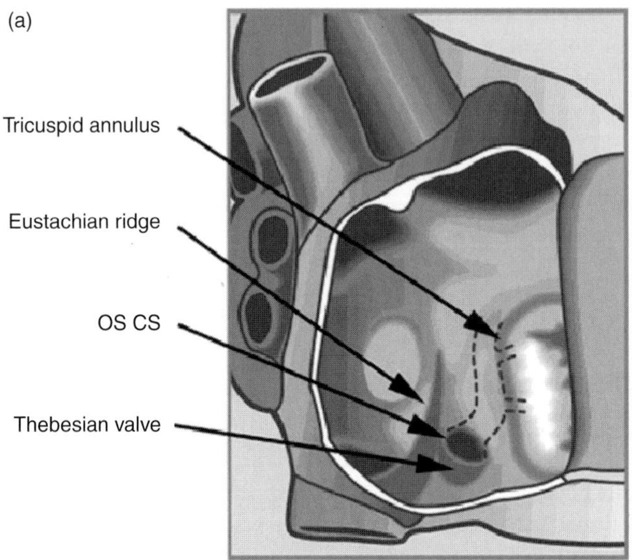

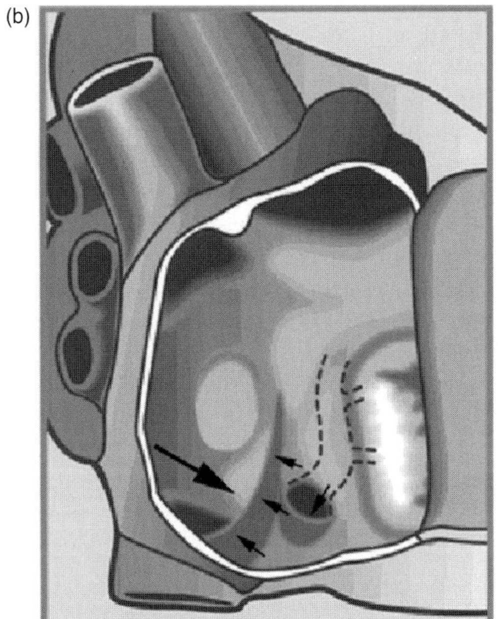

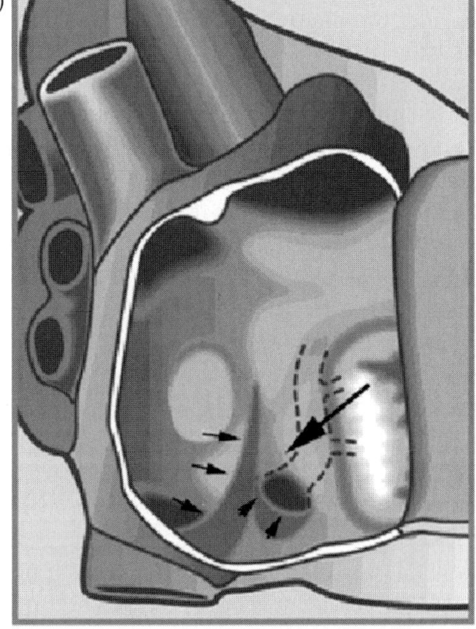

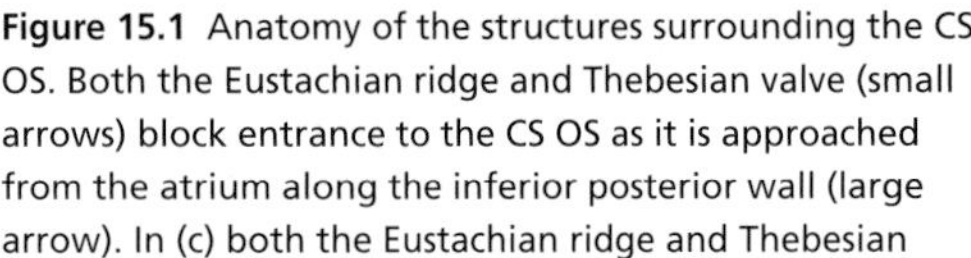
Figure 15.1 Anatomy of the structures surrounding the CS OS. Both the Eustachian ridge and Thebesian valve (small arrows) block entrance to the CS OS as it is approached from the atrium along the inferior posterior wall (large arrow). In (c) both the Eustachian ridge and Thebesian valve (small arrows) direct the tip of the guide into the CS OS as it is approached from the posterior superior tricuspid annulus (large arrow). (Used by permission of Ellenbogen, KA, Kay, GN, Wilkoff BL, 2004.)

facilitate engaging the CS OS during withdrawal (retrograde approach) from the right ventricle with counterclockwise torque of the guide catheter (Figure 15.1(c)). Thus, several guide catheters have been designed to approach the OS from the posterior – superior tricuspid annulus.

Identification of the OS can be facilitated by both electrical or contrast mapping of the area. Several guide catheters allow the use of a steerable electrophysiologic catheter to map for CS electrograms. Once located, the catheter can be advanced into the CS and the guide advanced over the catheter that is subsequently removed.

Contrast mapping of the area of the CS OS is another alternative. Using this method, the tip of the guide is advanced across the tricuspid annulus and directed posterior with 20–30° of counterclockwise torque. A 2–3 ml injection of contrast outlines the trabeculae and confirms the location of the guide in the right ventricle. Gradual withdrawal of the guide catheter with additional counterclockwise torque, while additional small injections of contrast, will identify the CS OS. The contrast first becomes trapped between the tricuspid valve and posterior wall of the right ventricle outlining the tricuspid annulus. The guide enters the right atrium at the superior–posterior aspect of the tricuspid annulus. Further injections of contrast delineate the sub-Eustachian space, thus allowing the identification of the exact location of the CS OS. After visualization of the OS, finer manipulation of the guide can then be performed to allow engagement and advancement into the CS.

Guide design is critical for advancement of the sheath into the body of the CS but more so with contrast-guided rather than electrogram-guided techniques. With electrical mapping, the guide merely follows the steerable EP catheter into the CS; since it uses the steerable nature and stiffness of the catheter to provide an internal guide for the sheath. DeMartino *et al.* [2] demonstrated that electrophysiology catheter techniques were superior to guide catheter techniques alone in gaining access to the CS. However, when using contrast mapping or guided techniques, the guide is usually either directly advanced into the CS or over a 0.035″ guidewire rather than over another catheter. Thus the guide design is important in successful CS cannulation. The presence of a large "proximal curve" is important. The addition of this curve to the guide places the guide tip above the CS on the tricuspid annulus or in the right ventricle rather than in the right atrium. Counterclockwise torque is then able to direct the "proximal curve" guide inferior, posterior, and toward the right atrium into the OS. Figure 15.2(a) and (b) demonstrate how, based on the anatomy of the right atrium, a catheter without a curve approaching the CS OS along the inferior–posterior wall of the right atrium will be deflected away from the OS by the Eustachian ridge and Thebesian valve. The addition of this proximal curve allows for the advancement of the guide into the ventricle and subsequent maneuvering into the sub-Eustachian space and OS. This curve could be added to standard multipurpose guides through shaping of the guide in a manner similar to shaping of a pacing stylet. However, as this procedure has evolved, a wide range of guide catheter shapes with this type of preformed curve have become commercially available for use.

Both modalities, electrogram based and contrast based, use different shaped guides and types of proximal curves to engage and cannulate the CS OS. When using the electrogram-based method, the outer guide surrounding the EP catheter relies more upon the curve of the EP catheter to provide its shape and support. Its advantage relies on its adjustability and use of intracardiac electrograms for guidance, but necessitates that the EP catheter is far enough within the CS to provide support over which the guide can be advanced into the CS OS.

Contrast-based CS cannulation is more dependent on the curve of the guide as it is used to directly engage the OS. The most commonly used systems all have a notable proximal curve, however, these curves vary in shape, point of anchor, and size. One of the earliest preformed guides used a large proximal curve designed to anchor the guide against the lateral wall and Eustachian ridge of the right atrium (SafeSheathCSG™, Figure 15.3). Though the size of the guide and curve vary, the anchor point remains the same to allow more stability and to prevent pushing the sheath out of the CS when advancing the lead. Alternatively, a different proximal curve design utilizes the superior vena cava/RA junction as its primary anchor point (RapidO™ Figure 15.3). This may help direct the tip upward into the CS when

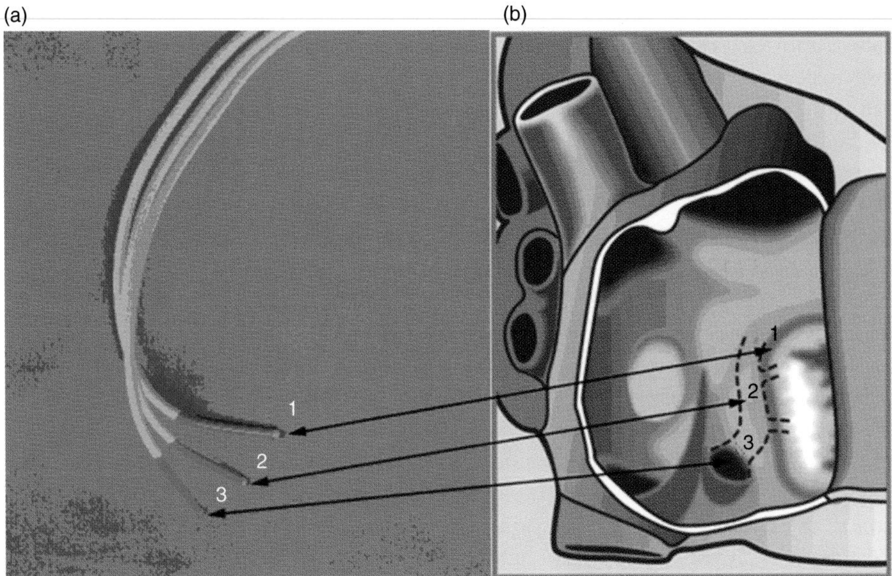

Figure 15.2 Effect of counterclockwise torque applied to a braided guide inside a peel away sheath. (a) Three positions of a guide with progressive application of torque are superimposed. (1) Initial counterclockwise torque at the hub of the guide directs the tip of the guide back. (2) With additional counterclockwise torque the guide tip can no longer move back. The torque thus directs the tip of the guide down and to the left. (3) As more counterclockwise torque is added, the tip of the guide continues to move down and to the left. In (2) and (3) the proximal section of the guide lifts off the surface (out of the plane of the illustration). (b) A drawing of the area of the CS OS demonstrate the relative position of the tip of the guide as torque is applied assuming an initial position on the posterior superior tricuspid annulus. (Used by permission of Ellenbogen, KA, Kay, GN, and Wilkoff, BL, 2004.)

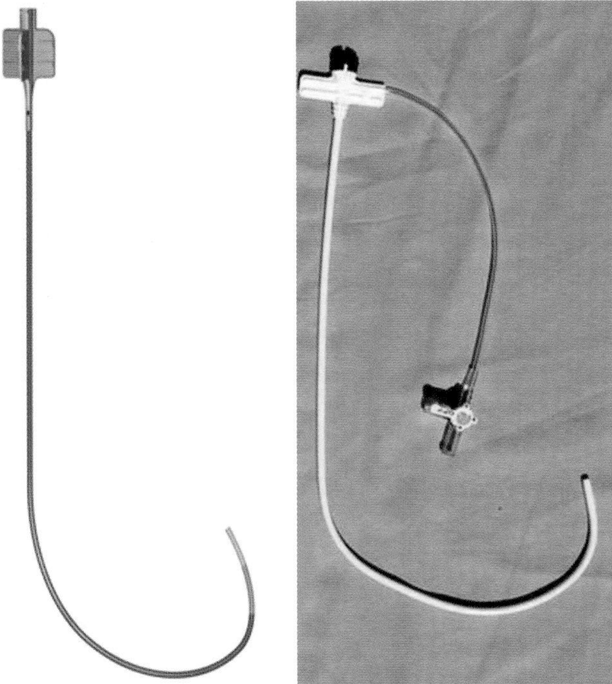

Figure 15.3 RapidO (left panel) shape as compared to the SafeSheathCSG (right panel) demonstrating the different curves. The RapidO curve is designed to anchor off the superior vena cava as compared to the SafeSheathCSG, which is designed to anchor off the lateral right atrium.

pulling back from the tricuspid annulus, however, it may be less stable in larger atria.

The CS ostium: difficult anatomy

The two most common anatomic variants that make it difficult to locate and cannulate the CS include a high or atypical ostium and an enlarged right atrium. Use of a contrast mapping, especially with a proximally curved guide, is often able to delineate atypical origins of the CS. Often, a high ostium will require walking the guide along the RA wall using intermittent injections of contrast. Though patients with this type of anatomic variants often require more contrast than those without, direct visualization of the CS opening provides the operator a target to direct the guide (either by adding or removing torque). Additionally, contrast will provide more information on how coaxial the guide is oriented within the CS OS for further advancement.

The presence of a large right atrium presents a challenge for both approaches, as both sheaths require a far enough reach to engage the OS. Using the electrically guided approach, the amount of curve at the end of the EP catheter can be adjusted by the operator, but in larger atriums, the location of the curve may be too distal. When using contrast-based approaches in large right atria, the sheath is often unable to cross the tricuspid valve into the right ventricle. The sheath then flails aimlessly within the right atria. One possible solution is to place a guidewire into the ventricle and then advance the sheath over the guidewire into the ventricle. Once in the ventricle, the sheath is more directable, and may be able to reach the CS OS. Also, there are several sheaths designed specifically for large right atria. These sheaths have a larger, gentler curve than standard sheaths providing the reach needed in these atria. Stability is another concern with large atria. Without sufficient stability, the force needed to advance an inner catheter or even the lead may force the entire sheath out into the atria dragging its contents with it. Though larger curves are available, consideration must be made as to the anchoring point of the sheath. Guides that use the RA/superior vena cava junction for the proximal curve anchor point are designed to angle up into the CS. Though this makes reaching the CS easier, it may not provide stability when advancing a catheter or lead. In contrast, the guides whose curve is designed to anchor against the lateral wall of the right atria provide excellent stability during advancement of the lead. However, in these guides, RA size/sheath match may be more of a concern. Usually, larger curved sheaths are required for patients with chronic atrial fibrillation.

CS Venography

Once the CS guide is placed within the CS, venography may be performed. Though occlusive venography is not always performed it is useful in delineating target veins (origin and destination), valves, strictures, collateral connections, and other specific anatomic details that permit optimal placement of LV pacing leads. The preferred approach to coronary venography utilizes a 4–6 French catheter inserted through the guide and positioned anywhere along the course of the CS for injection of contrast with or without occluding CS blood flow. The commonly used venographic catheter is relatively stiff 4–6 French, with a single injection lumen, and an inflatable balloon located about 1 cm from the tip. Balloon inflation blocks blood flow into the right atrium, and permits contrast visualization of the entire venous tree directly, or indirectly through collateral venous channels. The risks of balloon venography include dissection, venous rupture, allergic reaction to contrast, and contrast nephrotoxicity in patients with renal insufficiency [3]. Use of low-pressure injection and dilution of the contrast with saline are other means by which complications may be reduced. Other precautions include careful avoidance of over inflating the balloon in a CS or branch with small diameter to prevent vessel rupture during injection. However, failure to visualize all the venous branches may produce suboptimal localization of the LV lead.

Image projections

Documenting a "roadmap" of the venous structure in at least two radiographic planes usually provides sufficient information to evaluate the course of the CS and its branches. Two views, with at least one in the LAO projection usually demonstrates all the possible cardiac venous targets, the site at which each LV vein enters into the CS, and the course of each vein and its tributaries. The standard LAO view (usually 30–45°) will demonstrate which vessels course to the posterior and lateral walls of the LV. The anterior–posterior (AP) projection removes overlap of the anterior–septal and anterior–lateral veins that can be seen in the right anterior oblique (RAO) projection. Adding a slight cranial or caudal angulation may help delineate the origin of the lateral branches off the CS. The LAO view usually foreshortens the view of the body of the tributary vein. Therefore, a venogram in another view permits precise localization in the subbranches for positioning and also reduces radiation exposure to the operator by avoiding the LAO projection. Fluoroscopy in the AP or RAO 15–30° projection best visualizes the course of LV veins from the CS to the apex of the ventricle. The LAO view facilitates entry into the cardiac vein from the CS; the AP or RAO guides advancement within the LV vein to the target site. Extending the fluoroscopic acquisition for a few seconds after contrast injection allows time for the contrast to reach all venous tributaries through collateral flow. Opacification of collaterals to posterior and posterior–lateral LV veins demonstrates potential target veins that would otherwise go unnoticed during injection of contrast beyond the point at which those veins enter the CS. Normal physiology dictates that all of the LV myocardium requires venous drainage. The inability to identify venous drainage from a large segment of the LV implies that venography failed to detect either the tributary from that segment, collateral flow from one segment to a vein draining an adjacent segment, or that failure to occlude the CS led to suboptimal contrast injection. Failure to utilize venography to guide LV lead implant can diminish the chance of a successful implant. One may fortuitously find LV veins without performing a venogram simply by probing for CS tributaries with a guidewire. However, the advantages of proper venography may outweigh its risks to the patient.

Cardiac venous anatomy

Cardiac venous anatomy varies greatly, perhaps more so than the anatomy of coronary arteries. We would classify LV venous drainage into four general types based upon the site along the mitral annulus where the posterior, posterior–lateral, and lateral LV veins enter the CS. The course of the anterior cardiac vein around the anterior aspect of the intraventricular groove and the aortic root follows a fairly consistent pattern in most individuals. The angle at which LV veins enter the CS varies greatly, ranging from very shallow (120–160°) to very acute angles (30–60°) with respect to the CS (Figure 15.4). The most acute angles of entry usually occur along the lateral and high-lateral CS, with the less acute angles usually along the posterolateral aspect of the atrioventricular groove. Superimposing a clock over the mitral annulus facilitates a nomenclature to describe the anatomic site where LV veins enter the CS as viewed by fluoroscopy at LAO 45°. The suggested nomenclature assigns the 7 o'clock position to the CS ostium and 11 o'clock to the junction of the anterior wall and septum.

The most commonly encountered coronary venous drainage pattern parallels the typical left-dominant coronary artery anatomy. The posterior

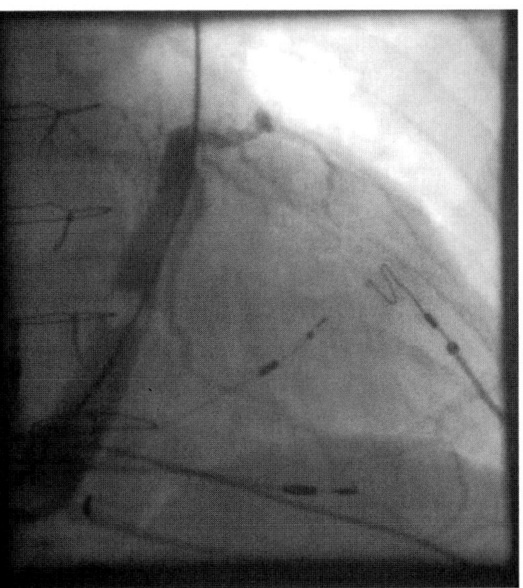

Figure 15.4 Demonstrating the angle of entry of the target LV vein into the CS is crucial to successful lead insertion. Entry of LV veins into the CS at acute angles present obstacles to LV lead insertion. The presence of strictures calls for selection of alternate veins or venoplasty to open access through obstructed veins. (Used by permission of Ellenbogen, KA, Kay, GN, and Wilkoff, BL, 2004.)

interventricular vein enters the CS within 1–2 cm of the ostium (6 o'clock). Occasionally, the posterior interventricular vein enters the RA through what appears to be a separate ostium. The posterior interventricular vein courses below the intraventricular septum, and often receives divisions draining the posterior and lateral segment of the LV. The posterior vein enters the CS near the point where the CS begins its upward course along the free-wall aspect of the mitral annulus (4–5 o'clock). The lateral vein usually enters the CS near the midpoint of the free wall of the LV (2–3 o'clock). The CS becomes the great cardiac vein as it courses across the anterior mitral annulus and around the aortic root (12 o'clock) before descending over the intraventricular septum toward the cardiac apex as the anterior cardiac vein. As the anterior cardiac vein courses to the apex, the anterolateral vein draining the high-lateral LV free-wall enters into the upper segment of the anterior cardiac vein. Injection of contrast at the lateral CS may not demonstrate any lateral vein draining the lateral LV wall. In this situation, collateral flow usually reveals the presence of a large posterolateral vein with divisions that parallel the CS slightly below the atrioventricular groove, and serve as venous drainage of the LV free-wall. This type of posterolateral vein may have a number of posterior–lateral and lateral divisions not seen during brief injections within the CS that also travel up the mid-lateral wall of the LV. Contrast injection through a catheter selectively inserted into the posterolateral vein trunk demonstrates all the possible divisions of the trunk that can serve as target veins. Occasionally, a single trunk may leave the CS at or near the 3 o'clock position and give superior and inferior divisions that serve as the lateral vein, posterolateral vein, and anterolateral vein (Figure 15.5).

Rarely, one may encounter a variety of anomalous CS and LV venous patterns including persistent left superior vena cavae that drain directly into the CS, persistent anterior drainage from the great cardiac vein to the RA, and multiple veins draining the LV at any one segment along the CS.

An anatomic description of coronary venous anatomy based upon flow through the vessel designates the proximal end of the vein as that near the capillary bed, with the distal portion entering the CS. Any coronary vein may demonstrate tortuous segments or multiple points of confluence along its course to the CS. The most distal segments of the veins, as they enter the CS, usually contain the most

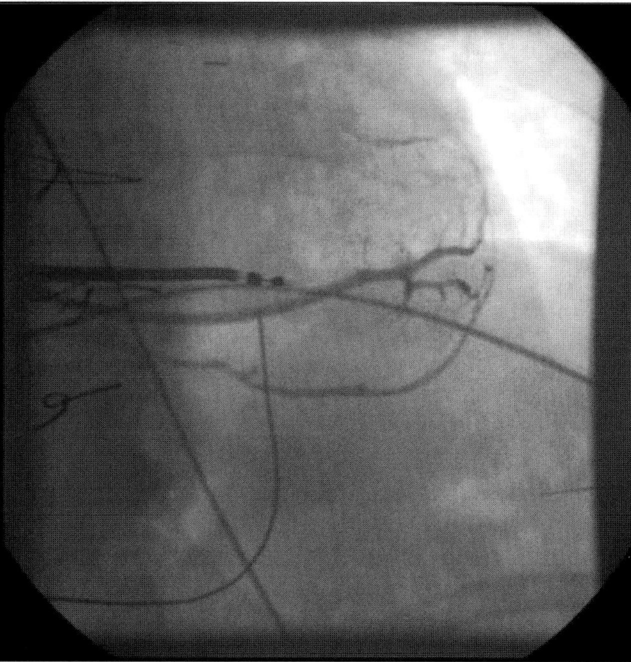

Figure 15.5 A large posterolateral venous trunk enters the CS and drains the large aspect of the LV free-wall. Absence of any lateral or anterolateral veins should herald the presence of such a posterolateral trunk. Proper positioning of the venogram balloon should demonstrate this access point to the lateral LV veins. (Used by permission of Ellenbogen, KA, Kay, GN, and Wilkoff, BL, 2004.)

tortuous segments. The proximal segments, near the ventricular apex, show confluence of small veins to form the main vein as it approaches the atrioventricular groove. The diameter of LV veins also varies from barely visible small veins to a large posterolateral vein or lateral vein with a diameter exceeding 4 mm. Venography often uncovers extensive collateral channels that connect the posterior interventricular vein, posterolateral vein, lateral vein, and anterolateral veins. The extent of collateral circulation in the venous circulation greatly exceeds that observed in coronary arteries. One may frequently pass a guidewire from the posterolateral vein to the anterolateral vein through one of the channels. The presence of rich collateral connections between the main LV veins produces greater access to potential pacing sites along the LV from different LV veins along the CS. The ability to use collateral veins to reach a desired pacing site may salvage an otherwise unsuccessful implant, when anatomic barriers prevent antegrade insertion of a pacing lead to the desired site.

Subselection and lead advancement

After engaging the CS OS with the guide, it should be advanced 2–3 cm into the CS. This allows sufficient stability for passage of the balloon angiography catheter, directable catheter, or even the lead itself into the CS. When using the electrical mapping system, the EP catheter is advanced into the CS first and the guide is advanced over the catheter that is subsequently removed. However, when using contrast mapping, the guide is first advanced into the right ventricle, turned counterclockwise while pulling back into the atrium near the OS of the CS. Using small puffs of contrast, the CS OS is identified and the guide is directly advanced into the CS ~2–3 cm. Valves either near the ostium of the CS (Thebesian valve) or well within the CS (valve of Vieussens) may obstruct proper entry of the guide catheter.

The Thebesian valve forms a flap-like cover over the CS OS and represents the posterior extension of the Eustachian ridge. A large Thebesian valve may prevent the guide catheter from engaging or entering the CS OS. Because of the direction and placement of this valve, approaching the ostium from the superior aspect of the RA makes CS placement more difficult. The Eustachian ridge acts like a roof, covering the entry to the CS from above. Approaching the CS with the guide catheter pointing up and posterior from the floor of the RA often avoids the obstruction created by the valve. The valve of Vieussens, commonly found near the site of entry of the posterolateral LV vein into the CS, interferes with proper advancement of the guide, catheter, wire, or lead into the CS. When encountering a valve of Vieussens, crossing the valve with a 0.035" guidewire may open the valve and allow catheter advancement without damage to the valve and potential dissection.

A small-diameter guidewire (0.025 mm) may be advanced through the balloon venogram catheter deep into the CS. The balloon catheter may then be advanced across strictures, curves, or valves found in the CS. Cautious advancement is essential regardless of methodology, in that forcing a guide catheter, wire, or mapping catheter into a valve can tear or perforate the CS. When resistance is met during advancement, injection of a small amount of contrast can reveal the presence of a valve, stricture, or kink in the vessel. Defining the cause of the obstruction allows the implanter to select a coated wire, a 0.025" guidewire, or an inner telescoping catheter to aide in crossing the obstruction. Desired position of the catheter within the CS is when its tip advances to the lateral aspect of the CS. A small injection of 2–3 cc of contrast through the catheter confirms the position, and detects any mural trauma or dissection. This test injection aids in ruling out a small tear or dissection of the CS prior to full injection thus reducing the probability of injecting a large contrast load into the extravascular space.

Once your guide is in ideal position and contrast venogram has demonstrated a target posterior or lateral branch, it must be decided if a wire can be advanced into the branch and distal to an ideal location. Ideally, an angioplasty wire is easily shaped and advanced into and distal within the target vein. Either the guide can be advanced over the wire or the actual LV lead can be loaded onto the wire and advanced through the guide and into the target location over the wire. This is the clear advantage of using a directional guide with a large enough inner diameter that allows for direct lead placement. If the angle into the lateral branch is too acute or if the vein is tortuous a directing catheter can be advanced through the guide. This catheter has a smaller inner diameter through which only the wire can pass. However, the variety of angles of the catheter allow for the wire to pass much easier around sharp bends. These catheters, when advanced over the wire into the lateral branch, provide stability. This stability allows for the guide to then be advanced into the lateral branch. The inner/directing catheter can be removed and the lead then placed over the wire into the lateral branch directly.

These inner/directing catheters are too small to allow for lead passage but do allow for a wire to be passed and placed within the lateral branch. The exchange of this catheter for the lead adds an additional step, but the shapes of these inner catheters allow for easier reach of many branches. Additionally, it provides the support needed to advance the guide into venous tributaries that branch off the CS. Once the guide has subselected the branch, the lead can be advanced into position and the system removed. Lead selection and choosing ideal positioning will be discussed in a later chapter.

Future venographic techniques

One of the most frustrating aspects of LV epicardial lead placement in the cardiac venous drainage system is the inability to plan the procedure due to the extreme variability in the venous anatomy. Perhaps the most promising technique in this regard is the use of Multislice CT imaging to preoperatively define the cardiac veins. The same techniques employed to define the coronary arteries, potentially a future replacement for invasive coronary angiography, are beginning to be use to preoperatively image the cardiac veins. Imaging with 16-slice imaging techniques have been used to define the size, length, angle of take off, and most importantly the presence or absence of veins in the posterior and lateral walls of the left ventricle [4]. With the advent of 40 and 64 slice imaging systems, diagnostic quality images can be obtained with 30 cc of angiographic dye given through a peripheral vein and with 5–10 s breath holds (Figure 15.6). It seems likely that patients without promising veins in the appropriate territory would be sent directly for surgical epicardial placement.

Alternatively, percutaneous epicardial lead placement via a subxiphoid pericardial needle puncture is likely to become a more flexible and powerful technique. This type of access, first described in Brazil by Dr Sosa for ablation of tachyarrhythmias, described by Dr Schweikert and Dr Natale in Chapter 25 in this text, is under development for permanent pacemaker lead placement [5, 6]. It seems likely that not only LV pacing leads, but RV, RA and LA, and potentially defibrillation leads could be placed using this technique. Perhaps,

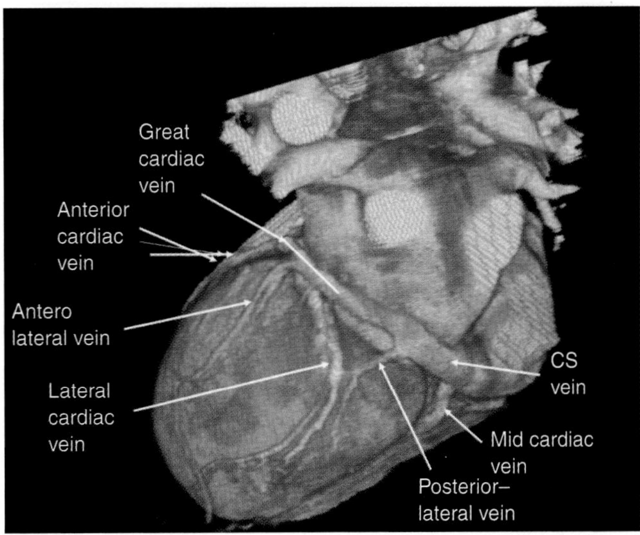

Figure 15.6 Labeled view of the epicardial cardiac veins obtained by surface rendered 16 slice CT scan of the heart after 100 cc of radiographic dye administration.

this will be a technique for failed transvenous attempts, for patients without targets visualized by multislice CT or potentially due to flexibility of lead placement as a primary technique for most patients.

Conclusion

In summary, the indications for implementation of biventricular pacing systems have increased dramatically in the United States. They have been proven to be effective in treating many of the symptoms of congestive heart failure. Placement of the LV pacing leads can be difficult and complex. Although the technology continues to improve, many cases remain challenging. Many factors contribute to this complexity including difficulty accessing the CS or variable coronary venous anatomy. Physicians implanting these devices should be familiar with various techniques and tools used to overcome these obstacles. A systematic approach to implanting biventricular pacing systems will improve success rates and procedural times. Fortunately, as the number of these device implants increase, technology will improve and expand as well.

References

1 Worley S, Leon A, Wilkoff BL. Anatomy and implantation techniques for biventricular devices. In: Ellenbogen KA, Kay GN, Wilkoff BL eds. *Device Therapy for Congestive Heart Failure*, Philadelphia, PA, WB Saunders, 2004; 118–231.

2 De Martino G, Sanna T, Dello Russo A *et al.* A randomized comparison of alternative techniques to achieve coronary sinus cannulation during biventricular implantation procedures. *J Interv Card Electrophysiol* 2004; **10**(3): 227–230.

3 Parfrey PS, Griffiths SM, Barrett BY *et al.* Contrast material-induced renal failure in patients with diabetes mellitus, renal insufficiency, or both: a prospective controlled study. *N Engl J Med* 1989; **320**(3): 43–49.

4 Sun JP, Greenberg NL, Grimm RA *et al.* Coronary venous anatomy by computed tomography in cardiac resynchronization therapy. *Circulation* 2004; **110**: 17, 1783.

5 Sosa E, Scanavacca M, d'Avila A, Pilleggi F. A new technique to perform epicardial mapping in the electrophysiology laboratory. *J Cardiovasc Electrophysiol* 1996; **7**(6): 531–536.

6 Schweikert RA, Saliba WI, Tomassoni G *et al.* Percutaneous pericardial instrumentation for endo-epicardial mapping of previously failed ablations. *Circulation* 2003; **108**(11): 1329–1335.

16

CHAPTER 16

New resynchronization lead systems and devices

Robert F. Rea, MD

Cardiac resynchronization therapy (CRT) used adjunctively with appropriate medical therapy provides additional improvement in congestive heart failure (CHF) symptoms and, in some studies, improved mortality especially when CRT capability is combined with an implantable defibrillator [1, 2]. For patients to realize the potential benefits of this therapy, however, the surgical procedure must be low risk and the delivery site of left ventricular (LV) pacing stable, anatomically appropriate, and free from extracardiac stimulation. In addition, the pulse generator must incorporate unique timing algorithms to maximize the percentage of time that LV pacing is delivered even in the face of irregular underlying native rhythms. Since even the most advanced pulse generator is useless without the ability to pace the LV correctly, I will start this review with a discussion of LV leads. I will then review changes in pulse generator technology. Finally, I will briefly discuss some emerging pacing technologies designed to improve CHF symptoms.

LV lead implantation success rates

Early in the cardiac resynchronization era, standard right ventricular (RV) pacing leads were placed in coronary veins. In some but not all cases, CS delivery guides were utilized. With the subsequent development of a dedicated LV pacing lead (Medtronic, model 2187) that had a more flexible curved distal segment LV lead implant times decreased by about 38% (Medtronic, unpublished data).

In the MIRACLE Trial [3], Medtronic model 2187 or 2188 LV pacing leads were used (Figure 16.1). These are both stylet driven leads; the 2187 is

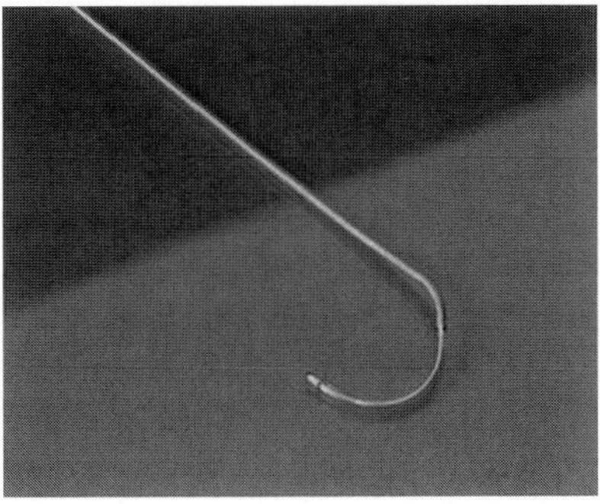
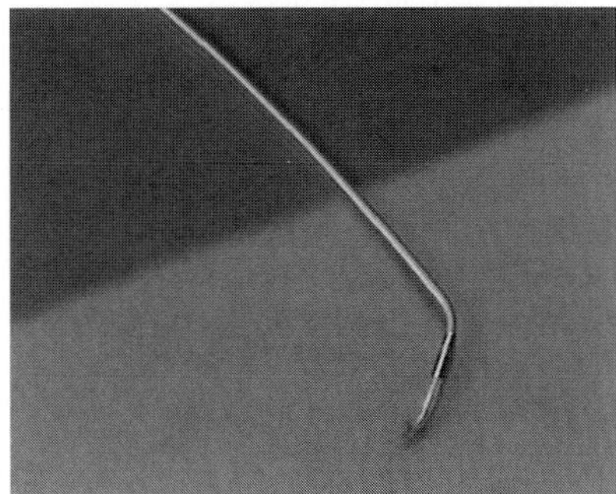

Figure 16.1 Medtronic 2187 (left) and 2188 (right) unipolar leads for LV pacing (Reproduced with permission from Medtronic).

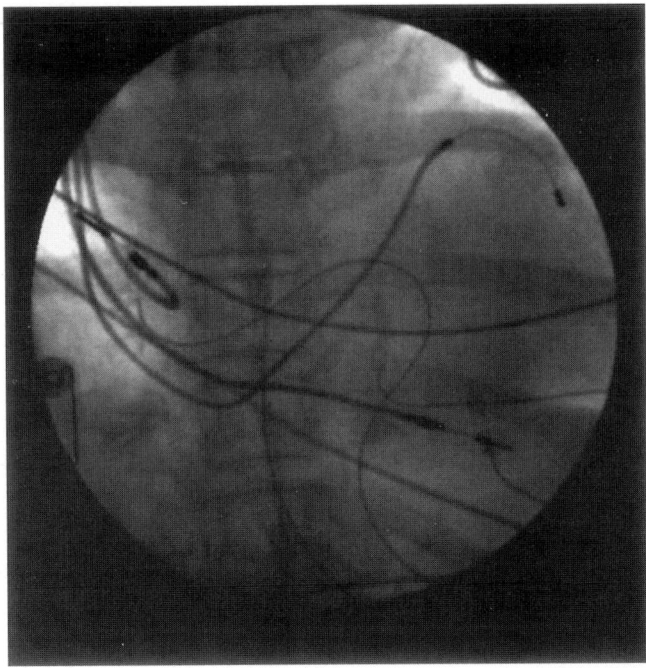

Figure 16.2 Left anterior oblique fluoroscopic image of a Medtronic 2187 lead positioned in a lateral coronary vein.

7 French size and the 2188 is 9 French. Important to implanters was the fact that the 2188 lead could not be passed though the coronary sinus (CS) guiding sheath supplied with the device/leads combination (which were investigational at the time). Other CS guides were in development at that time and not readily available.

Successful LV lead placement was achieved in 92% of patients. With the model 2187 lead, however, there was an 8% dislodgement rate. Extracardiac stimulation, typically phrenic nerve, resulted in lead repositioning in 2% and device reprogramming in 0.5%. Figure 16.2 shows fluoroscopy of a 2187 lead in a relatively proximal portion of a lateral coronary vein.

In a subsequent study of CRT pacing (Medtronic InSync III), an over-the-wire LV lead model 4193 was used. This is a 6.2 French lead through which an angioplasty wire can be passed (Figure 16.3). This smaller caliber lead can be threaded over the angioplasty wire into small and more distal tributaries of the coronary venous system as shown in Figure 16.4. Overall successful LV lead implant was achieved in 95% of patients. And, as hoped, with the over-the-wire technology the dislodgement rate of 3.4% was significantly lower than with the larger stylet-driven 2187 lead (8%). Extracardiac stimulation, however, required repositioning in 0.8% or reprogramming (or turning off of LV output) in 8.8% (Medtronic, unpublished data).

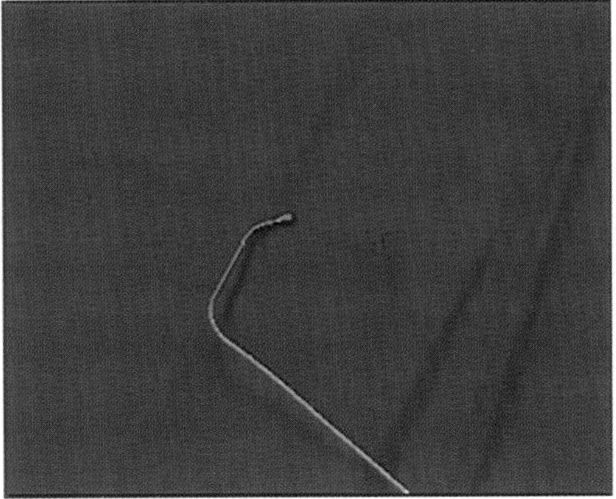

Figure 16.3 Medtronic 4193 over-the-wire LV pacing lead (Reproduced with permission from Medtronic).

The contrasting successes and limitations of these two types of leads illustrate an important consideration in LV lead design. More proximally located larger diameter leads may dislodge more frequently but as they do not pass close to the more distally located phrenic nerve they produce extracardiac stimulation less frequently.

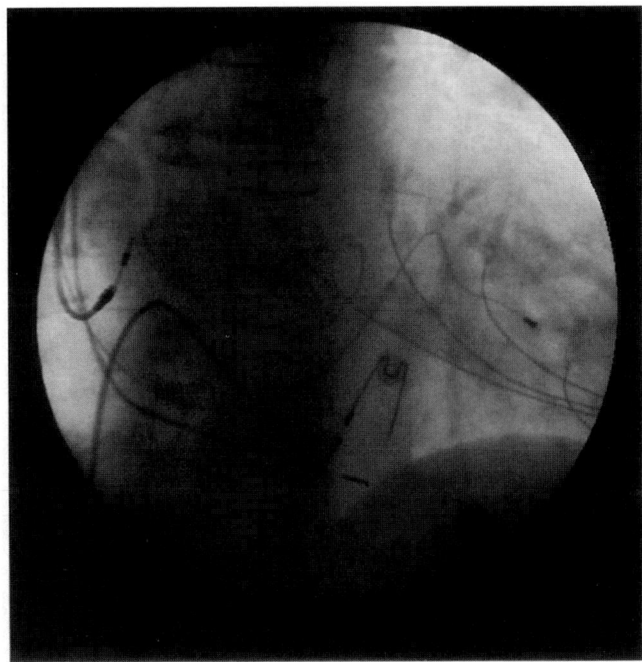

Figure 16.4 Left anterior oblique fluoroscopic image of a Medtronic 4193 lead positioned in a lateral coronary vein. See text for discussion.

Newer LV lead design

The ability to pass leads substantially more distally and in smaller and angulated vein tributaries has provided operators with more options in terms of lead placement. This flexibility was recognized as increasingly important as a substantial number of patients failed to derive clinical benefit from CRT devices [4]. Early acute hemodynamic studies employing epicardial LV lead placement [5] suggested that the mid-lateral to posterolateral LV provided the best. Subsequent studies using tissue-Doppler measurements of myocardial contraction have shown that highly targeted LV lead placement in regions of greatest dyssynchronous contraction [4, 6] may be required for optimal clinical effect. It was also recognized that prolongation of the QRS interval, a criterion for enrollment in all major randomized trials, might be a relatively blunt instrument for discerning potential responders to CRT [7]. These observations led to increasingly more critical approach to positioning of the LV lead. Along with this it was recognized that alternative approaches to the problem of extracardiac stimulation were needed.

Since coronary vein leads do not have myocardial trabeculae in which to lodge, many manufacturers have relied on shaping of the distal portion of the lead for fixation.

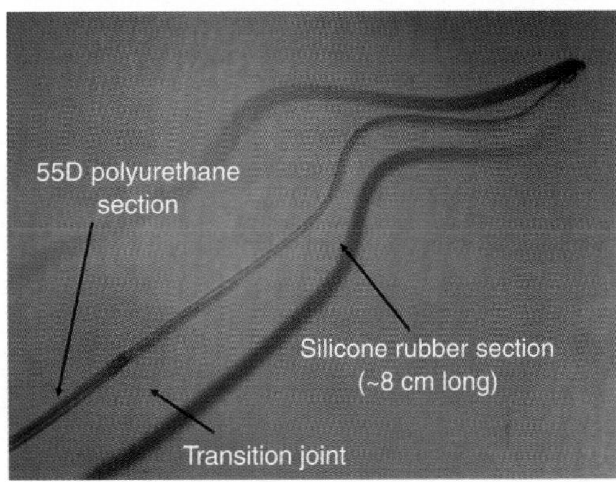

Figure 16.5 St. Jude Medical model 1056K LV pacing lead. See text for discussion (Reproduced with permission from St. Jude Medical).

The St. Jude model 1056K LV lead (Figure 16.5) has a 5.6 French polyurethane body and a 5.0 French silicone distal portion. It is a unipolar lead with an IS-1 connecting pin. For stabilization with the coronary vein the tip is S-shaped and designed prop itself on opposite walls of the vein of interest. Currently, a bipolar version of this lead is under investigation.

The Guidant Easytrak 3 (Figure 16.6) has a 6.0 French polyurethane body and a 5.7 French silicone distal portion. After removal of the guidewire or stylet, it develops a helical terminal portion with the intent of "bunching-up" in the coronary vein. The Guidant Easytrak 2 (Figure 16.7) has a 6.0 French polyurethane body and a 5.4 French silicone distal portion and is a straight lead. Two important changes were introduced in the Easytrak 2 and 3. First, the larger distal diameter of these leads (the first Easytrak was 4.5 French at the tip) was developed in part to allow more proximal lead stabilization in the coronary vein. Second, the two new leads are bipolar. In conjunction with the Renewal pulse generator this permits programming of LV output polarity so as to minimize the likelihood of extracardiac stimulation. LV pacing options are shown in Figure 16.8. Two dedicated bipolar and two extended bipolar configurations are programmable. Combined with independently programmable RV and LV outputs this feature provides a number of options for software-based solutions to extracardiac stimulation.

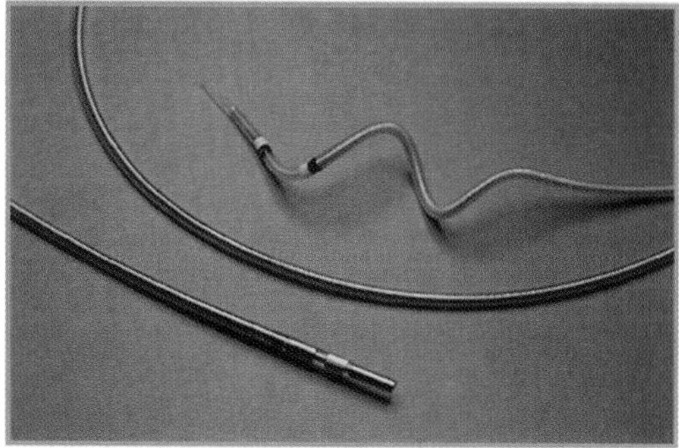

Figure 16.6 Guidant Easytrak 3 LV pacing lead. See text for discussion (Reproduced with permission from Guidant).

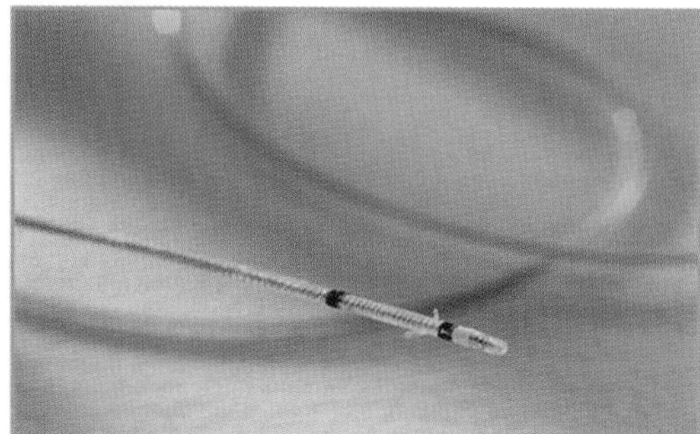

Figure 16.7 Guidant Easytrak 2 LV pacing lead. See text for discussion (Reproduced with permission from Guidant).

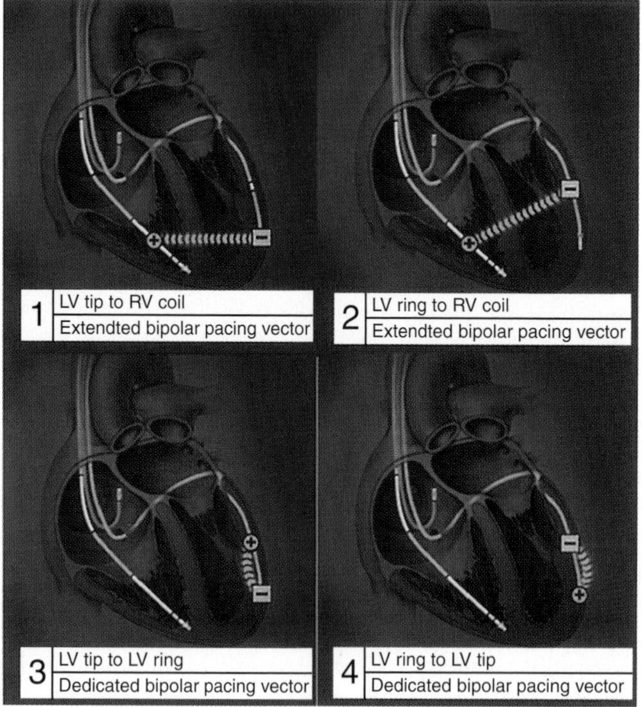

Figure 16.8 Diagram illustrating how LV pacing configuration may be programmed in Guidant CRT devices (Reproduced with permission from Guidant).

Medtronic has recently introduced the 4194 lead for LV pacing. It has a 6.2 French body tapering to a 5.4 French tip (Figure 16.9). Like the new Easytrak leads it has the capability for bipolar pacing. Different, however, is the construction of the proximal electrode as shown in Figure 16.10. It is a coil rather than an annular electrode and has a substantial (38 mm^2) surface area. This lead in conjunction with current Medtronic CRT-P and CRT-D devices offers programmable LV output polarities and configurations. ELA has an LV lead (Situs UW28D) under investigation in the United States that uses a novel endovascular stabilization mechanism (Figure 16.11). The 5 French lead body has a silicone "screw" applied to the lead that increases the external diameter initially to 7 French. The Situs UC28D (Figure 16.12) has two turns in the distal lead body, a steroid eluting ring electrode and a less than circumferential more distal ring electrode designed to stimulate the epicardial LV musculature. At the tip is an angulated silicone "horn" designed to aid in lead stabilization.

Features of new resynchronization devices

Programmable V–V timing

Available earlier in CRT pacemakers and now being released in CRT defibrillators is the ability to deliver pacing impulses to the RV and LV sequentially, rather than simultaneously. In a small observational study, improved tissue-Doppler indices of resynchronization and echocardiographic estimates of ejection fraction have been demonstrated with RV–LV timing offset with some suggestion that the etiology of heart failure may play a role in choice of RV versus LV preactivation [8]. In another study [9], stroke volume determined from the aortic velocity time integral was maximized by changing RV–LV impulse timing. With a V–V delay of ±40 ms, stroke volume was maximized at discharge. At 3 month follow-up, the optimized V–V timing was nearly the same in 27 of 34 patients indicating relative stability of the initial programming. LV was preactivated in 21 of

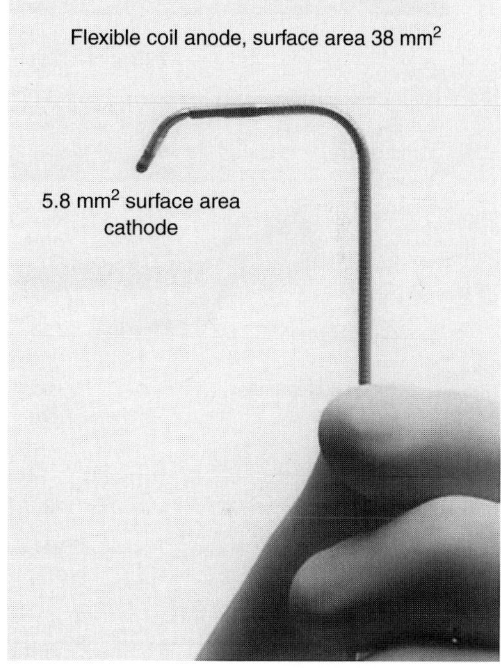

Figure 16.9 Medtronic 4194 LV bipolar pacing lead (Reproduced with permission from Medtronic).

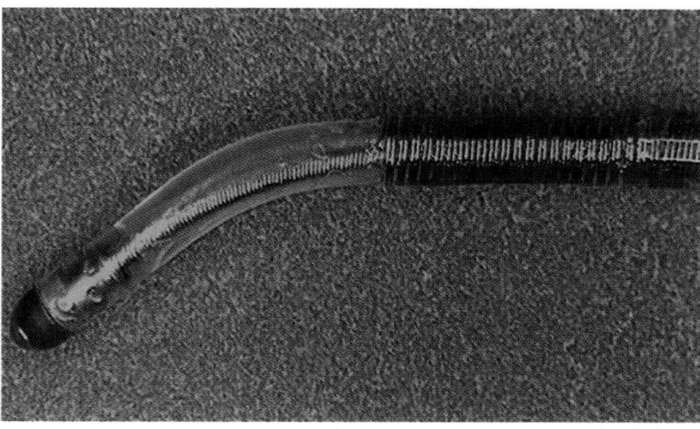

Figure 16.10 Close-up view of Medtronic 4194 lead showing detail of proximal coil electrode (Reproduced with permission from Medtronic).

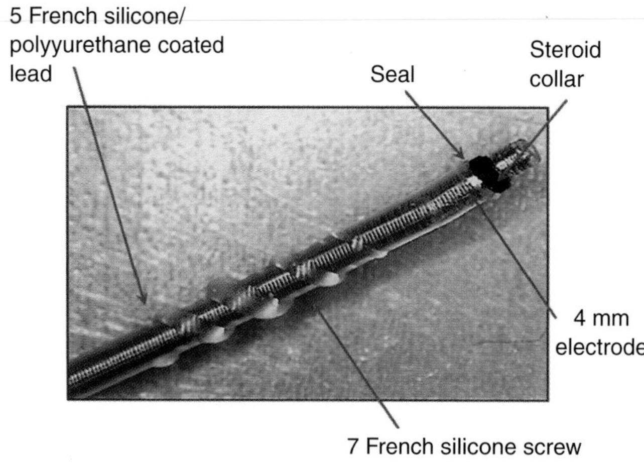

Figure 16.11 ELA Situs UW28D LV pacing lead (investigational in the United States). See text for discussion (Reprinted with permission from ELA).

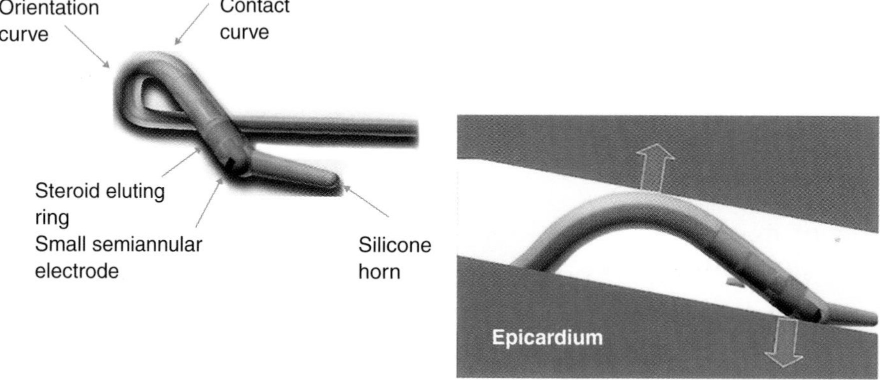

Figure 16.12 ELA Situs UC28D LV pacing lead (investigational). See text for discussion (Reprinted with permission from ELA).

34 patients at discharge and 17 of 34 at the 3 month follow-up. Despite this there was no discernible change in clinical status between patients that did and did not undergo V–V timing optimization in this small sample size. The exact mechanism by which this effect is achieved is unclear but likely reflects optimization of LA–LV activation time. Further study is warranted especially with deliberate pacing of the right atrium, as interatrial conduction times vary with spontaneous and paced atrial rhythms depending on atrial lead location.

Maximizing biventricular pacing

In a pacemaker clinic, providers are typically pleased if an implanted device is utilized minimally as this improves battery longevity. And in the case of DDD/R pacers and ICDs there is an increasing trend toward minimizing the amount of time the RV is paced so as to minimize device-related dyssynchrony. With CRT devices the opposite is the case: any situation that results in less than ~90% delivery of synchronizing pacing (biventricular or LV) can be deleterious.

Ventricular ectopic beats can potentially interfere with biventricular pacing by simple inhibition of pacing output as is seen in VVI/DDD pacers and ICDs. In many CRT devices, however, a sensed ventricular event can initiate right-left or biventricular pacing outputs (programmable) in an attempt to maintain synchronous ventricular activation. Another mechanism by which ventricular ectopic beats may interfere with delivery of CRT is shown in Figure 16.13. In a standard pacemaker, a premature

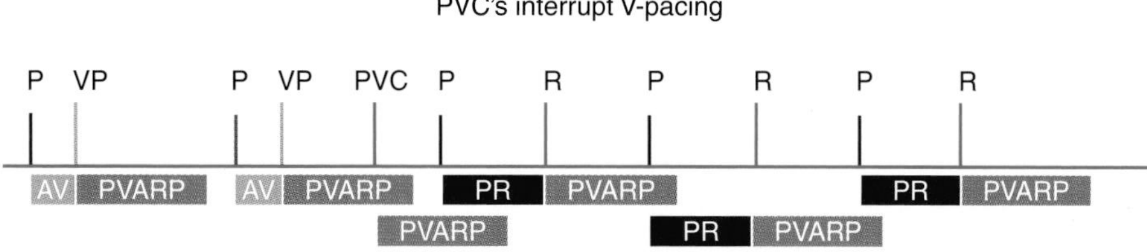

Figure 16.13 Diagram illustrating how a premature ventricular contraction (PVC) can interfere with delivery of ventricular pacing. P = sensed atrial event; R = sensed ventricular event; PR = P-R interval; VP = ventricular paced event; PVARP = postventricular atrial refractory period.

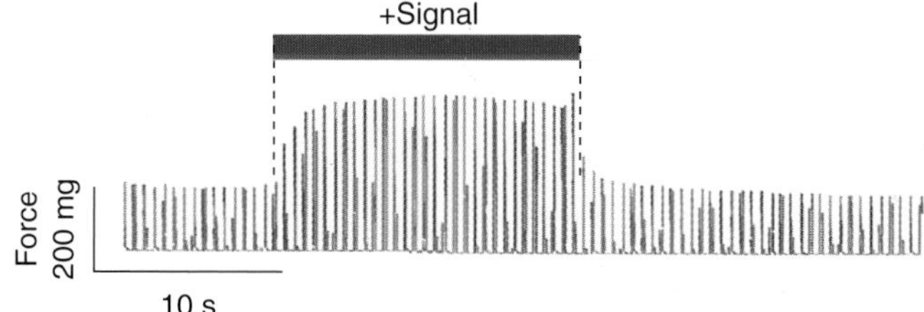

Figure 16.14 Illustration of the effect of cardiac contractility modulating signal on force generated in isolated heart muscle. During delivery of the signal, force generated per impulse more than doubles (Reprinted with permission from Dan Burkho, MD, PhD).

ventricular contraction (PVC) initiates extension of the postventricular atrial refractory period (PVARP) so as to minimize the possibility of a pacemaker-mediated tachycardia. This may bring the next sensed atrial event inside the PVARP. This refractory atrial event is not tracked and a conducted rather than paced ventricular event may occur. This could initiate another PVARP that encompasses the next atrial event triggering another conducted ventricular event and so on. To circumvent this problem in many CRT devices, after a programmed number of ventricular sensed events, which follow atrial refractory sensed events, the PVARP is shortened to allow atrial tracking and resume biventricular pacing.

Atrial fibrillation (AF) is common in CRT recipients and conduction of AF to the ventricles above the programmed rate could inhibit delivery of resynchronization therapy. In some patients it may be necessary to prescribe atrioventricular nodal blocking drugs or ablate the conduction system to enable the device to assume control of the ventricles. There are, however, pacing algorithms in current devices that attempt to pace the ventricles slightly faster than the conducted rate. The average ventricular response rate during a mode-switch for AF is calculated over a short time interval. The pacing rate is then adjusted upward until conducted beats are eliminated. When this is achieved, the pacing rate is decreased slightly until conducted beats reemerge. The rate is then adjusted upward slightly once again. With this iterative algorithm the pacemaker may assume substantial control of the ventricles even during relatively rapidly conducted AF and help to ensure consistent delivery of CRT.

Cardiac contractility modulation

A novel and currently investigational approach to improving cardiac contractility with pacing is referred to as cardiac contractility modulation (CCM). The concept behind the device is illustrated in Figure 16.14. In isolated heart muscle, subthreshold stimuli increase the force of contraction, an effect which likely is a dependent on calcium ion flux [10].

Whereas available devices for resynchronization depend on leads that pace the left ventricle, with the CCM device subthreshold stimulation pulses are delivered to the septal aspect of the right ventricle. Lead positions are shown in Figure 16.15. Two RV leads are placed; one is directed

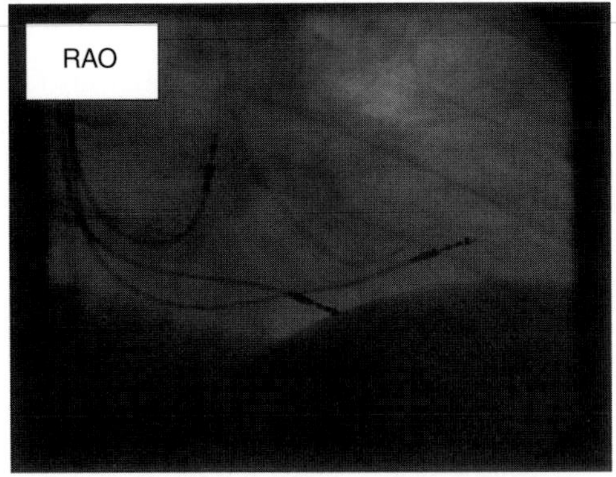

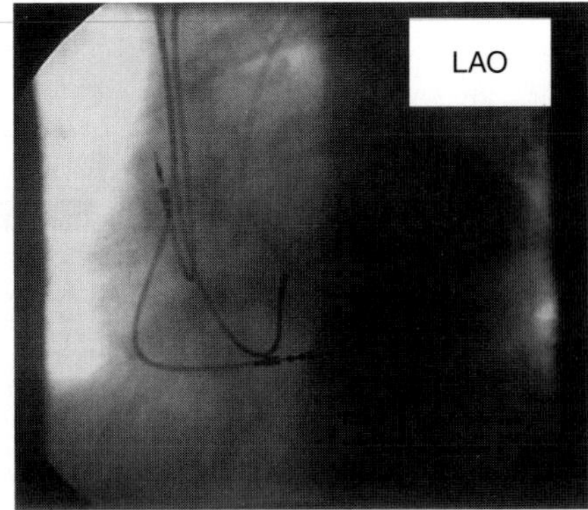

Figure 16.15 Right anterior oblique (RAO) and left anterior oblique (LAO) images of location of leads for delivery of cardiac contractility modulating signal. Note separation of the two leads and the course of the septal RV lead (lateral to medial) (Reprinted with permission from Impulse Dynamics).

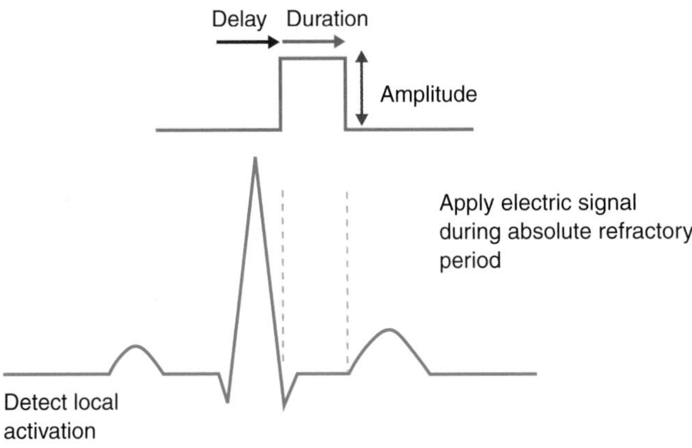

Figure 16.16 Timing of delivery of CCM signals. See text for discussion (Reprinted with permission from Dan Burkhoff, MD, PhD).

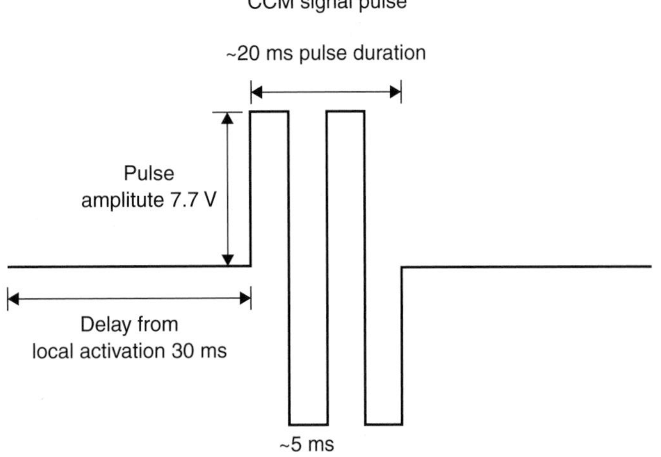

Figure 16.17 Diagram of cardiac contractility modulating signals. Note the large amplitude and prolonged duration of the pulse (Reprinted with permission from Dan Burkhoff, MD, PhD).

into the septum for delivery of the CCM pulses and the other is located a distance away for sensing. Pulses are delivered during the absolute refractory period in order to avoid local capture as shown in Figure 16.16. And as shown in Figure 16.17, the pulses are of substantial amplitude and duration. Since this results in a large current drain, the device is programmed to deliver the pacing therapy for a limited number of hours each day. It was considered that this therapy might be delivered via an LV epicardial lead but this resulted in patient discomfort likely as a result of stimulation of epicardial nociceptors with the large amplitude long duration pulses.

Despite the fact that the impulses are delivered to the septum it appears that global LV function is improved and preliminary data from investigational implants in Europe is encouraging. In the United States, the device is early in its investigational phase.

References

1 Bradley DJ, Bradley EA, Baughman KL *et al.* Cardiac resynchronization and death from progressive heart failure: a meta-analysis of randomized controlled trials. *JAMA* 2003; **289**(6): 730–740.

2 Bristow MR, Saxon LA, Boehmer J *et al.* Cardiac-resynchronization therapy with or without an implantable defibrillator in advanced chronic heart failure. *N Engl J Med* 2004; **350**(21): 2140–2150.

3 Abraham WT, Fisher WG, Smith AL *et al.* Cardiac resynchronization in chronic heart failure. *N Engl J Med* 2002; **346**(24): 1845–1853.

4 Mehra MR, Greenberg BH. Cardiac resynchronization therapy: caveat medicus! *J Am Coll Cardiol* 2004; **43**(7): 1145–1148.

5 Auricchio A, Stellbrink C, Sack S *et al.* The Pacing Therapies for Congestive Heart Failure (PATH-CHF) study: rationale, design, and endpoints of a prospective randomized multicenter study. *Am J Cardiol* 1999; **83**(5B): 130D–135D.

6 Sogaard P, Hassager C. Tissue Doppler imaging as a guide to resynchronization therapy in patients with congestive heart failure. *Curr Opin Cardiol* 2004; **19**(5): 447–451.

7 Pitzalis MV, Iacoviello M, Romito R *et al.* Cardiac resynchronization therapy tailored by echocardiographic evaluation of ventricular asynchrony. *J Am Coll Cardiol* 2002; **40**(9): 1615–1622.

8 Sogaard P, Egeblad H, Pedersen AK *et al.* Sequential versus simultaneous biventricular resynchronization for severe heart failure: evaluation by tissue Doppler imaging. *Circulation* 2002; **106**(16): 2078–2084.

9 Mortensen PT, Sogaard P, Mansour H *et al.* Sequential biventricular pacing: evaluation of safety and efficacy. *PACE* 2004; **27**(3): 339–345.

10 Burkhoff D, Shemer I, Felzen B *et al.* Electric currents applied during the refractory period can modulate cardiac contractility *in vitro* and *in vivo*. *Heart Fail Rev* 2001; **6**(1): 27–34.

17

CHAPTER 17

New indications for pacing

David L. Hayes, MD

Many times during the evolution of the discipline of cardiac pacing, some experts believed that the ultimate level of pacing technology and sophistication had been reached and that no further advances would be possible. If the technological evolution of cardiac pacing were to cease, it would be unlikely that device indications for this technique would expand; however, the opposite has been realized. Continued advancements in pacing technology have led to broader applicability of the technique, including the development of specialized devices for specific disease states. Cardiac resynchronization therapy (CRT) devices are the best example of a specialized pacing device that has markedly increased the indications for implantable cardiac devices.

This chapter will discuss the potential for current pacing indications to be expanded, newer indications for cardiac pacing and CRT, and how continued sophistication may extend the applicability of existing devices for existing indications.

Broadening of current pacing indications

Several single-center investigations and ongoing trials may affect the current indications for pacing. In the most recent American College of Cardiology/American Heart Association/North American Society of Pacing and Electrophysiology guidelines for pacemakers and implantable cardioverter defibrillators (ICDs) [1], Mobitz I atrioventricular (AV) block is a Class III indication for pacing (i.e. pacing not indicated unless the patient has symptoms secondary to hemodynamic compromise as a result of effective AV dissociation). However, a recent publication reported a decreased survival rate for patients with Mobitz I block who were not paced compared with a group that received permanent pacemakers [2]. Of 147 patients, 61 were believed to have symptoms attributable to bradycardia and 90 patients were paced. At 5 years of follow-up, patients with Mobitz I AV block who were not paced had lower overall mean ± SD survival (53.5% ± 6.7%) than that expected for the general population (68.6%; $p < .001$). Patients with Mobitz I AV block who received pacemakers had better overall mean ± SD 5 year survival (76.3% ± 4.5%) than those not paced (53.5% ± 6.7%; $p = .001$). The investigators concluded that Mobitz I block is associated with morbidity and mortality in patients older than 45 years. On the basis of their results, the investigators suggested that, during clinical assessment, pacemakers should be considered for such patients, even if symptomatic bradycardia or organic heart disease is not present [2]. If this study is validated by others, an expansion of the current guidelines should be considered.

The current pacing guidelines are based on the patient having a symptomatic bradycardia or an asymptomatic rhythm that is thought to place the patient at high risk for developing a potentially symptomatic bradycardia [1]. Two ongoing areas of investigation may expand the current list of cardiogenic symptoms that would indicate the need for pacing, especially in the elderly population. The Syncope and Falls in the Elderly Pacing and Carotid Sinus Evaluation 2 (SAFE PACE 2) [3] study is under way to assess pacing therapy for carotid sinus hypersensitivity (CSH). In the precursor to this study, SAFE PACE 1 [4], nonaccidental falls were strongly associated with cardioinhibitory CSH. The study recommended that patients with CSH be referred for cardiovascular assessment. Falls in these patients previously may have been considered either orthopedic or neurogenic in origin. If SAFE PACE 2 confirms the earlier findings, clinicians must be more alert to falls that occur without clearcut cause and may not currently result in consideration of the patient for pacing therapy.

Bradycardia usually is defined as heart rate <60 beats per minute (bpm); however, clinicians generally do not ascribe symptoms to bradycardia unless the heart rate is <40 bpm. Emerging evidence suggests that less profound bradycardia may be the cause of more diffuse symptoms, such as fatigue, vague dizziness, or light-headedness, in the elderly. The number of candidates for pacemakers might increase considerably if "significant" bradycardia were to be redefined according to the age of the patient.

Pacing for sleep-disordered breathing

Sleep disorders are being diagnosed with increasing frequency and are associated with multiple comorbid conditions in addition to daytime somnolence and fatigue. Systemic and pulmonary hypertension, bradyarrhythmias, tachyarrhythmias, and congestive heart failure (CHF) all have been linked to sleep disorders. An in-depth discussion of sleep disorders is beyond the scope of this text, but many excellent sources exist [5–7]. However, for the purpose of discussing the potential for pacing applications in patients with sleep disorders, the two types of sleep apnea syndrome, "obstructive" and "central" sleep apnea, must be defined. In obstructive sleep apnea, the upper airway is obstructed, with normal central control; in central sleep apnea, hypoventilation is a result of a central (neural) mediation. Some patients may have both types of sleep apnea.

The prevalence of sleep apnea and related disorders appears to be high in patients who are candidates for implantable cardiac devices, especially those who are candidates for CRT. A group of 88 patients with pacemakers or CRT devices who were not known to have sleep apnea were evaluated with polysomnography (PSM). Of the 88 patients, 50 (57%) had sleep-disordered breathing by PSM, including 50% of patients with dilated cardiomyopathy, 63% of patients with AV block, and 58% of patients with sinus node dysfunction [8].

An initial study by Garrigue *et al.* [9] has been the focus of considerable interest in the potential application of pacing in patients with sleep disorders. This study included 15 patients with central or obstructive sleep apnea who had a permanent pacemaker functioning in a P-synchronous ventricular pacing mode. Pacemakers had been implanted for the treatment of symptomatic sinus bradycardia. PSM was performed on three consecutive nights, the first night for baseline evaluation, and, in random order, 1 night each in spontaneous rhythm and dual-chamber pacing mode with atrial overdrive (overdrive was accomplished by programming the device 15 bpm faster than the patient's mean nocturnal sinus rate). In this group of 15 patients with sleep apnea syndrome, the investigators concluded that atrial overdrive pacing significantly decreased the number of episodes of central or obstructive sleep apnea. In addition, they did not observe a significant decrease in total sleep time.

In another small study, investigators compared sleep indices from PSM in patients with DDD pacemakers using either the VVI or the DDD pacing mode [10]. They reported a decrease in sleep disturbance and an improvement in sleep efficacy with the DDD mode compared with the VVI pacing mode. Notably, sleep apnea syndrome improved with DDD pacing in four patients with an apneic/hypopneic index (AHI) of 15 or higher. A subsequent study of 15 patients with obstructive sleep apnea and normal left ventricular (LV) function did not show any decrease in apnea or hypopnea with atrial overdrive pacing [11].

Results are still pending from the BREATHE (Base Rest Rate Elevation for Apnea Therapy) study. This multicenter trial will assess the effect of an increased pacing rate during rest in patients with pacemakers and documented sleep apnea or hypopnea [12].

Results are encouraging for the subset of patients with CHF and sleep apnea syndromes. Specifically, several investigators have reported CRT as a therapy for patients with sleep apnea [13, 14]. Both studies included patients who received CRT for standard indications [13, 14]. Each of the studies showed a significant prevalence of apnea in these CRT patients, who were not initially suspected of having apnea. In one study, CRT resulted in a decrease of the AHI from 49 ± 36 to 14 ± 10 ($p = .01$), and nocturnal oxygen saturation improved significantly from 85% ± 6% to 91% ± 5% ($p = .02$) in patients with central sleep apnea [13]. In patients with central sleep apnea and Cheyne–Stokes respiration, Sinha *et al.* [14] demonstrated that CRT resulted in significant decrease in the AHI ($p < .001$) and the Pittsburgh Sleep Quality Index ($p < .001$). They also reported an improvement in minimal oxygen saturation (SaO_2min) with CRT ($p < .001$). Patients without central sleep apnea had no significant change in AHI or SaO_2min.

Regardless of the long-term therapeutic role of pacing for sleep-disordered breathing, pacemakers will undoubtedly have a role in the diagnosis of these disorders. Pacemakers currently available in the European market are capable of measuring apneic and hypopneic episodes. Given the prevalence of sleep disorders in certain populations, pacemaker monitoring could provide a reliable screening method for sleep disturbances.

Cardiac contractility modulation

Whether as a potential stand-alone application for the treatment of CHF or adjunctive to CRT, cardiac contractility modulation (CCM) has been the subject of great interest. CCM is defined as nonexcitatory electrical cardiac stimulation delivered at the time of absolute myocardial refractoriness for the purpose of enhanced cardiac contractility [15–17].

Animal and human studies to date suggest that such electrical modulation may have potential as a long-term implantable therapy [18, 19]. In a study of 25 patients with drug-refractory New York Heart Association (NYHA) Class III heart failure, of both ischemic and idiopathic etiologies, a CCM pulse generator was implanted and stimuli were delivered via two right ventricular (RV) leads [20]. Acute effect was evaluated by measuring the time derivative of LV pressure (dP/dt). After implantation, the CCM generator was activated for 3 h per day over an 8-week period. The CCM system was implanted successfully in 23 of 25 patients enrolled. The clinical status of the patients' heart failure improved significantly, as determined by change in NYHA functional class. NYHA class improved from Class III to Class II in 15 patients and to Class I in 4 patients ($p < .000001$). LV ejection fraction also improved from 22% ± 7% to 28% ± 8% ($p = .0002$), and quality of life, as assessed by the Minnesota Living with Heart Failure Score, improved from 43 ± 22 to 25 ± 18 ($p = .001$). The 6-min walk test increased from 411 ± 86 m to 465 ± 81 m ($p = .02$). Although these data should be considered preliminary, they suggest that CCM by delivery of intermittent nonexcitatory electrical stimuli holds promise for ameliorating symptoms in patients with drug-refractory NYHA Class III heart failure and for increasing LV performance in these Class III patients with significant systolic dysfunction [20].

A randomized clinical trial under way in the United States, the Optimizer III Trial, will assess the efficacy of CCM with a permanently implanted pulse generator that will stimulate for 5 h per day for a period of 6 months. It is unknown when initial results are anticipated.

CCM therapy also has been used adjunctively with biventricular pacing in an acute study with temporary CCM application in six patients with heart failure. Although this study had multiple limitations, CCM was shown to augment the effects of biventricular pacing acutely, with improvements in pulse pressure, LV end-systolic pressure, and LV dP/dt [21].

Is there potential for expansion of CRT indications?

CRT is now established as an effective therapeutic tool in a subset of patients with CHF. Indications for CRT that are widely accepted or mandated by US Food and Drug Administration labeling include Class III or IV NYHA heart failure, ejection fraction less than 30%, normal sinus rhythm, optimized medical therapy, and QRS longer than 120 ms. Ongoing evaluations may expand CRT indications by challenging all of the "current" indications.

A substantial amount of data demonstrates that selecting patients for CRT on the basis of intraventricular dyssynchrony is superior to selecting by QRS width alone. Patients with clinical CHF and a normal surface QRS width may still have considerable intraventricular dyssynchrony and benefit from CRT. QRS width should not be ignored, however. QRS longer than 120 ms usually implies some degree of intraventricular dyssynchrony. To offer therapy only if the QRS meets certain criteria would deprive a subset of patients of a proven therapy.

Should functional class specify who receives CRT? The overwhelming majority of patients included in clinical trials of CRT have been in NYHA functional Class III or IV heart failure. Functional Class II patients were enrolled in CONTAK CD [22] and MIRACLE ICD [23], and a few Class II patients were included in other trials, but, overall, the data with Class II patients are limited.

Stages of the "disease progression" classification of CHF are described as follows: stage A, the first indications of any disease process; stage B, dysfunction and remodeling; stage C, CHF; and stage D, terminal CHF and death [24]. Current CRT indications include only patients in stages C and D. If the goal of CRT is to reverse the pathophysiologic sequelae of the underlying cardiomyopathic process, initiation of CRT earlier in the process, at the first sign of LV dysfunction and remodeling, may prevent subsequent remodeling.

Several trials are under way or in developmental stages to assess the effects of CRT during earlier stages of the disease process. One trial under way, the REVERSE (REsynchronization reVErses Remodeling in Systolic left vEntricular dysfunction) trial, will evaluate patients with NYHA Class I or II symptoms or those who were previously symptomatic but are currently without symptoms. Criteria include LV ejection fraction ≤45% and documented ventricular dyssynchrony.

Normal sinus rhythm as a criterion for CRT has already been challenged. Given the substantial incidence of atrial fibrillation in patients with advanced CHF, application of CRT in this patient population has been a natural progression. Randomized trial data assessing CRT in patients with chronic atrial fibrillation are still limited, but many practitioners advocate the use of CRT in this subset of patients. The application of CRT in patients with less serious LV dysfunction and patients with normal systolic function but diastolic dysfunction has not been addressed.

Many potential augmentations of current CRT devices may benefit disease management. Although not actually an expanded "indication" of therapy, additional disease management tools may encourage some physicians to apply this approved therapy more broadly. Devices already are available that can detect RV pressure changes and can be used to derive dP/dt and pulmonary artery pressures. Direct measurement of pulmonary artery pressures also is possible [25, 26]. Direct measurement or estimation of left atrial and LV pressures has been investigated and may provide even more specific information for use in the management of heart failure [27, 28].

Pulmonary edema and congestion may presage overt CHF. Increasing pulmonary edema can be detected with intrathoracic impedance changes that can be measured with standard pacing and ICD leads [29]. As heart failure progresses, ventricular wall thickness and myocardial conduction velocity also may change. These measurements can be monitored by paced ventricular evoked response and could be incorporated into a CRT device [30]. Heart failure exacerbation might also be predicted by a change in mixed venous oxygen saturation that could be monitored by the CRT system [28].

Randomized, controlled trials and small studies of CRT have shown a decrease in functional mitral regurgitation after CRT. In the MIRACLE trial, the decrease in mitral regurgitation was shown to be sustained at 6 months of follow-up [31]. If a patient presents with severe functional mitral regurgitation but does not meet criteria for CRT in terms of LV dysfunction or functional class, should CRT be considered? If CRT is considered as a therapeutic method for functional mitral regurgitation, should lead placement be altered or standard biventricular lead positions, RV and lateral LV, be used? The answers to these questions are yet to be determined, but a pacing indication for functional valvular regurgitation is possible.

Role of pacing in atrial fibrillation

Multiple approaches have been advocated for the decrease or prevention of atrial fibrillation by pacing techniques. Dual-site [32] and alternate-site pacing, specifically atrial–septal pacing [33], have been advocated for decreasing the burden of atrial fibrillation and flutter. No approach has emerged as being superior to the others.

In addition to the proposed change in implantation technique, multiple pacing algorithms have been used to decrease or prevent atrial fibrillation. Available algorithms include: (1) pacing that responds to premature atrial contractions (i.e. the atrial pacing rate is incremented in the presence of premature atrial contractions); (2) atrial overdrive pacing to consistently maintain the atrial pacing rate above the intrinsic atrial rate; and (3) a post-mode-switch algorithm to pace at a faster atrial rate after the pathologic atrial rhythm is terminated and the original dual-chamber pacing mode resumed. Several completed clinical trials demonstrate some benefit of atrial pacing algorithms [34, 35] and others are in progress.

Despite many investigations of alternate-site and dual-site atrial pacing and atrial pacing algorithms, the benefit of any or all of the above remains controversial. Further detail regarding these investigations will not be provided in this chapter, but investigations of present and future pacing techniques for the decrease or prevention of atrial fibrillation will undoubtedly continue.

An entirely different consideration for pacing applications in the treatment of atrial fibrillation is that of neuromodulation. The data for neuromodulation are limited at this time. In an animal study, selective AV nodal vagal stimulation produced graded slowing of the ventricular rate response during atrial fibrillation without AV nodal ablation. This approach was hemodynamically superior to AV nodal ablation and subsequent regular or irregular ventricular pacing [36]. Whether such vagal stimulation can be sustained over long periods of time remains to be demonstrated [37]. Nonetheless, when considering new indications for pacing in the broadest sense, the potential application of neuromodulation to alter atrial fibrillation or other arrhythmias is exciting.

Summary

Cardiac resynchronization therapy is an example of how electrical stimulation can be applied to a disease and can achieve significant results in a relatively short period of time. All the potential applications of pacing have not yet been considered, but many may be as successful as CRT. New indications for pacing could expand substantially if noncardiac stimulation is considered for the treatment of cardiac disorders, specifically, the use of neural stimulation to effect cardiac control.

References

1 Gregoratos G, Abrams J, Epstein AE *et al.* ACC/AHA/NASPE 2002 Guideline update for implantation of cardiac pacemakers and antiarrhythmia devices: summary article: a report of the American College of Cardiology/American Heart Association Task Force on Practice Guidelines (ACC/AHA/NASPE Committee to update the 1998 pacemaker guidelines). *Circulation* 2002; **106**: 2145–2161.

2 Shaw DB, Gowers JI, Kekwick CA *et al.* Is Mobitz type I atrioventricular block benign in adults? *Heart* 2004; **90**: 169–174.

3 Kenny RA, Seifer C. SAFE PACE 2 Syncope and falls in the elderly pacing and carotid sinus evaluation: a randomized control trial of cardiac pacing in older patients with falls and carotid sinus hypersensitivity. *Am J Geriatr Cardiol* 1999; **8**: 87.

4 Kenny RA, Richardson DA, Steen N *et al.* Carotid sinus syndrome: a modifiable risk factor for nonaccidental falls in older adults (SAFE PACE). *J Am Coll Cardiol* 2001; **38**: 1491–1496.

5 Lee-Chiong TL Jr. Sleep and sleep disorders: an overview. *Med Clin North Am* 2004; **88**: xi–xiv.

6 Parish JM, Somers VK. Obstructive sleep apnea and cardiovascular disease. *Mayo Clin Proc* 2004; **79**: 1036–1046.

7 Young T, Peppard PE, Gottlieb DJ. Epidemiology of obstructive sleep apnea: a population health perspective. *Am J Respir Crit Care Med* 2002; **165**: 1217–1239.

8 Defaye P, Garrigue S, Pepin J-L *et al.* Prevalence of sleep apnea in a population of DDD and CRT patients. *Heart Rhythm* 2004; **1**: S133.

9 Garrigue S, Bordier P, Jais P *et al.* Benefit of atrial pacing in sleep apnea syndrome. [Erratum in *N Engl J Med* 2002; **346**: 872.] *N Engl J Med* 2002; **346**: 404–412.

10 Mizutani N, Waseda K, Asai K *et al.* Effect of pacing mode on sleep disturbance. *J Artif Organs* 2003; **6**: 106–111.

11 Garrigue S, Defaye P, Poezevara MS *et al.* Can atrial overdrive pacing prevent pure obstructive sleep apnea? *Heart Rhythm* 2004; **1**: S81.

12 St. Jude Medical [homepage on the Internet]. St. Jude Medical, Inc. c2004 [cited 2004 Sept. 15]. Available from: http://www.sjm.com/resources/clinicalstudies.aspx

13 Seidl K, Rameken M, Becker T *et al.* Cardiac resynchronization therapy improves sleep related breathing disorders in patients with chronic heart failure. *J Am Coll Cardiol* 2004; **43**(Suppl.): 152A–153A.

14 Sinha AM, Skobel EC, Breithardt OA *et al.* Cardiac resynchronization therapy improves central sleep apnea and Cheyne–Stokes respiration in patients with chronic heart failure. *J Am Coll Cardiol* 2004; **44**: 68–71.

15 Pappone C, Vicedomini G, Salvati A *et al.* Electrical modulation of cardiac contractility: clinical aspects in congestive heart failure. *Heart Fail Rev* 2001; **6**: 55–60.

16 Pappone C, Rosanio S, Burkhoff D *et al.* Cardiac contractility modulation by electric currents applied during the refractory period in patients with heart failure secondary to ischemic or idiopathic dilated cardiomyopathy. *Am J Cardiol* 2002; **90**: 1307–1313.

17 Augello G, Santinelli V, Vicedomini G *et al.* Cardiac contractility modulation by nonexcitatory electrical currents: the new frontier for electrical therapy of heart failure. *Ital Heart J* 2004; **5**(Suppl.): 68S–75S.

18 Morita H, Suzuki G, Haddad W *et al.* Long-term effects of non-excitatory cardiac contractility modulation electric signals on the progression of heart failure in dogs. *Eur J Heart Fail* 2004; **6**: 145–150.

19 Pappone C, Augello G, Rosanio S *et al.* First human chronic experience with cardiac contractility modulation by nonexcitatory electrical currents for treating systolic heart failure: mid-term safety and efficacy results from a multicenter study. *J Cardiovasc Electrophysiol* 2004; **15**: 418–427.

20 Stix G, Borggrefe M, Wolpert C *et al.* Chronic electrical stimulation during the absolute refractory period of the myocardium improves severe heart failure. *Eur Heart J* 2004; **25**: 650–655.

21 Pappone C, Vicedomini G, Ioricchio ML *et al.* Application of nonexcitatory electrical signals combined with biventricular pacing improves hemodynamic parameters in heart failure patients beyond the improvement achieved by biventricular pacing alone. *PACE* 2000; **23**(Pt II): 590.

22 Lozano I, Bocchiardo M, Achtelik M *et al.* (the VENTAK CHF/CONTAK CD Investigators Study Group) Impact of biventricular pacing on mortality in a randomized crossover study of patients with heart failure and ventricular arrhythmias. *PACE* 2000; **23**(Pt 2): 1711–1712.

23 Young JB, Abraham WT, Smith AL *et al.* (for The Multicenter InSync ICD Randomized Clinical Evaluation (MIRACLE ICD) Trial Investigators) Combined cardiac resynchronization and implantable cardioversion defibrillation in advanced chronic heart failure: the MIRACLE ICD Trial. *JAMA* 2003; **289**: 2685–2694.

24 Hunt SA, Baker DW, Chin MH *et al.* ACC/AHA guidelines for the evaluation and management of chronic heart failure in the adult: executive summary: a report of the American College of Cardiology/American Heart Association Task Force on Practice Guidelines (Committee to Revise the 1995 Guidelines for the Evaluation and Management of Heart Failure). *Circulation* 2001; **104**: 2996–3007.

25 Magalski A, Adamson P, Gadler F *et al.* Continuous ambulatory right heart pressure measurements with an implantable hemodynamic monitor: a multicenter, 12-month follow-up study of patients with chronic heart failure. *J Card Fail* 2002; **8**: 63–70.

26 Adamson PB, Magalski A, Braunschweig F *et al.* Ongoing right ventricular hemodynamics in heart failure: clinical value of measurements derived from an implantable monitoring system. *J Am Coll Cardiol* 2003; **41**: 565–571.

27 Kar S, Aragon J, McClean D *et al.* Chronic implantation of left atrial pressure monitor accurately measures left atrial pressure in porcine model. *J Am Coll Cardiol* 2004; **43**(Suppl.): 208A.

28 Bennett TD, Taepke RT, Cinbis C *et al.* Chronic performance of a new implantable pressure and oxygen saturation sensor in canines (abstract). *J Card Fail* 2003; **9**(Suppl.): S48.

29 Wang L, Yu C-M, Chau E *et al.* Prediction of CHF hospitalization by ambulatory intrathoracic impedance measurement in CHF patients is feasible using pacemaker or ICD lead systems. *PACE* 2003; **26**(Pt II): 959.

30 Ebner E, Kratschmer H, Danilovic D *et al.* Ventricular evoked response as clinical marker for hemodynamic changes in dilative cardiomyopathy. *PACE* 2004; **27**: 166–174.

31 St John Sutton MG, Plappert T, Abraham WT *et al.* (for the Multicenter InSync Randomized Clinical Evaluation (MIRACLE) Study Group) Effect of cardiac resynchronization therapy on left ventricular size and function in chronic heart failure. *Circulation* 2003; **107**: 1985–1990.

32 Saksena S, Prakash A, Ziegler P *et al.* (for the DAPPAF Investigators) Improved suppression of recurrent atrial fibrillation with dual-site right atrial pacing and antiarrhythmic drug therapy. *J Am Coll Cardiol* 2002; **40**: 1140–1150.

33 Padeletti L, Michelucci A, Pieragnoli P *et al.* Atrial septal pacing: a new approach to prevent atrial fibrillation. *PACE* 2004; **27**(Pt 2): 850–854.

34 Carlson MD, Ip J, Messenger J *et al.* (for the Atrial Dynamic Overdrive Pacing Trial (ADOPT) Investigators) A new pacemaker algorithm for the treatment of atrial

fibrillation: results of the Atrial Dynamic Overdrive Pacing Trial (ADOPT). *J Am Coll Cardiol* 2003; **42**: 627–633.

35 Lee MA, Weachter R, Pollak S *et al.* (for the ATTEST Investigators) The effect of atrial pacing therapies on atrial tachyarrhythmia burden and frequency: results of a randomized trial in patients with bradycardia and atrial tachyarrhythmias. *J Am Coll Cardiol* 2003; **41**: 1926–1932.

36 Zhuang S, Zhang Y, Mowrey KA *et al.* Ventricular rate control by selective vagal stimulation is superior to rhythm regularization by atrioventricular nodal ablation and pacing during atrial fibrillation. *Circulation* 2002; **106**: 1853–1858.

37 DiMarco JP. Selective vagal stimulation for rate control in atrial fibrillation. *Circulation* 2002; **106**: 1746–1747.

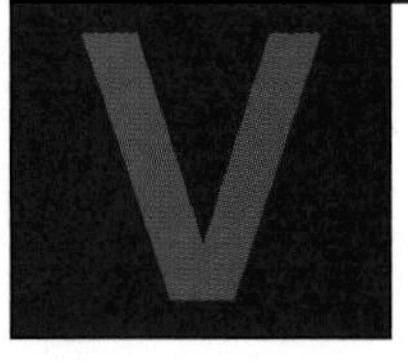

PART V

Advances in implantable defibrillators

18

CHAPTER 18

Implantable defibrillator sensing and discrimination algorithms

Kelly Richardson, MD, *Amin Al-Ahmad,* MD, *&*
Paul J. Wang, MD

As technology continues to advance, detection and appropriate treatment for ventricular tachycardia (VT) and ventricular fibrillation (VF) has remained the central task of implantable defibrillators. Discrimination of VT from supra ventricular tachycardia (SVT) has emerged as one of the most important enhancements of basic defibrillator function, resulting in better patient care and increased comfort [1]. While seemingly at odds with each other, sensing and discrimination algorithms are able to work in a coordinated fashion improving overall outcome. Proper functioning of the implantable cardioverter defibrillator (ICD) is dependent on reliable sensing of ventricular depolarizations for discrimination to take place [2]. The sensing and detection are a two part integrated system incorporated into the devices although each has separate distinct functions. This chapter will focus on sensing and detecting as well as discrimination algorithms for classification of tachyarrhythmias.

Sensing and detection mechanisms

The clinical efficacy of ICD depends on its ability to accurately sense and detect intracardiac signals. The variability and relative small amplitude of the signals in VF compared with signals in sinus rhythm present a particular challenge for sensing and detection algorithms. Sensing is performed using sense amplifiers, filters, and rectifiers. The incoming electrogram is amplified, filtered and rectified, and then compared with the sensing threshold. A set of RR intervals is then given to the detection algorithm for processing.

There are several challenges that detection algorithms face (Table 18.1). They must detect ventricular events of low and fluctuating amplitude while avoiding oversensing in sinus rhythm. In addition, sensing errors due to the combination of bradycardia and tachycardia therapy also must be avoided [3]. The intracardiac signal is first filtered and then rectified by making all of the components of the signal positive in deflection. A fixed gain system has difficulty in avoiding T-wave oversensing while preserving adequate VF sensing. There are several strategies that help avoid these difficulties. Ventricular refractory periods are used to avoid double counting of ventricular events although double counting rarely may still be seen.

Table 18.1 Automatic adjustable sensing threshold: effect of programmable sensitivity and initial sensing threshold percentage.

Undersensing
Fluctuating amplitude R-waves
Oversensing necessitating less-sensitive setting
Oversensing
Large T-wave signals
short-QT (early repolarization time)
Wide delayed depolarization component with double counting

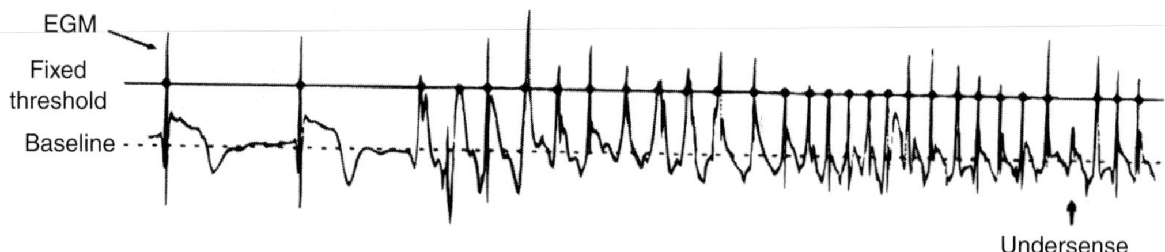

Figure 18.1 Automatic gain adjustment. Automatic gain adjustment algorithm adjusts the amplitude or gain of the signal while using a fixed sensing threshold. One undersensed beat is noted. EGM = electrogram (Reprinted from [4], with permission.)

These refractory periods are not usually sufficient to avoid sensing of repolarization signals. Since the amplitude of the repolarization signal seems to be proportional to the amplitude of the depolarization event, a general strategy is to keep the sensing threshold relatively high to avoid T-wave sensing. Overtime, smaller and smaller R-waves may be detected. There are two major time-dependent methods of detecting ventricular events: automatic adjusting threshold or sensitivity and automatic gain adjustment (Figure 18.1).

Using automatic adjustable sensitivity, once the first QRS is detected, the sensing threshold decreases over time. The decay function may be linear, exponential, or polynomial decay function. The initial threshold after sensing of the QRS complex may be proportional to the R-wave amplitude but constrained by the programmed ventricular sensitivity. For example, the ventricular sensitivity may start as 75% of the ventricular electrogram peak up to eightfold times the programmed ventricular sensitivity. Thus, for a programmed ventricular sensitivity of 0.3 mV, any R-wave of 3.2 mV or greater will result in an initial sensitivity of 2.4 mV but any lower amplitude R-wave will be 75% of the electrogram peak to a minimum value of 0.3 mV (Table 18.2).

Sensing abnormalities often depend on the programmed sensitivity and the relative size of the predominant R-wave and T-wave amplitudes. Cycle length changes are associated with a fluctuation in R-wave amplitude increasing the possibility of R-wave undersensing [5]. For large R-waves the initial sensing threshold will be larger, and the greatest problem will be fluctuating R-waves, that is, small R-waves alternating with large R-waves, a condition seen in some polymorphic VTs, such as torsade de pointes or even VF. Dekker *et al.* reported a case of complete failure of sensing VF due to cyclical high-amplitude signals with undersensing of subsequent lower amplitude signals [6]. Endocardial R-wave alternans during VT may also interfere with adequate sensing [7]. The primary difficulty with a less sensitive programmed setting occurs when there are lower amplitude signals, particularly with fluctuating amplitude since a large R-wave will result in a high initial sensing threshold. Such a situation may occur when there is evidence of oversensing, requiring programming of a less sensitive setting. At a less sensitive programmed setting, small amplitude signals may occasionally be undersensed, but this is usually in a setting also of a small R-wave amplitude in sinus rhythm, necessitating a new lead placement. Modifications of the current algorithms may be needed to address the issue of fluctuating R-wave amplitude, particularly in an alternating pattern. R-wave undersensing also has been reported due to an electrogram width algorithm that required two consecutive points above the programmed sensitivity threshold [8]. T-wave oversensing occurs when the T-waves are relatively large in amplitude compared with the R-wave. Specific entities, such as hypertrophic cardiomyopathy, hyperkalemia [9], and short-QT syndrome, may be at increased risk of having T-wave oversensing [10]. Use of morphologic criteria may also prevent T-wave oversensing [11]. Because most devices use the same sensing algorithms for bradycardia pacing as tachycardia detection, it is possible for oversensing to result in failure to pace, even resulting in asystole [12, 13] (Table 18.3).

Table 18.2 Challenges for detection.

Example of effect of programmed sensitivity with maximum initial sensing threshold of eight-fold programmed sensitivity	
For 0.3 mV sensitivity	
R-wave > 3.2 mV	Initial sensing threshold is 2.4 mV
0.3 mV < R-wave < 3.2 mV	Initial sensing threshold is 75% of peak
For 1.2 mV sensitivity	
R-wave > 12. 8 mV	Initial sensing threshold is 9.6 mV
1.2 mV < R-wave < 12.8 mV	Initial sensing threshold is 75% of peak
Example of effect of programmable initial percent of peak	
75%	
R-wave > 6 mV	Initial sensing threshold is 3 mV
2 mV < R-wave < 6 mV	Initial sensing threshold is 75% of peak
R-wave < 2 mV	Initial sensing threshold is 1 mV
50%	
R-wave > 6 mV	Initial sensing threshold is 3 mV
2 mV < R-wave < 6 mV	Initial sensing threshold is 50% of peak
R-wave < 2 mV	Initial sensing threshold is 1 mV

Table 18.3 Troubleshooting sensing abnormalities.

Strategy	*Limitation*
Oversensing of T-wave	
Increase ventricular refractory period	Frequently may result in undersensing
Program sensitivity to less sensitive value	May result in undersensing
Increase time to onset of sensing decay	May result in undersensing
Diaphragmatic oversensing	
Program sensitivity to less sensitive value	May result in undersensing; requires testing
New lead placement	
Undersensing QRS	
Program sensitivity to more sensitive value	May result in oversensing; may already be set to most sensitive value
New lead placement	
Double-counting QRS	
Lengthen ventricular refractory period	
Program sensitivity to less sensitive value	May not prevent double counting
New lead placement	May not prevent double counting

The decay in the sensing threshold may begin immediately after the end of the ventricular refractory period or may start after a programmable delay following the end of the ventricular refractory period. When the decay is delayed, the initial sensing threshold is kept constant during the delay period (Figure 18.2) [14]. Programming the delay can be particularly useful when oversensed events occur after the sensed refractory period. The maximal sensitivity is reached when the decay curve reaches the programmed sensitivity and no ventricular sensed event has occurred. Some ICDs have a separate sensitivity for pacemaker bradycardia function from that used with ventricular tachyarrhythmia detection. Sensing may also be modified by programming the sensing ventricular refractory period. Refractory periods are important in preventing double counting of each QRS

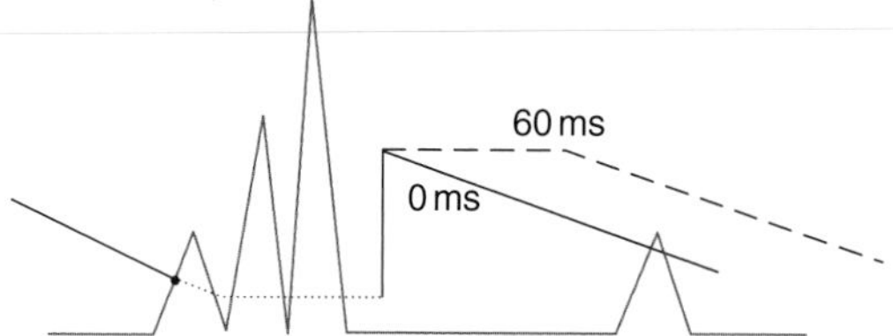

Figure 18.2 Programmable adjustment of delay in decay. The programmable decay delay will keep the sensitivity threshold constant for the programmed duration. (Reprinted from [14], with permission.)

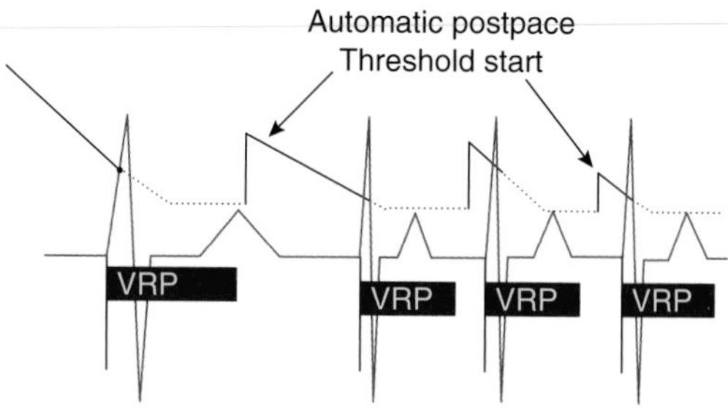

Figure 18.3 Ventricular refractory period during pacing. The ventricular refractory period shortens during pacing to permit improved sensing during pacing. The threshold start is adjusted for each pacing cycle. VRP = ventricular refractory period. (Reprinted from [14], with permission.)

complex. However, caution is used when significantly extending the ventricular refractory period since significant ventricular undersensing during ventricular tachyarrhythmias may occur.

Paced ventricular events present a particular challenge since there are no ventricular sensed events with which to compare. It is particularly important to avoid sensing the ventricular event resulting from capture and also to be able to detect ventricular arrhythmias occurring soon after a paced event. The refractory period following a paced event is accordingly longer than for sensed events. In some devices this is called a blanking period rather than a refractory period. Following a paced event, the initial sensing threshold is usually a fixed value. In some devices, this value may vary according to the pacing rate in an attempt to adjust for the changes in QT interval with pacing (Figure 18.3) [50]. As the pacing rate increases, the initial sensing threshold will decrease and the decay delay will shorten. In some algorithms, the ventricular refractory period decreases during pacing to promote appropriate sensing [15]. The combination of undersensing resulting in pacing during the onset of a tachyarrhythmia and a VT just faster than the pacing may lead to a delay in tachyarrhythmia detection. Such a potential for interaction has led many manufacturers to require a separation in the maximum pacing rate and the slowest ventricular tachyarrhythmia detection rate.

Redetection is the term used to indicate sensing algorithms following first delivered therapy. Sensing abnormalities can occur following ICD shock [16] but advances in both lead characteristics and ICD sensing systems have made postshocking sensing abnormalities uncommon [17, 18].

Most devices use feed-through filters and other filtering processes to decrease the likelihood of electromagnetic interference causing oversensing. However, as new electronic devices are introduced into society, there is a new possibility that electromagnetic interference will result in oversensing. As an example, recently devices, such as neuromuscular electrical stimulators, have been shown to cause atrial and ventricular oversensing, but testing these devices first in individual patients may permit their safe use [19–21]. Similarly sensing of myopotentials can result in inappropriate ICD discharges [22]. Care must be taken to avoid oversensing during electromagnetic sources, such as arc welding [23, 24]. Future sensing algorithms may also enhance the ability to prevent oversensing while maintaining the ability to sense VF.

Rhythm discrimination algorithms

Discrimination algorithms were first implemented in single-chamber devices; however, with the introduction of dual-chamber devices, dual-chamber discriminators are now available [25].

Single-chamber discriminators

Ventricular rate

Ventricular rate remains the basic criterion for ventricular tachyarrhythmia detection in ICDs. However, a significant incidence of inappropriate therapy for sinus tachycardia (ST) and atrial arrhythmias has led to important discriminators being introduced. Therefore, enhancements such as rate stability and onset have been developed to help differentiate atrial fibrillation (AF) and sinus rhythm from VT. Nonetheless, all ICDs use the ventricular rate as a first criterion. The criterion is most commonly set as a number of consecutive short intervals or as a percentage of ventricular intervals within in a sliding window.

Sudden onset

Sudden onset criterion primarily differentiates sinus rhythm from VT/VF. Generally, ST gradually increases in rate whereas VT or VF has a sudden onset. Using this enhancement, a percentage of the cycle length or an interval in milliseconds may be selected. The sudden onset criteria compare an interval at the start of tachycardia to an average of the previous intervals to determine if the onset was sudden or gradual. It may also detect a sudden shortening of the ventricular interval at the onset. If the onset is gradual then tachyarrhythmia therapy is inhibited. However, sudden onset criteria are unable to distinguish a supraventricular tachyarrhythmia from ventricular tachyarrhythmias. In addition, a VT that develops during the ST may not exhibit a large enough change in intervals. Also, if multiple premature ventricular contractions occur before the onset of the tachycardia it may hinder determination of sudden onset.

Ventricular rate stability

Rate stability criterion measures the variability in the beat-to-beat intervals during a sensed tachycardia. Most monomorphic VTs have a variability in intervals of <30–60 ms. AF and polymorphic VTs have a wider variability from beat to beat. Several different rate stability algorithms may be used but all are approximations of variability of the intervals. The stability index may use criteria, such as the running average of intervals, the standard deviation of intervals, or the number of cycles outside mean $\pm$ 1 SD.

Most commonly the rate stability index is used to separate AF from monomorphic VT. In such cases, greater variability in ventricular intervals results in a classification as supraventricular, inhibiting therapy. In other cases, greater variability may be used in a VT zone to indicate a polymorphic VT that is less likely to be terminated with antitachycardia pacing, resulting in therapy being advanced to shock therapy. Limitations of the stability criteria include the inability to distinguish rapid AF from polymorphic VT. In addition, at faster rates AF tends to have less variability of ventricular response.

Studies have shown that using stability and sudden onset enhanced detection criteria, which enhances specificity in detecting VT leading to less inappropriate shocks for SVT. Importantly, the improved detection for SVT did not lead to any undersensing or delayed sensing of VT [26].

Electrogram characteristics

Discrimination algorithms based on electrogram characteristics provide a useful means of distinguishing supraventricular from ventricular rhythms. Like the appearance of the QRS complex on the surface ECG, intracardiac electrogram morphology may reflect changes in the activation sequences that occur when activation originates in the ventricles compared with the atrium. One of the simplest algorithms is the estimation of QRS width using the rate (near-field) or shock (far-field) electrograms. However, this parameter has significant limitations as a rhythm discriminator in sensitivity and specificity [27–29].

Various algorithms have been developed that compare morphologic characteristics of a template derived in sinus rhythm with the one that is obtained during a tachycardia [30]. The overall morphology of the QRS can be monitored and compared with a template. In addition, it may be possible to examine the timing or appearance of the electrograms. The electrogram morphology may be assessed by creating a morphology template in sinus rhythm and comparing it with the electrogram morphology during a tachyarrhythmia. Peak alignment is the first step in comparing the electrogram morphology and introduces a potential difficulty when alignment is not straightforward.

There are several different possible methods of comparing morphologies. One method involves finding the dominant peaks and calculating the area of the peaks. The similarity of the electrograms may be calculated by determining the percent differences in the areas of the peaks. The St. Jude morphology algorithm analyzes specific feature points within the electrogram (Figure 18.4) [32]. The largest four

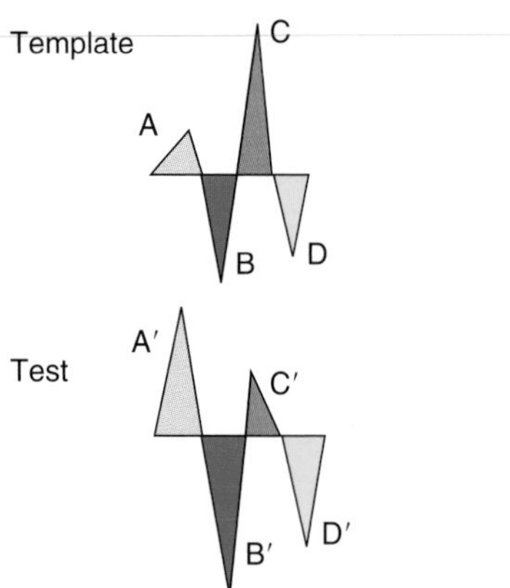

Figure 18.4 Morphology discrimination algorithm. Area of each of four dominant peaks are compared in the template and test complexes. (Reprinted from [31], with permission.)

contiguous peaks are used. The polarity of the highest or dominant peak in the tachycardia complex is compared with the template complex. The sum of the differences of the corresponding areas of interest is calculated. The smaller the sum of these differences the larger the percentage match score. In single-chamber devices the above-mentioned criterion can be combined in a wide range of algorithms providing multiple different sensitivities and specificities for differentiating SVT from VT [33]. Correctly identifying the rhythm as VT is defined as sensitivity and correctly defining the episode as SVT is defined as specificity. One study, using morphology discrimination alone resulted in a sensitivity and specificity of 77% and 71%, respectively [34]. When morphology discrimination [35] was combined with sudden onset the sensitivity increased to 99.5%, but the specificity decreased to 48%. Another study demonstrated that the use of the three discriminators, morphology discrimination, sudden onset, and stability in a "2 of 3" diagnostic logic gave a specificity of 90.9% and sensitivity of 96% for spontaneous arrhythmias. Another study in 25 patients implanted with a St. Jude Ventritex that used a ventricular depolarization complex morphology for morphology discrimination exhibited a specificity of 98% and a sensitivity of 66% and a diagnostic accuracy of 80% [36]. All episodes of AF were correctly diagnosed as SVT. Overall, morphology discrimination exhibits a high specificity and sensitivity when combined with sudden onset and stability.

The Medtronic WAVELET algorithm uses wavelet transforms to compare the sinus template with the tachycardia template (Figure 18.5). Templates are created by averaging up to 6 beats. The template consists of the wavelet-based waveform description, normalization factor, and position and sign of waveform peak. When the VT counter reaches 3 (VF counter reaches 4) the ICD initiates electrogram collection. Then the positive and negative peak is aligned to the template. Using Haar-wavelet transform data compression, 48 samples of the QRS complex are collected and applied, describing the QRS complex. Wavelet coefficients are filtered decreasing computational effort and filtering noise. The unknown QRS is sampled, aligned and filtered, and then compared. The match percentage is calculated and nominally set at 70%. Continuous classification is based on an 8 beat sliding window. If three of the eight are classified as SVT then it withholds therapy.

In a study by Swerdlow *et al.* [37], the wavelet algorithm was assessed for temporal and postural stability as well as accuracy of SVT–VT discrimination in 23 patients. For the most part, percent match in baseline rhythms was stable despite changes in body position, walk versus rest, isometric exercise, and over time. A nominal threshold match of 70% was used for the study. Sensitivity for correctly defining VT was 100%. Specificity for rejection of SVT was 78%. Inappropriate detection of SVT as VT were caused by electrogram truncation, myopotential interference with low-amplitude electrograms, waveform alignment error, and rate-dependent aberrancy. All but rate dependent aberrancy was corrected with changes in programming. This change could have improved specificity as the first three causes resulted in 69% of the inappropriate classification. Since this initial study, a larger study of the performance of this algorithm has been completed. In this study, a total of 1342 of 1352 (99.3%) of episodes of sustained VT or VF were successfully detected. The wavelet resulted in a reduction in inappropriate therapy in 534 of 885 episodes (60.3%). This large study demonstrates the utility of this algorithm in improving detection in a single-chamber device.

Other algorithms utilize the ability to detect differences in the time of arrival of wavefronts at different electrograms. This concept is analogous

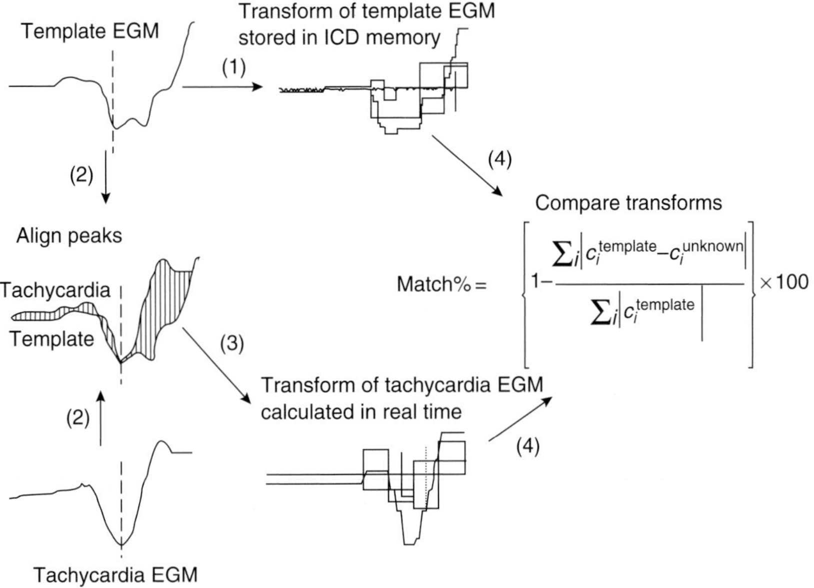

Figure 18.5 WAVELET discrimination algorithm.

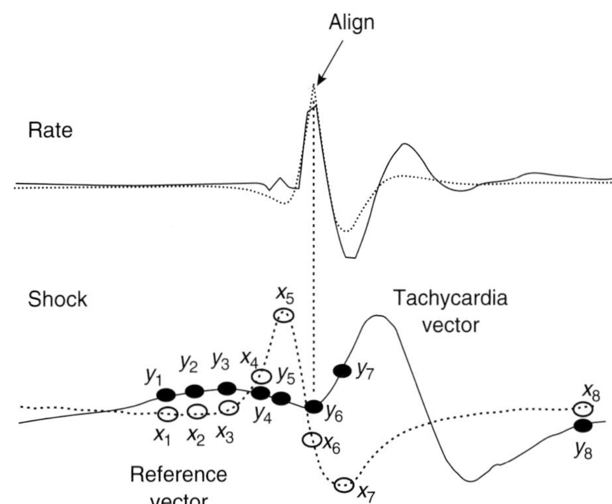

Figure 18.6 Rhythm ID rhythm discrimination algorithm utilizing time of arrival at two electrodes. The rate and shock channel electrogram are aligned by fiducial points. *x* points indicate the reference or template values and *y* indicate the tachycardia values. (Reprinted from *J Cardiovasc Electrophysiol* [38], with permission.)

to using the time of arrival of sound at each ear to determine the direction from which a sound originates. The Guidant Rhythm ID algorithm calculates a coefficient of correlation between the reference and the tachycardia electrograms termed VTC (vector and timing correlation) (Figure 18.6). In these devices the ICD periodically and automatically saves a reference vector using the shock and rate electrograms. The shock channel vector is aligned with the rate channel vector fiducial point. Eight features of the shock channel vector are selected. During the tachycardia, the amplitude of each of the time locations with respect to the fiducial point are measured. The product-moment correlation coefficient is calculated. A sliding window of 10 complexes is used. When eight or greater of these complexes are felt to be abnormal, the tachycardia is classified as ventricular in origin. In an early study of this algorithm, Gold *et al.* [38], observed that 35 out of 36 supraventricular episodes

Table 18.4 Comparison of algorithm features.

	Primary Usefulness	*Limitations*
Single chamber		
Sudden onset	Distinguishes ST	SVT or VT during ST is difficult; cannot distinguish SVT from VT
Stability	Distinguishes AF from monomorphic VT	Polymorphic VT may be unstable; (ST) with PVCs may be unstable
Electrogram characteristics	Distinguishes SVT from VT	Template may fluctuate, affected by posture, bundle-branch block
Dual chamber		
Atrial and ventricular events	Distinguishes VT from ST or SVT	Undersensing or oversensing; 1 : 1 is difficult
A-V Association/Relationship	Distinguishes VT from ST or SVT	Undersensing or oversensing; 1 : 1 is difficult
Chamber of Origin	Distinguishes SVT from VT	Undersensing or oversensing

Notes:
SVT = supraventricular tachycardia; ST = sinus tachycardia; VT = ventricular tachycardia; PVCs = premature ventricular contractions; AF = atrial fibrillation.

were correctly classified, yielding a specificity of 97% and all 81 ventricular episodes were correctly classified (100% sensitivity).

Atrial and ventricular discriminators

In dual-chamber devices an atrial lead is present that allows the comparison of atrial and ventricular activity, further enhancing rhythm discrimination [25, 39]. The atrial information can be used in several ways described in further detail below. A comparison can be made between the number of atrial and ventricular events during tachycardia. Atrial and ventricular association or dissociation can be analyzed and used. The number and relative position(s) of atrial sensed events between ventricular events can be incorporated into the analysis. The R-wave morphology can be analyzed and the effect of premature stimulation can be analyzed (Table 18.4).

Chamber of origin

This criterion found in ELA devices [40] analyzes the first tachycardia interval (Figure 18.7). If it begins with an atrial event, the rhythm is classified as an SVT. If the ventricular event begins without a preceding atrial event, then the rhythm is classified as VT. Atrial undersensing limits the usefulness of this algorithm.

Atrial versus ventricular events

The comparison of ventricular and atrial rates ($V>A$) is one of the most useful discriminators based on relative rates alone. If there are more ventricular activations than atrial activations then the rhythm is VT. However, undersensing of atrial events during a supraventricular arrhythmia may lead to the incorrect diagnosis of VT [41]. There are limitations to classifying the rhythm as supraventricular if there are more atrial events than ventricular events. For example, there may be oversensing of the ventricle signal on the atrial channel, leading to 1 : 1 sensing. Similarly, underlying atrial arrhythmias during VT limits the usefulness of $A>V$ algorithms.

Atrioventricular relationship

The relationship of the atrium and the ventricle during a tachycardia is one of the most powerful relationships available. The device can analyze the timings of the activity in the atria and ventricle to help differentiate if the tachycardia began independently in the ventricle or originates in the atria. This criterion monitors the PP interval, the PR interval, and the RR help to categorize the tachycardia as supraventricular or ventricular in origin. The beat-to-beat relation between the *A* and *V* are compared using PR stability, establishing a relationship between the atrium and the ventricle. Rhythms in which there is a 1 : 1 atrial–ventricular (AV) relationship present the greatest challenges since both supraventricular and ventricular arrhythmias may have this relationship.

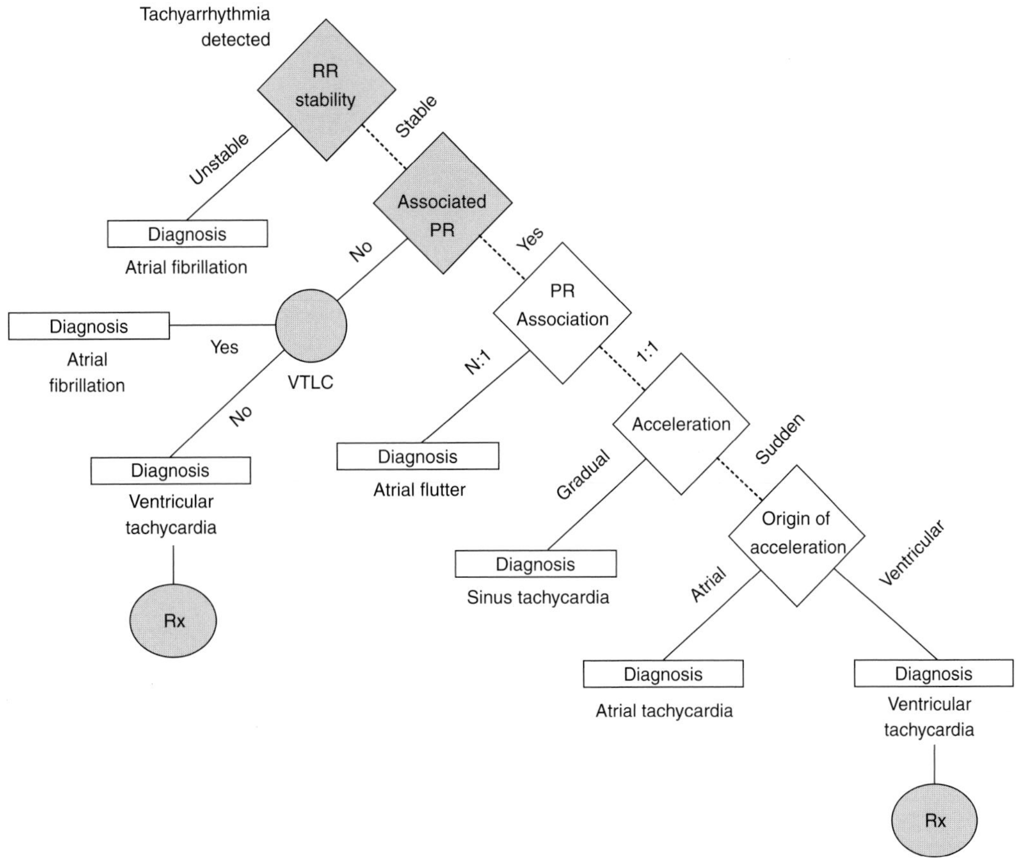

Figure 18.7 PARAD+ Rhythm discrimination algorithm. See text for discussion. (Reprinted from *EUROPACE* [25], with permission.)

Specific algorithms

With dual-chamber devices, multiple different algorithms applying the above-mentioned criterion have been created to help differentiate SVT from VT (Table 18.5). Studies comparing algorithms in different devices has found that specificity is increased by using PR association, atrial onset, and timing of the atrial event relative to the ventricular event [42]. If rate and stability alone are used, many stable supraventricular arrhythmias are misclassified as VT; however, most cases of AF are correctly classified. Other systems use hierarchical approach with AV rate branch feature utilizing morphology analysis, onset, and stability criteria [43]. A neural network classification system has also been proposed to classify arrhythmias based on atrial–ventricular relationship [44].

The Biotronik SMART (Figure 18.8) [45] detection algorithm utilizes average heart rate, rate stability, and beat-to-beat relation between the atria and the ventricle [46]. The algorithm is created with branches. Initially, the ventricular rate and atrial rate are compared. If the ventricular rate is faster than the atrial rate then VT is classified and therapy is initiated. If the ventricular and atrial rates are equal, then the rhythm is monitored based on stability. If the RR is stable, but the PP is unstable, then AV dissociation can be assumed and the rhythm is classified as VT. If the ventricular and atrial rhythms are stable, then the algorithm analyzes the PR interval. Sudden onset is classified as VT and gradual onset as SVT. If the RR interval is unstable, the rhythm is classified based on stability of the PR: stable is SVT, unstable is VT. Lastly, if the ventricular rate is slower than the atrial rate, classification is based on ventricular stability. If the RR is

Table 18.5 Comparison of individual algorithm sets.

	Biotronik (SMART)	*ELA (PARAD +)*	*Guidant (Rhythm ID)*	*Medtronic (PR Logic)*	*St. Jude (MD + A/V)*
Sudden onset	+	+		+	+
Rate stability	+	+	+	+	+
Electrogram characteristics			+		+
A/V events	+		+		+
AV relationship	+	+		+	
Chamber of Origin		+			

Notes:
MD = morphology discrimination; A/V = atrial and ventricular events.

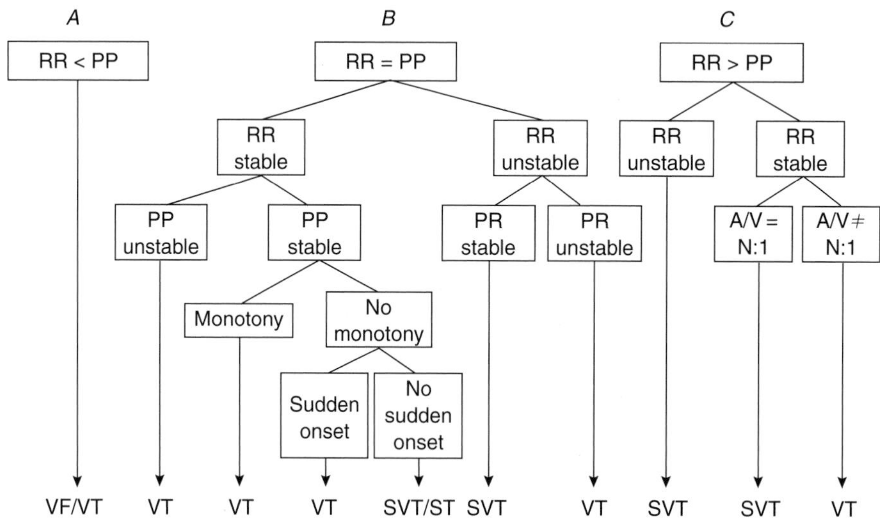

Figure 18.8 SMART Rhythm discrimination algorithm. Algorithm based on relative atrial and ventricular rates, stability, monotony, and sudden onset. SVT = supraventricular tachycardia, VT = ventricular tachycardia, A/V = atrial/ventricular ratio, ST = sinus tachycardia. (Reprinted from *J Cardiovasc Electrophysiol* [46], with permission.)

unstable, then it suggests some association between the atrium and ventricle classifying the rhythm as an SVT. If the RR is stable, then the device measures multiplicity to determine if an integral conduction relationship exists between the ventricle and the atrium.

There are several different decision tree algorithms that classify the rhythm based on AV relationship. The Medtronic PR Logic (Figure 18.9) incorporates data regarding the timing of the atrial event with the RR interval. The RR interval is divided into different zones that are used to classify the rhythm. For example, atrial events shortly before the next R-wave are classified as supraventricular or junctional while atrial events shortly after the R-wave are more likely to be ventricular. AV dissociation criteria may be met when there are no atrial events between the RR interval or the second longest and the second shortest of the previous eight AV intervals, which differ by more than 40 ms.

Owing to misclassification of 1 : 1 tachycardias, three enhancements were added to PR Logic – programmable 1 : 1 VT–ST boundary, enhanced far-field R-wave criterion, and enhanced transition counter. The VT–ST boundary allows programming of the percentage of the antegrade and retrograde zones so that the atrial event is more likely to fall within the antegrade zone if the PR interval is long. In doing so, VT therapy will be withheld. This enhancement was developed to address SVTs with long PR intervals. The downside

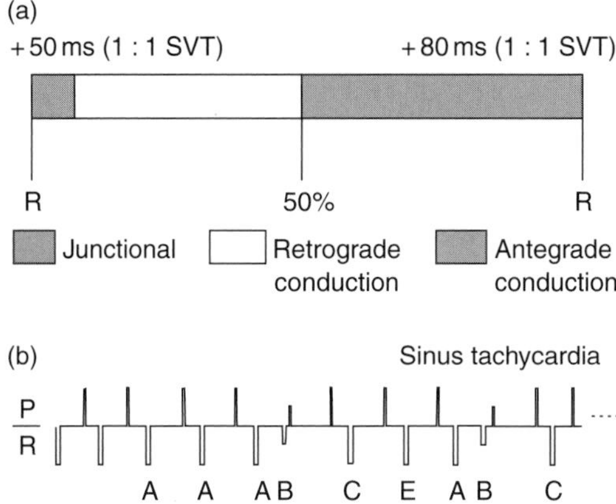

Figure 18.9 PR Logic atrial–ventricular relationship algorithm. Retrograde and Antegrade zones are used to classify the rhythm as ventricular or supraventricular, respectively.

of increasing the antegrade zone is the potential for decreasing sensitivity for VT with consistent 1 : 1 retrograde conduction. The transition counter allows PR logic to reclassify different types of SVTs. If PR logic is unable to classify the SVT, then VT detection is met and therapy is delivered. Previously, the transition counter was 6 beats, but more recently it has been increased to 10 beats to improve the ability to reject SVTs with transitions between SVT definitions.

The ELA PARAD+ algorithm examines a combination of stability, AV association, acceleration, the chamber of acceleration, and a long ventricular cycle detector (Figure 18.7) algorithm, RR stability is used as initial screening algorithm, with unstable rhythms being considered to be AF and stable rhythms being further classified. If PR association is absent, then the presence of a long cycle is used to classify the rhythm as AF and the absence of a long cycle is used to detect VT. If PR association is present, more atrial than ventricular events is classified as atrial flutter. A PR association of 1 : 1 is further classified based on acceleration. If the acceleration is gradual, the rhythm is classified as ST. A sudden acceleration is further classified based on the chamber of acceleration origin. Very simply, if the atrium is the chamber of acceleration the rhythm is classified as an atrial tachycardia (AT) and if the ventricle is the chamber of acceleration the rhythm is classified as a VT. Sadoul *et al.* [40] examined the performance of this algorithm. It demonstrates a high specificity and sensitivity. The algorithm performs well with very high sensitivity and a specificity of 89.2% and 91.6% on an episode and patient basis, respectively.

A review of sustained arrhythmias showed that ST or AT with long PR intervals and ST or AT with intermittent atrial oversensing of R-waves are the most common causes of inappropriate therapy, accounting for 56.5% of such events [47] (Figure 18.10). Therefore, an adaptive ST algorithm was created using P- and R-wave interval information. Using a combination of 1 : 1 AV conduction patterns, gradual changes in PR intervals, and gradual changes in intrinsic PR intervals, evidence for ST is established. Any deviation from 1 : 1 conduction or abrupt changes in RR or intrinsic PR intervals excludes ST. The algorithm applies four steps outlined below. The first step is establishing 1 : 1 AV conduction using the methods described above in PR logic. The 1 : 1 conduction updates the AV conduction counter that summarizes the recent history. A 1 : 1 conduction is classified if the majority of RR intervals are 1 : 1 or if the last four RR intervals were 1 : 1. The second step requires classification of the RR interval as expected or not expected. The expected range is composed of an estimate of the RR intervals ± estimate of the variability of the RR intervals. RR intervals are classified as unexpected and evidence against ST. The third step is determining if the PR interval is expected. For this step, RR intervals that contain paced events are excluded. The PR interval expected range is computed and applied similar to the expected RR range. PR intervals shorter or longer than expected exclude ST. The fourth and final step is accumulating evidence of ST. Expected PR and RR intervals supply separate and independent information. During intermittent pacing and ectopy the intervals may be classified as unexpected; therefore, determinations of expected intervals are summarized on a beat-to-beat basis. Specific beat patterns over time establish ST via an evidence counter similar to the current PR logic counters. When the ST evidence counter is ≥ 6, VT/VF therapy is withheld. The SVT limit parameter, SVT counter and transition encounter are the same.

This adaptive-interval-based algorithm was compared with the standard ST algorithm using

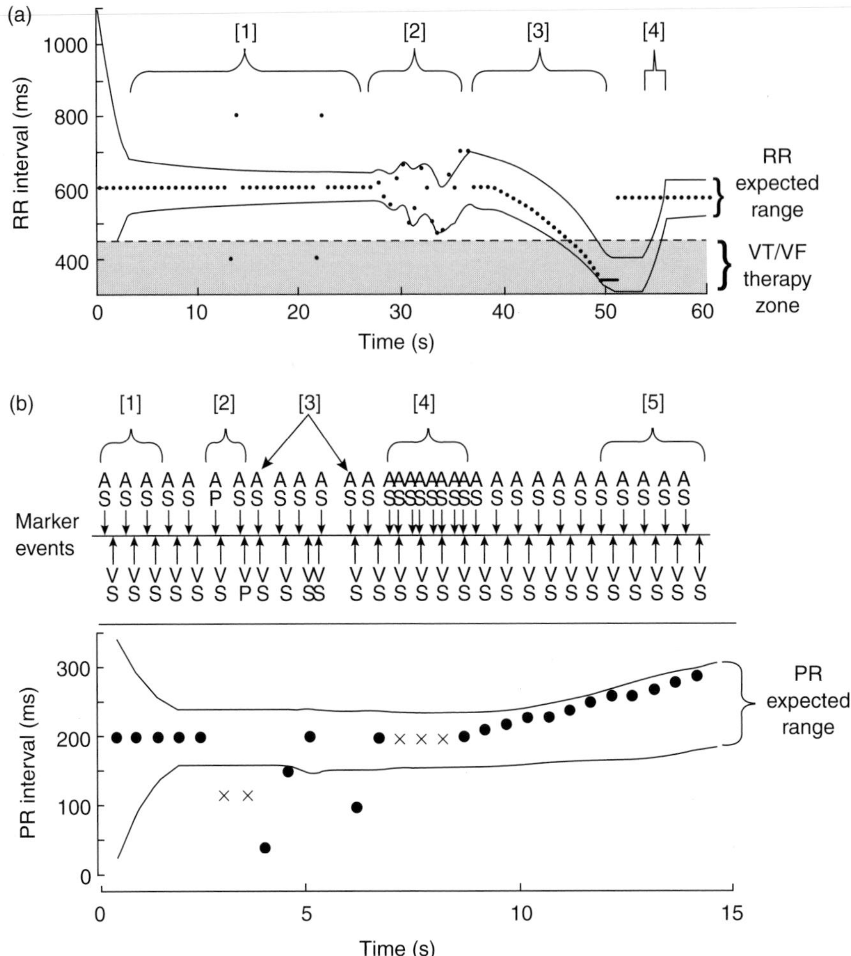

Figure 18.10 Adaptive interval algorithm for ST detection. (a) Expected RR range. During period 1, the two premature ventricular beats and the resulting pause result in intervals outside the expected range. During period 2, stable heart rate acceleration occurs. During period 4, there is sudden acceleration with RR intervals outside the expected range. (b) Expected PR range. "X" indicates PR intervals outside the expected range. (Reprinted from *PACE* [47], with permission.)

three different databases: 684 spontaneous VT/VF episodes; 216 spontaneous SVT episodes that received VT/VF therapy; 320 spontaneous ST/AT episodes that appropriately had therapy withheld. The adaptive algorithm had equivalent sensitivity for allowing VT/VF therapy. The net benefit of the adaptive algorithm for withholding therapy for those SVTs that received inappropriate therapy was 35.2%. The largest improvement was in appropriately classifying ST/AT with long PR intervals and ST/AT with atrial far-field R-wave oversensing. The adaptive algorithm has some weaknesses. It may not withhold therapy for sudden onset atrial tachyarrhythmias, rhythms with variable PR interval (Wenckebach or dual AV node physiology), or rhythms with high density of ectopic beats. Patients with VT that initiates during ST or high-rate atrial pacing may have their therapy delayed.

Retrograde conduction from the ventricle may be used for tachyarrhythmia discrimination. DiGregorio *et al.* demonstrated that the unipolar atrial electrogram shape and lag time between the onset of the proximal and the distal unipolar electrograms accurately identified retrograde conduction [48]. Correlation waveform analysis of atrial electrograms has also been shown to be able to distinguish antegrade and retrograde conduction [49].

Failing to sense VT as SVT can have extremely deleterious outcomes. Therefore, as a safety mechanism, many current devices have a rate duration safety net. If the tachycardia continues for a certain period of time within the VT zone, then the device will implement therapies for the VT zone. One study showed that the rate duration safety along with sudden onset and stability resulted in appropriate management in most patients [50].

Although dual-chamber sensing provides important data for rhythm classification, comparative data demonstrating the superiority of atrial and ventricular discrimination algorithms are limited. In one study by Deisenhofer *et al.*, dual-chamber rhythm discrimination algorithms did not offer benefits in avoiding inappropriate therapies due to supraventricular arrhythmias compared with single-chamber devices [51]. Most of these failures resulted from intermittent atrial sensing problems demonstrating that atrial sensing errors can also negatively affected by tachycardia classification. Hintringer *et al.* on the other hand, showed that algorithms incorporating atrial and ventricular relationship improved rhythm discrimination [42]. A large-scale randomized study comparing the available single- and dual-chamber algorithms is lacking.

Conclusions

The development of new algorithms has improved ventricular sensing and rhythm discrimination. Current algorithms for ventricular detection have made undersensing of VF uncommon. Undersensing of VT only rarely occurs due to problems such as fluctuating R-wave amplitudes. Oversensing problems such as oversensing T-waves or double counting the QRS still occur but algorithms may be adjusted to decrease this likelihood. Rhythm discrimination algorithms have made significant advances in distinguishing supraventricular arrhythmias from ventricular arrhythmias. However, inappropriate therapy remains a challenge in many patients. Full utilization of existing algorithms and the development of new methods will further decrease this problem in the future.

References

1 Cannom DS, Prystowsky EN. The evolution of the implantable cardioverter defibrillator. *PACE* 2004; **27**(3): 419–431.

2 Bhatia A, Cooley R, Berger M *et al.* The implantable cardioverter defibrillator: technology, indications, and impact on cardiovascular survival. *Curr Probl Cardiol* 2004; **29**(6): 303–356.

3 Callans DJ, Hook BG, Kleiman RB, Mitra RL, Flores BT, Marchlinski FE. Unique sensing errors in third-generation implantable cardioverter-defibrillators. *J Am Coll Cardiol* 1993; **22**(4): 1135–1140.

4 Olson W. Tachyarrhythmia sensing and detection. In: Singer I, ed. *Implantable Cardioverter-Defibrillators.* Futura Publishing Company, Armonk, NY, 1994: 77.

5 Callans DJ, Hook BG, Marchlinski FE. Effect of rate and coupling interval on endocardial R wave amplitude variability in permanent ventricular sensing lead systems. *J Am Coll Cardiol* 1993; **22**(3):746–750.

6 Dekker LR, Schrama TA, Steinmetz FH, Tukkie R. Undersensing of VF in a patient with optimal Rwave sensing during sinus rhythm. *PACE* 2004; **27**(6 Pt 1): 833–834.

7 Jongnarangsin K, Mela T. Implantable cardioverter defibrillator sensing failure due to endocardial R wave electrical alternans. *J Cardiovasc Electrophysiol* 2002; **13**(7): 702–704.

8 Eberhardt F, Peters W, Bode F, Wiegand UK. R wave undersensing caused by an algorithm intended to enhance sensing specificity in an implantable cardioverter defibrillator. *PACE* 2003; **26**(8): 1776–1777.

9 Koul AK, Keller S, Clancy JF, Lampert R, Batsford WP, Rosenfeld LE. Hyperkalemia induced T wave oversensing leading to loss of biventricular pacing and inappropriate ICD shocks. *PACE* 2004; **27**(5): 681–683.

10 Schimpf R, Wolpert C, Bianchi F *et al.* Congenital short QT syndrome and implantable cardioverter defibrillator treatment: inherent risk for inappropriate shock delivery. *J Cardiovasc Electrophysiol* 2003; **14**(12): 1273–1277.

11 Duru F, Bauersfeld U, Candinas R. Avoiding inappropriate ventricular tachycardia detection due to T-wave oversensing in an implantable cardioverter defibrillator: a novel application of the electrogram width criterion. *Europace* 2001; **3**(1): 80–84.

12 Cossu SF, Hsia HH, Simson MB, Hanna MS, Clyne CA. Inappropriate pauses during bradycardia pacing in a third-generation implantable cardioverter defibrillator. *PACE* 1997; **20**(9 Pt 1): 2271–2274.

13 Curwin JH, Roelke M, Ruskin JN. Inhibition of bradycardia pacing caused by far-field atrial sensing in a third-generation cardioverter defibrillator with an automatic gain feature. *PACE* 1996; **19**(1): 124–126.

14 St.JudeMedical. Sensing slide collection.

15 Ellenbogen KA, Edel T, Moore S *et al.* A prospective randomized-controlled trial of ventricular fibrillation detection time in a DDDR ventricular defibrillator. Ventak AV II DR Study Investigators.[erratum appears in PACE 2000 **23**(11 Pt 1): viii]. *PACE* 2000; **23**(8): 1268–1272.

16 Callans DJ, Swarna US, Schwartzman D, Gottlieb CD, Marchlinski FE. Postshock sensing performance in transvenous defibrillation lead systems: analysis of detection and redetection of ventricular fibrillation. *J Cardiovasc Electrophysiol* 1995; **6**(8): 604–612.

17 Ellis JR, Martin DT, Venditti FJ, Jr. Appropriate sensing of ventricular fibrillation after failed shocks in a transvenous cardioverter-defibrillator system. *Circulation* 1994; **90**(4): 1820–1825.

18 Isbruch FM, Block M, Bocker D *et al.* Improved sensing signals after endocardial defibrillation with a redesigned integrated sense pace defibrillation lead. *PACE* 1996; **19**(8): 1211–1218.

19 Crevenna R, Stix G, Pleiner J *et al.* Electromagnetic interference by transcutaneous neuromuscular electrical stimulation in patients with bipolar sensing implantable cardioverter defibrillators: a pilot safety study. *PACE* 2003; **26**(2 Pt 1): 626–629.

20 Crevenna R, Wolzt M, Fialka-Moser V *et al.* Long-term transcutaneous neuromuscular electrical stimulation in patients with bipolar sensing implantable cardioverter defibrillators: a pilot safety study. *Artif Organs* 2004; **28**(1): 99–102.

21 Glotzer TV, Gordon M, Sparta M, Radoslovich G, Zimmerman J. Electromagnetic interference from a muscle stimulation device causing discharge of an implantable cardioverter defibrillator: epicardial bipolar and endocardial bipolar sensing circuits are compared. *PACE* 1998; **21**(10): 1996–1998.

22 Deshmukh P, Anderson K. Myopotential sensing by a dual chamber implantable cardioverter defibrillator: two case reports. *J Cardiovasc Electrophysiol* 1998; **9**(7): 767–772.

23 Embil JM, Geddes JS, Foster D, Sandeman J. Return to arc welding following defibrillator implantation. *PACE* 1993; **16**(12): 2313–2318.

24 Fetter JG, Benditt DG, Stanton MS. Electromagnetic interference from welding and motors on implantable cardioverter-defibrillators as tested in the electrically hostile work site. *J Am Coll Cardiol* 1996; **28**(2): 423–427.

25 Aliot E, Nitzsche R, Ripart A. Arrhythmia detection by dual-chamber implantable cardioverter defibrillators. A review of current algorithms. *Europace* 2004; **6**(4): 273–286.

26 Schaumann A, von zur Muhlen F, Gonska BD, Kreuzer H. Enhanced detection criteria in implantable cardioverter-defibrillators to avoid inappropriate therapy. *Am J Cardiol* 1996; **78**(5A): 42–50.

27 Favale S, Nacci F, Galati A *et al.* Electrogram width parameter analysis in implantable cardioverter defibrillators: Influence of body position and electrode configuration. *PACE* 2001; **24**(12): 1732–1738.

28 Duru F, Schonbeck M, Luscher TF, Candinas R. The potential for inappropriate ventricular tachycardia confirmation using the intracardiac electrogram (EGM) width criterion. *PACE* 1999; **22**(7): 1039–1046.

29 Unterberg C, Stevens J, Vollmann D, Hasenfuss G, Buchwald AB. Long-term clinical experience with the EGM width detection criterion for differentiation of supraventricular and ventricular tachycardia in patients with implantable cardioverter defibrillators. *PACE* 2000; **23**(11 Pt 1): 1611–1617.

30 Greenhut SE, Deering TF, Steinhaus BM, Ingram JL, Camp SR, DiCarlo LA. Separation of ventricular tachycardia from sinus rhythm using a practical, real-time template matching computer system. *PACE* 1992; **15**(11 Pt 2): 2146–2153.

31 St.JudeMedical. Morphology discrimination slide set. 2004

32 Michaud GF, Li Q, Costeas X, Stearns R, Estes M III, Wang PJ. Correlation waveform analysis to discriminate monomorphic ventricular tachycardia from sinus rhythm using stored electrograms from implantable defibrillators. *PACE* 1999; **22**(8): 1146–1151.

33 Boriani G, Occhetta E, Pistis G *et al.* Combined use of morphology discrimination, sudden onset, and stability as discriminating algorithms in single chamber cardioverter defibrillators. *PACE* 2002; **25**(9): 1357–1366.

34 Gronefeld GC, Schulte B, Hohnloser SH *et al.* Morphology discrimination: a beat-to-beat algorithm for the discrimination of ventricular from supraventricular tachycardia by implantable cardioverter defibrillators. *PACE* 2001; **24**(10): 1519–1524.

35 Leenhardt A, Hamdaoui B, Di Fusco S *et al.* [Brugada syndrome]. Archives des Maladies du Coeur et des Vaisseaux 2003; 96 Spec No 4:30–37.

36 Boriani G, Biffi M, Frabetti L, Lattuca JJ, Branzi A. Clinical evaluation of morphology discrimination: an algorithm for rhythm discrimination in cardioverter defibrillators. *PACE* 2001; **24**(6): 994–1001.

37 Swerdlow CD, Brown ML, Lurie K *et al.* Discrimination of ventricular tachycardia from supraventricular tachycardia by a downloaded wavelet-transform morphology algorithm: a paradigm for development of implantable cardioverter defibrillator detection algorithms. *J Cardiovasc Electrophysiol* 2002; **13**(5): 432–441.

38 Gold MR, Shorofsky SR, Thompson JA *et al.* Advanced rhythm discrimination for implantable cardioverter defibrillators using electrogram vector timing and correlation. *J Cardiovasc Electrophysiol* 2002; **13**(11): 1092–1097.

39 DiCarlo L, Jenkins JM, Caswell S, Morris M, Pariseau B. Tachycardia detection by antitachycardia devices: present

limitations and future strategies. *J Interventional Cardiology* 1994; 7(5): 459–472.

40 Sadoul N, Jung W, Jordaens L *et al.* Diagnostic performance of a dual-chamber cardioverter defibrillator programmed with nominal settings: a European prospective study. *J Cardiovasc Electrophysiol* 2002; **13**(1): 25–32.

41 Glotzer TV, Radoslovich GA, Neglia J, Zimmerman JM. Variability of atrial sensing during exercise in a patient with a dual chamber ICD caused inappropriate ICD discharges. *PACE* 1999; **22**(12): 1838–1841.

42 Hintringer F, Schwarzacher S, Eibl G, Pachinger O. Inappropriate detection of supraventricular arrhythmias by implantable dual chamber defibrillators: a comparison of four different algorithms. *PACE* 2001; **24**(5): 835–841.

43 Bailin SJ, Niebauer M, Tomassoni G, Leman R. The Photon I. Clinical investigation of a new dual-chamber implantable cardioverter defibrillator with improved rhythm discrimination capabilities. *J Cardiovasc Electrophysiol* 2003; **14**(2): 144–149.

44 Leong PH, Jabri MA. MATIC – an intracardiac tachycardia classification system. *PACE* 1992; **15**(9): 1317–1331.

45 Theuns D, Klootwijk AP, Kimman GP, Szili-Torok T, Roelandt JR, Jordaens L. Initial clinical experience with a new arrhythmia detection algorithm in dual chamber implantable cardioverter defibrillators. *Europace* 2001; 3(3): 181–186.

46 Sinha AM, Stellbrink C, Schuchert A *et al.* Clinical experience with a new detection algorithm for differentiation of supraventricular from ventricular tachycardia in a dual-chamber defibrillator. *J Cardiovasc Electrophysiol* 2004; **15**(6): 646–652.

47 Stadler RW, Gunderson BD, Gillberg JM. An adaptive interval-based algorithm for withholding ICD therapy during sinus tachycardia. *PACE* 2003; **26**(5): 1189–1201.

48 Di Gregorio F, al-Bunni M, Bulla V *et al.* Retroconduction selective recognition in wide-dipole floating atrial sensing. The Multicenter Study Group. *PACE* 1997; **20**(11): 2817–2824.

49 Saba S, Gorodeski R, Yang S *et al.* Use of correlation waveform analysis in discrimination between anterograde and retrograde atrial electrograms during ventricular tachycardia. *J Cardiovasc Electrophysiol* 2001; **12**(2): 145–149.

50 Brugada J. Is inappropriate therapy a resolved issue with current implantable cardioverter defibrillators? *Am J Cardiol* 1999; **83**(5B): 40D–44D.

51 Deisenhofer I, Kolb C, Ndrepepa G, Schreieck J, Karch M, Schmieder S *et al.* Do current dual chamber cardioverter defibrillators have advantages over conventional single chamber cardioverter defibrillators in reducing inappropriate therapies? A randomized, prospective study. *J Cardiovasc Electrophysiol* 2001; **12**(2): 134–142.

19

CHAPTER 19

Arrhythmia prevention and termination algorithms

Gregory Engel, MD, *Paul J. Wang*, MD, & *Amin Al-Ahmad*, MD

Ventricular arrhythmia prevention

Since the development of the implantable cardioverter defibrillator (ICD), termination of malignant ventricular tachyarrhythmias using shock or pacing therapy has been achievable. This therapy can cause a significant amount of pain and mental anguish to patients. In addition, termination of arrhythmias may require several shocks or may be unsuccessful. Development of methods to prevent ventricular tachyarrhythmias is therefore of paramount importance.

One obvious potential intervention that the ICD can be used to effect is that of heart rate. Although heart rate is an important factor in the development of arrhythmias and pacing may be able to prevent arrhythmias in certain situations, several factors limit the role of pacing to prevent ventricular tachycardias (VTs). Ventricular and His-Purkinje tissue refractoriness are modified by heart rate and bradycardia-dependent arrhythmias (early after-depolarizations or reentry) can theoretically be prevented by increasing heart rate. However, increased heart rate can theoretically increase the risk of arrhythmias due to delayed after-depolarizations and triggered activity. Heart rate is also an indicator of autonomic nervous system tone that is important in arrhythmogenesis but pacing tends to shift the autonomic balance toward a sympathetic predominance that is likely to have an unfavorable effect [1]. Premature ventricular and atrial contractions (PVCs and PACs) that occur at critical coupling intervals are also important in initiating arrhythmias but the optimal way to use pacing to prevent these initiating complexes from occurring is unclear. These factors significantly limit the ability of pacing alone to prevent arrhythmias.

Advances in microprocessor technology have allowed the development of advanced and complex pacing algorithms capable of arrhythmia prevention [2]. Multiple investigators have attempted to design algorithms to try to overcome these limitations and use pacing to prevent arrhythmia initiation. Many factors must be considered including: the relationship of heart rate to arrhythmia initiation, frequency and coupling interval of initiating complexes, the presence of long–short intervals and short–long–short intervals, and initiation patterns of bradycardia-dependent arrhythmias.

Overdrive pacing

Overdrive suppression using continuous pacing slightly above the patients spontaneous rates can be effective in significantly decreasing the frequency of ventricular ectopy and nonsustained VT. It can prevent bradycardia-dependent ventricular activity and has been shown to be useful in some cases of drug refractory VT [3].

Patients with the congenital long-QT syndrome are especially prone to ventricular tachyarrhythmias following pauses. Pauses alone or short–long–short sequences appear to be responsible for most of the episodes of torsade de pointes in congenital long-QT syndrome [4]. It is especially important to avoid shocks in these patients as they can lead to recurrent bursts of torsades. Overdrive pacing combined with beta blockade has been demonstrated to be effective in preventing pauses and decreasing episodes of torsades [5, 6]. A review of patients with acquired long-QT syndrome revealed that episodes of torsades were optimally prevented when pacing rates were greater than 70 beats per minute (bpm) [7].

More recently, the approach of overdrive pacing to suppress ventricular arrhythmias has been attempted in patients who are not affected by the long-QT syndrome. In a study of 23 patients with an ICD, detection of VT or nonsustained VT triggered overdrive pacing at a rate of 90 bpm for a mean time of 61 s. This intervention seemed to result in a significant reduction in episodes of nonsustained VT and a trend in the reduction in episodes of VT [8]. Further studies are needed prior to routine adoption of this strategy for ventricular tachyarrhythmia prevention.

Ventricular rate stabilization

Rate stabilization algorithms (also called rate smoothing) can be triggered by variations in rate that may cause changes in pacing intervals. Rate stabilization algorithms can be triggered when the rate changes dramatically from one beat to the next, for example, with atrial or ventricular premature contractions. The goal of rate stabilization algorithms is to decrease symptoms related to dramatic rate variations. Rate stabilization can also prevent short–long–short sequences that may predispose to arrhythmias. When this type of algorithm is programmed "on," the device will initiate atrioventricular (AV) pacing at a programmed percentage of the preceding R–R interval and can be programmed to increase or decrease. The ability to attenuate or prevent rate variations makes this algorithm appealing as a potential method to prevent ventricular tachyarrhythmias.

Rate smoothing algorithms have been evaluated in two large studies to date. A prospective crossover study of 309 patients, using an intention to treat analysis, showed a 35% risk reduction in arrhythmias with rate stabilization. However, in a Cox model adjusted for confounding variables, there was only an 8% nonsignificant relative risk reduction [9]. The PREVENT study was a randomized multicenter prospective crossover study designed to evaluate the use of a rate smoothing algorithm for the prevention of VT [10]. One-hundred fifty-three patients were evaluated during 3 months with the rate smoothing algorithm on and 3 months with it off. There was a significant reduction in episodes of sustained VT from 358 without to 145 with rate smoothing turned on. Episodes of VT clearly following a short–long–short sequence were decreased from 100 without to 40 with rate smoothing. Interestingly, there was no statistically significant reduction in VT episodes per patient [11].

Although no proarrhythmic effects were seen in the PREVENT study, there are possibilities for abnormal ICD function with ventricular rate stabilization algorithms, such as AV sequential pacing during sustained VT [12].

Based on the data supporting the use of these algorithms to suppress VT, the Ventricular Arrhythmia Suppression Trial (VAST) is currently underway. This trial is a randomized, single blinded, crossover design that randomizes patients to rate smoothing "on" versus "off". The data from this trial, once completed, may shed some additional light on the use of rate smoothing algorithms for arrhythmia prevention.

Future directions in arrhythmia prevention

As we learn more about the hemodynamic consequences of pacing in patients who are at risk for VT, future uses of pacing to prevent VT may rely on biventricular pacing [13, 14]. Biventricular pacing has been shown to decrease the frequency of ventricular ectopy, decrease appropriate ICD shocks, and decrease the inducibility of ventricular arrhythmias during programmed electrical stimulation as well [15–17].

While the use of pacing to prevent VT may have its limitations, future use of the ICD for arrhythmia prevention may involve nontraditional uses of the ICD. For example, combining ICD technology with that of a pulsatile drug pump that allows for release of an antiarrhythmic agent may be useful in decreasing the amount of ventricular arrhythmias. Other technologies that may show promise for the prevention of ventricular tachyarrhythmias include thoracic spinal cord stimulation. In experimental animal models of ischemic heart failure, thoracic spinal cord stimulation has been shown to decrease the incidence of ventricular tachyarrhythmias [18]. Combining this technology with ICD technology either directly or with device-to-device communication may be useful in the future.

One major challenge for the prevention of ventricular arrhythmias is the ability to predict episodes before they occur. This would help limit the intervention to the times that are higher risk than others for the development of arrhythmias.

Several investigators are evaluating methods to detect changes in the arrhythmogenic substrate immediately prior to arrhythmia onset, allowing for the possibility of predicting VT before it starts and initiating preventative therapy at those critical times. In a retrospective analysis of device-detected tachycardia in 923 ICD patients, Zhou *et al.* [19] found that sustained ventricular arrhythmias were temporally related to the amount of nonsustained episodes of VT in that the sustained episodes were likely to occur on the same day or within a 3 day window. By using a metric of nonsustained episodes of VT, a statistical likelihood of sustained VT may be calculated and once this likelihood achieves a threshold value the ICD can perhaps initiate preventative therapies.

Using signal processing techniques, several methods have been developed for long-term risk stratification for mortality. Decreased heart rate variability (HRV) is a risk factor for mortality in patients with cardiac disease. In addition to a long-term increase in risk, assessment of the nonlinear dynamic parameters of HRV have been shown to change prior to the onset of VT [20, 21]. Another method for predicting arrhythmic events is the modified Karhunen–Loeve transformation that identifies a core pattern of cardiac cycles and then tracks changes in, and identifies progressive destabilization of, the cardiac rhythm [22]. Other currently used risk markers for ventricular arrhythmias such as T-wave alternans and heart rate turbulence once this technology advances for potential real-time assessment may be used in ICDs to predict ventricular arrhythmias.

As more insight is gained on the mechanisms of ventricular tachyarrhythmias and as we become more able to predict the occurrence of these rhythm abnormalities, future ICD may have the ability to reliably predict and prevent ventricular arrhythmias.

Ventricular arrhythmia termination

The primary function of the current generation ICD is not to prevent VT or VF (ventricular fibrillation) but to treat these arrhythmias with either rapid overdrive pacing or shock.

The standard approach is tiered therapy, allowing different responses for ventricular arrhythmias with different characteristics. Devices capable of tiered therapy provided a significant advance in therapy beginning in the early 1990s [23]. Painless antitachycardia pacing (ATP) can be used as the initial response to terminate slower, organized VT. If unsuccessful, this can be followed by shock therapy, this can be programmed depending on the defibrillation threshold to minimize charge time and maximize battery life. Faster ventricular tachyarrhythmias often require high-energy shocks as initial therapy.

Pacing to terminate VT

Current generation ICDs utilize ATP to overdrive VT. The goal is to competitively pace the ventricle at a faster rate than the VT in order to interrupt the reentry circuit and, thereby, terminate the abnormal rhythm. ATP uses bursts of high-output pacing pulses delivered through the ventricular pacing electrode. The advantage of ATP is that it is painless, quick, and limits battery drain. It is therefore a good technique to be used for a first attempt at termination of VT. Often, patients are unaware that an abnormal rhythm has occurred and that it has been treated with overdrive pacing.

Antitachycardia pacing can take the form of fixed, autodecremental, or adaptive burst pacing. Fixed burst pacing is delivered at a constant cycle length. In autodecremental pacing, the initial stimulus is delivered at a percentage of the VT cycle length and each subsequent cycle length becomes shorter, thereby accelerating the pacing rate. Adaptive burst pacing utilizes adjusted cycle lengths usually at about 80–90% of that of the VT. Most sustained monomorphic VT, especially in patients with coronary artery disease, is due to reentry and can be terminated by pacing [24]. Excitable gaps within the reentrant circuit allow for the access and block of the circuit required for successful termination of VT [25–28].

Several studies have evaluated the different ATP modalities [24, 29–45]. ATP has been found to be highly efficacious with success rates over 90%, especially in patients with VT cycle lengths over 300 ms [37, 39, 41, 42, 44, 46]. Most devices use either autodecremental or adaptive burst pacing. Both techniques have been shown to have similar efficacy and safety [29, 31, 33, 36, 40].

Although it is often successful in terminating an arrhythmia, overdrive pacing can accelerate the tachycardia or induce VF. Early attempts to use pacemakers for treatment of VT were severely limited by these hazards [47, 48]. Acceleration is seen in up to 10% of treatment episodes [39, 44, 49]. Therefore, all devices that attempt overdrive pacing must have defibrillation available as a backup.

Tachycardia cycle length is a major determinant of pace termination with ATP [35]. The critical paced cycle length required for termination during overdrive pacing is directly related to the refractory period of the circuit. An experimental study of induced VT demonstrates that tachycardia is entrained when the paced cycle length is significantly longer than the relative refractory period of the circuit while termination of the tachycardia only occurs when it is significantly shorter [28]. Evaluation of registry information on patients with ICDs shows that there is no significant difference in pacing termination when coupling intervals range from 80% to 99% of the spontaneous cycle length [39]. Paced cycle lengths of <80% of the VT cycle length are rarely used due to a much higher rate of acceleration [24]. A randomized evaluation of adaptive burst pacing algorithms suggests that 91% of the VT cycle length is more effective than a lower cycle length (81%) [41]. The only independent predictors of pacing termination were the coupling interval and a longer tachycardia cycle length (slower VT). This study also showed that longer pacing trains (15 versus 7 beats) were more effective but this was in exchange for a higher acceleration rate. Other studies have also shown that the acceleration risk increases when longer pulses are used [45, 50] while no differences in termination or acceleration with a range of 6–15 pulses were found by Nasir *et al.* [39].

Fine tuning of the ATP algorithm for each individual based on inducible VT is of limited value because spontaneous episodes of VT are usually slower and more easily convertible than VT induced by programmed electrical stimulation [51]. In addition, patients who are not inducible can develop spontaneous monomorphic VT. The most important consideration in using ATP is hemodynamic tolerance of the VT. As rate is the most important factor in hemodynamic stability during VT, ATP is usually reserved for slower VT while faster VT with a higher risk of syncope is usually treated initially with cardioversion. However, there is more recent evidence to suggest that fast VT (240–320 ms cycle length) can be effectively treated with ATP with a low incidence of acceleration and syncope [52]. When it is possible to safely make use of ATP, it is clear that it is effective and patient tolerance of the device is greatly improved [53]. Since ATP may have variable success in termination of VT, and may be the cause of VT acceleration, some devices have the feature of turning ATP "off" if ATP fails repeatedly [54]. This will then limit the amount of time the individual is in VT as the device will treat with therapies that have been effective, rather than those that are not.

With the increased prevalence of biventricular pacing for heart failure, investigators have also begun to evaluate ATP performed by biventricular devices. A study of over 200 patients has demonstrated that the rates of sensing and termination with biventricular devices are comparable to right ventricular devices [55]. One study using an animal model has suggested that biventricular ATP may be superior to single ventricle ATP in certain circumstances [56]. In a retrospective evaluation of the 89 patients in the InSync ICD study, there was a statistically significant higher success rate for termination of VT when ATP was programmed to biventricular as compared with right ventricular [57]. With increasing insight into the use of biventricular ATP, this feature will likely be an option in future biventricular ICD systems.

Cardioversion and defibrillation

If ATP fails to terminate a ventricular tachyarrhythmia, the device will then utilize shock therapy after redetection. This can be programmed in some cases as a synchronized shock (cardioversion) where it is synchronized to a ventricular sensed event or an asynchronous shock. Successive therapies are delivered up to 4–6 times in cases of failure to terminate with one shock before the device completes its therapeutic algorithm.

Early ICDs were "committed" to delivering therapy once the tachyarrhythmia was detected while current ICDs are capable of continued detection during the charging period and are "noncommitted." Current ICDs will reconfirm the presence of the tachyarrhythmia before shock delivery for the first therapy. After the delivery of the first therapy, they may become "committed" after redetection and subsequent therapies. After charging, when the programmed energy is reached, most ICDs will attempt to synchronize with the leading edge of a ventricular sensed event but will deliver an asynchronous shock if it is unable to synchronize.

Cardioversion or defibrillation require depolarization of the majority of the cells in the ventricle, many of which may be as much as 10 cm from the distal tip of the electrode. Therefore, successful therapy requires much higher energies than pacing. Voltages up to 100 times greater than the ICD battery voltage may be required. To achieve this, capacitors store charge prior to delivering the therapy. The time required to charge the capacitor (5–10 s) accounts for most of the delay between detection of the arrhythmia and delivery of therapy. Charge time is linearly related to the voltage being delivered and lengthens as the battery voltage is depleted. The current standard is the biphasic shock waveform, with reversal of shock polarity along a truncated exponential waveform. It is a simple system that provides adequate defibrillation safety margins for the vast majority of patients. Switching from monophasic to biphasic shock waveforms in the 1980s [58–60] was a significant breakthrough but more recent efforts to make adjustments in the biphasic waveforms to reduce defibrillation requirements have had limited success [61–63].

Electrical energy exceeding 1–2 joules (J) generally causes skeletal and diaphragmatic muscle depolarization and is painful to a conscious patient. Most ICD discharge is in the range of 10–40 J. A 96% probability of successful defibrillation has been demonstrated with a safety margin of 7 J [64] and some recent investigations have also suggested that a 5 J safety margin may be adequate for device implantation [65–67]. There is also evidence to suggest that a single successful shock 15 J below the maximum output is a safe testing method at implantation [68]. Owing to the pain induced, testing of ICDs after implantation is routinely performed using either conscious sedation or general anesthesia.

Low-energy cardioversion

The use of low-energy cardioversion, in addition to saving battery life as described above, also reduces capacitance time and, thereby, reduces time to therapy. Autodecremental overdrive pacing and low-energy defibrillation have been shown to have similar efficacy [69]. It is important to note that even low-energy shocks do not eliminate the pain felt by the patient. As low-energy cardioversion and ATP were shown to have similar efficacy and similar rates of VT acceleration, ATP has been the preferred technique for VT as it has the advantages of less patient discomfort, battery drain, and atrial proarrhythmia [70]. Others have argued that there still may be a role for low-energy cardioversion for treatment of fast VT which is inherently less responsive to ATP. A third detection and therapy zone programmed to treat fast VT with intervals of 270–330 ms using 3 or 5 J biphasic shocks has been shown to have high success rates, comparable to treatment of slow VT with pacing algorithms [71].

Low-energy termination of VF

As opposed to low-energy cardioversion of VT, low-energy defibrillation of VF has not generally been found to be successful. Localized membrane depolarization requires limited amounts of energy but termination of VF requires much higher energies to depolarize a critical mass of tissue. It is hypothesized that wavefront synchronization is an important aspect of VF termination and large amount of energy is required to ensure that large areas of myocardium are depolarized to avoid continued VF [72]. Optimizing shock timing has produced only a maximal 20% reduction in defibrillation thresholds [73, 74]. Evidence of excitable gaps during VF have led to attempts at pace termination of VF [75]. Although animal studies have shown that it is possible to capture VF and terminate it, the efficacy of this approach is limited [76]. As there are no effective alternatives and VF is inherently a hemodynamically unstable rhythm, ICDs are programmed to deliver a high-energy shock as soon as possible after VF is detected.

Future directions in arrhythmia termination

While the ICD will always be tasked with termination of ventricular tachyarrhythmias, new technologies will emerge that will enable us to do this more efficiently and with a higher efficacy. We may also have a "smarter" ICD, one that not only is more simple to program, but one that might learn to modify therapies such that only successful therapies are used.

Many of the issues that are the cause of problems in today's defibrillator may be solved with newer generations. A major issue that continues to plague ICD therapy is that of painful shocks. An ideal ICD would be able to provide adequate defibrillation without pain or with less painful shocks.

Another area for future development of ICD treatment is in the area of treating electromechanical dissociation (EMD). EMD is a common cause of sudden death after VT or VF is appropriately treated with shock [77, 78]. Techniques to treat EMD, such as use of medium voltage therapy may have some promise for development in future ICDs [79].

The ICD has been responsible for saving countless lives since its inception. Future developments will undoubtedly improve this valuable medical device.

References

1 Chiladakis JA, Kalogeropoulos A, Manolis AS. Autonomic responses to single- and dual-chamber pacing. *Am J Cardiol* 2004; **93**(8): 985–989.

2 Roth JA *et al.* Implementation of a new DDDR algorithm for tachycardia prevention and treatment utilizing an implantable RAM-based software-controlled pacemaker. *J Electrocardiol* 1992; **24**: 136–145.

3 Fisher JD *et al.* Antiarrhythmic effects of VVI pacing at physiologic rates: a crossover controlled evaluation. *PACE* 1987; **10**(4 Pt 1): 822–830.

4 Viskin S *et al.* Mode of onset of torsade de pointes in congenital long QT syndrome. *J Am Coll Cardiol* 1996; **28**(5): 1262–1268.

5 Dorostkar PC *et al.* Long-term follow-up of patients with long-QT syndrome treated with beta-blockers and continuous pacing. *Circulation* 1999; **100**(24): 2431–2436.

6 Eldar M *et al.* Permanent cardiac pacing in patients with the long QT syndrome. *J Am Coll Cardiol* 1987; **10**(3): 600–607.

7 Pinski SL, Eguia LE, Trohman RG. What is the minimal pacing rate that prevents torsades de pointes? Insights from patients with permanent pacemakers. *PACE* 2002; **25**(11): 612–1615.

8 Yee R *et al.* Pacing Algorithm for ventricular arrhythmic prevention in patients with implantable cardioverter-defibrillator. *PACE* 2003; **26**: 1038 abstracts.

9 Gronefeld GC *et al.* Ventricular rate stabilization for the prevention of pause dependent ventricular tachyarrhythmias: results from a prospective study in 309 ICD recipients. *PACE* 2002; **25**(12): 1708–1714.

10 Fromer M, Wietholt, D. Algorithm for the prevention of ventricular tachycardia onset: the prevent study. *Am J Cardiol* 1999; **83**(5B): 45D–47D.

11 Wietholt D *et al.* Prevention of sustained ventricular tachyarrhythmias in patients with implantable cardioverter-defibrillators – the PREVENT study. *J Interv Card Electrophysiol* 2003; **9**(3): 383–389.

12 Barold SS. Ventricular rate stabilization algorithm of ICD causing dual chamber pacing during ventricular tachycardia. *J Interv Card Electrophysiol* 2003; **9**(3): 397–400.

13 Wilkoff BL *et al.* Dual-chamber pacing or ventricular backup pacing in patients with an implantable defibrillator: the Dual Chamber and VVI Implantable Defibrillator (DAVID) Trial. *JAMA* 2002; **288**(24): 3115–3123.

14 Whang W *et al.* Heart failure and the risk of shocks in patients with implantable cardioverter defibrillators: results from the Triggers of ventricular Arrhythmias (TOVA) study. *Circulation* 2004; **109**(11): 1386–1391.

15 Walker S *et al.* Usefulness of suppression of ventricular arrhythmia by biventricular pacing in severe congestive cardiac failure. *Am J Cardiol* 2000; **86**(2): 231–233.

16 Higgins SL *et al.* Biventricular pacing diminishes the need for implantable cardioverter defibrillator therapy. Ventak CHF Investigators. *J Am Coll Cardio*, 2000; **36**(3): 824–827.

17 Kowal R *et al.* Biventricular pacing reduces the induction of monomorphic ventricular tachycardia: a potential mechanism for arrhythmia supression. *Heart Rhythm* 2004; **1**(3): 295–300.

18 Issa Z *et al.* Thoracic spinal cord stimulation reduces the risk of ischemic ventricular arrhythmias in a post-infarction heart failure canine model. *Heart Rhythm* 2004.

19 Zhou X *et al.* Incidence of nonsustained and sustained ventricular tachyarrhythmias in patients with an implantable cardioverter defibrillator. *J Cardiovasc Electrophysiol*, 2004; **15**(1): 14–20.

20 Meyerfeldt U *et al.* Heart rate variability before the onset of ventricular tachycardia: differences between slow and fast arrhythmias. *Int J Cardiol* 2002; **84**(2–3): 141–151.

21 Zimmermann M. Variation of sympathetic balance before the onset of repetitive monomorphic idiopathic ventricular tachycardia. *Heart Rhythm* 2004; abstracts.

22 Shusterman V *et al.* Multidimensional rhythm disturbances as a precursor of sustained ventricular tachyarrhythmias. *Circ Res* 2001; **88**(7): 705–712.

23 Bardy GH *et al.* Clinical experience with a tiered-therapy, multiprogrammable antiarrhythmia device. *Circulation* 1992; **85**(5): 1689–1698.

24 Almendral J *et al.* The importance of antitachycardia pacing for patients presenting with ventricular tachycardia. *PACE* 1993; **16**(3 Pt 2): 535–539.

25 Almendral JM *et al.* Analysis of the resetting phenomenon in sustained uniform ventricular tachycardia: incidence and relation to termination. *J Am Coll Cardiol* 1986; **8**(2): 294–300.

26 Almendral JM *et al.* Resetting response patterns during sustained ventricular tachycardia: relationship to the excitable gap. *Circulation* 1986; **74**(4): 722–730.

27 Stamato NJ *et al.* The resetting response of ventricular tachycardia to single and double extrastimuli: implications for an excitable gap. *Am J Cardiol* 1987; **60**(7): 596–601.

28 Callans DJ *et al.* Characterization of return cycle responses predictive of successful pacing-mediated termination of ventricular tachycardia. *J Am Coll Cardiol* 1995; **25**(1): 47–53.

29 Calkins H *et al.* Comparison of fixed burst versus decremental burst pacing for termination of ventricular tachycardia. *PACE* 1993; **16**(1 Pt 1): 26–32.

30 Charos GS *et al.* A theoretically and practically more effective method for interruption of ventricular tachycardia: self-adapting autodecremental overdrive pacing. *Circulation* 1986; **73**(2): 309–315.

31 Cook JR *et al.* Comparison of decremental and burst overdrive pacing as treatment for ventricular tachycardia associated with coronary artery disease. *Am J Cardiol* 1992; **70**(3): 311–315.

32 Fisher JD *et al.* Mechanisms for the success and failure of pacing for termination of ventricular tachycardia: clinical and hypothetical considerations. *PACE* 1983; **6**(5 Pt 2): 1094–1105.

33 Gillis AM *et al.* A prospective randomized comparison of autodecremental pacing to burst pacing in device therapy for chronic ventricular tachycardia secondary to coronary artery disease. *Am J Cardiol* 1993; **72**(15): 1146–1151.

34 Hammill SC *et al.* Termination and acceleration of ventricular tachycardia with autodecremental pacing, burst pacing, and cardioversion in patients with an implantable cardioverter defibrillator. Multicenter PCD Investigator Group. *PACE* 1995; **18**(1 Pt 1): 3–10.

35 Ip JH *et al.* Determinants of pace-terminable ventricular tachycardia: implications for implantable antitachycardia devices. *PACE* 1991; **14**(11 Pt 2): 1777–1181.

36 Kantoch MJ, Green MS, Tang AS. Randomized cross-over evaluation of two adaptive pacing algorithms for the termination of ventricular tachycardia. *PACE* 1993; **16**(8): 1664–1672.

37 Leitch JW *et al.* Reduction in defibrillator shocks with an implantable device combining antitachycardia pacing and shock therapy. *J Am Coll Cardiol* 1991; **18**(1): 145–151.

38 Naccarelli GV *et al.* Influence of tachycardia cycle length and antiarrhythmic drugs on pacing termination and acceleration of ventricular tachycardia. *Am Heart J* 1983; **105**(1): 1–5.

39 Nasir N Jr *et al.* Spontaneous ventricular tachycardia treated by antitachycardia pacing. Cadence Investigators. *Am J Cardiol* 1997; **79**(6): 820–822.

40 Newman D, Dorian P, Hardy J. Randomized controlled comparison of antitachycardia pacing algorithms for termination of ventricular tachycardia. *J Am Coll Cardiol* 1993; **21**(6): 1413–1418.

41 Peinado R *et al.* Randomized, prospective comparison of four burst pacing algorithms for spontaneous ventricular tachycardia. *Am J Cardiol* 1998; **82**(11): 1422–1425, A8–A9.

42 Porterfield JG *et al.* Conversion rates of induced versus spontaneous ventricular tachycardia by a third generation cardioverter defibrillator. The VENTAK PRx Phase I Investigators. *PACE* 1993; **16**(1 Pt 2): 170–173.

43 Roy D *et al.* Termination of ventricular tachycardia: role of tachycardia cycle length. *Am J Cardiol* 1982; **50**(6): 1346–1350.

44 Trappe HJ, Klein H, Kielblock B. Role of antitachycardia pacing in patients with third generation cardioverter defibrillators. *PACE* 1994; **17**(3 Pt 2): 506–513.

45 Wietholt D *et al.* Clinical experience with antitachycardia pacing and improved detection algorithms in a new

implantable cardioverter-defibrillator. *J Am Coll Cardiol*, 1993; **21**(4): 885–894.

46 Grosse-Meininghaus D *et al*. Efficacy of antitachycardia pacing confirmed by stored electrograms. A retrospective analysis of 613 stored electrograms in implantable defibrillators. *Z Kardiol* 2002; **91**(5): 396–403.

47 Hartzler GO. Treatment of recurrent ventricular tachycardia by patient-activated radiofrequency ventricular stimulation. *Mayo Clin Proc* 1979; **54**(2): 75–82.

48 Fisher JD *et al*. Long-term efficacy of antitachycardia pacing for supraventricular and ventricular tachycardias. *Am J Cardiol* 1987; **60**(16): 1311–1316.

49 Sharma V, DeGroot PJ, Wathen MS. Incidence and characteristics of type-2 breaks in response to antitachycardia pacing therapy in implantable cardioverter defibrillator patients. *J Cardiovasc Electrophysiol* 1156; **14**(11): 1156–1162.

50 San Roman Sanchez D *et al*. Determining factors of acceleration in sustained monomorphic ventricular tachycardias in response to bursts of stimuli. *Rev Esp Cardiol* 1992; **45**(7): 438–446.

51 Rosenqvist M. Antitachycardia pacing: which patients and which methods? *Am J Cardiol* 1996; **78**(5A): 92–97.

52 Wathen, MS *et al*. Shock reduction using antitachycardia pacing for spontaneous rapid ventricular tachycardia in patients with coronary artery disease. *Circulation* 2001; **104**(7): 796–801.

53 Mehta D *et al*. Comparison of clinical benefits and outcome in patients with programmable and nonprogrammable implantable cardioverter defibrillators. *PACE* 1992; **15**(9): 1279–1290.

54 Medtronic Inc. Marquis DR 7274 Reference Manual. 2002: pp. 139–143.

55 Bocchiardo M *et al*. Efficacy of biventricular sensing and treatment of ventricular arrhythmias. *PACE* 2000; **23**(11 Pt 2): 1989–1991.

56 Byrd IA *et al*. Comparison of conventional and biventricular antitachycardia pacing in a geometrically realistic model of the rabbit ventricle. *J Cardiovasc Electrophysiol* 2004; **15**(9): 1066–1077.

57 Heintze J *et al*. Efficacy of anti-tachycardia pacing in biventricular and right ventricular pacing. *Heart Rhythm* 2004; abstracts.

58 Chapman PD *et al*. Comparative efficacy of monophasic and biphasic truncated exponential shocks for nonthoracotomy internal defibrillation in dogs. *J Am Coll Cardiol* 1988; **12**(3): 739–745.

59 Jones JL, Jones RE. Improved defibrillator waveform safety factor with biphasic waveforms. *Am J Physiol* 1983; **245**(1): H60–H65.

60 Winkle RA *et al*. Improved low energy defibrillation efficacy in man with the use of a biphasic truncated exponential waveform. *Am Heart J* 1989; **117**(1): 122–127.

61 Malkin RA. Large sample test of defibrillation waveform sensitivity. *J Cardiovasc Electrophysiol* 2002; **13**(4): 361–370.

62 Matula MH *et al*. Biphasic waveforms for ventricular defibrillation: optimization of total pulse and second phase durations. *PACE* 1997; **20**(9 Pt 1): 2154–2162.

63 Mouchawar G *et al*. ICD waveform optimization: a randomized, prospective, pair-sampled multicenter study. *PACE* 2000; **23**(11 Pt 2): 1992–1995.

64 Strickberger SA *et al*. Probability of successful defibrillation at multiples of the defibrillation energy requirement in patients with an implantable defibrillator. *Circulation* 1997; **96**(4): 1217–1223.

65 Ahern TS *et al*. Device interaction – antitachycardia pacemakers and defibrillators for sustained ventricular tachycardia. *PACE* 1991; **14**(2 Pt 2): 302–307.

66 Gold MR *et al*. Efficacy and temporal stability of reduced safety margins for ventricular defibrillation: primary results from the Low Energy Safety Study (LESS). *Circulation* 2002; **105**(17): 2043–2048.

67 Mann DE *et al*. The Low Energy Safety Study (LESS): rationale, design, patient characteristics, and device utilization. *Am Heart J* 2002; **143**(2): 199–204.

68 Gold MR *et al*. Safety of a single successful conversion of ventricular fibrillation before the implantation of cardioverter defibrillators. *PACE* 2003; **26**(1 Pt 2): 483–486.

69 Bardy GH *et al*. A prospective randomized repeat-crossover comparison of antitachycardia pacing with low-energy cardioversion. *Circulation* 1993; **87**(6): 1889–1896.

70 Estes NA III *et al*. Antitachycardia pacing and low-energy cardioversion for ventricular tachycardia termination: a clinical perspective. *Am Heart J* 1994; **127**(4 Pt 2): 1038–1046.

71 Neglia JJ *et al*. Evaluation of a programming algorithm for the third tachycardia zone in a fourth-generation implantable cardioverter-defibrillator. *J Interv Card Electrophysiol* 1997; **1**(1): 49–56.

72 Pak HN *et al*. Synchronization of ventricular fibrillation with real-time feedback pacing: implication to low-energy defibrillation. *Am J Physiol Heart Circ Physiol* 2003; **285**(6): H2704–H2711.

73 Jones J *et al*. Can shocks timed to action potentials in low-gradient regions improve both internal and out-of-hospital defibrillation? *J Electrocardiol* 1998; **31** (Suppl.): 41–44.

74 Kidwai BJ *et al*. Optimization of transthoracic ventricular defibrillation – biphasic and triphasic shocks, waveform rounding, and synchronized shock delivery. *J Electrocardiol* 2002; **35**(3): 235–244.

75 KenKnight BH *et al*. Regional capture of fibrillating ventricular myocardium. Evidence of an excitable gap. *Circ Res* 1995; **77**(4): 849–855.

76 Newton JC *et al.* Pacing during ventricular fibrillation: factors influencing the ability to capture. *J Cardiovasc Electrophysiol* 2001; **12**(1): 76–84.
77 Mitchell LB *et al.* Sudden death in patients with implantable cardioverter defibrillators: the importance of post-shock electromechanical dissociation. *J Am Coll Cardiol* 2002; **39**(8): 1323–1328.
78 Grubman EM *et al.* Cardiac death and stored electrograms in patients with third-generation implantable cardioverter-defibrillators. *J Am Coll Cardio* 1998; **32**(4): 1056–1062.
79 Rosborough JP, Deno DC. Electrical therapy for pulseless electrical activity. *PACE* 2000; **23**: 591, abstracts.

CHAPTER 20

New lead designs and lead-less systems

Kenneth A. Ellenbogen, MD, *Bruce D. Gunderson*, MS, & *Mark A. Wood*, MD

The implantable cardioverter defibrillator (ICD) has become the standard of care for the treatment of patients with life threatening and potentially life-threatening ventricular tachyarrhythmias [1]. As the use of ICDs evolves to include patients with less advanced forms of cardiac disease, ICD leads have been subjected to increased scrutiny of both their short- and long-term performance [2]. It is likely that we will see more problems with lead failures (Figure 20.1).

The introduction of ICDs into the clinical arena in the 1980s required nontransvenous implantation. Defibrillation and sensing functions of the ICD were performed via separate lead systems. ICD sensing was typically performed initially by two unipolar epicardial electrodes and then later by a bipolar transvenous right ventricular electrode. The defibrillation function was performed by two large or small epicardial patches placed directly on the surface of the heart.

Stambler *et al.* [3] was one of the earliest investigators to draw attention to the long-term reliability and performance of sensing leads as part of an ICD system. The investigators summarized the sensing/pacing lead complications with a single manufacturer's ICD. In this trial, 60% of patients had a transvenous sensing lead, all ICD generators were implanted in the abdomen. They studied 302 consecutive patients with a mean follow-up of 380 days. In this study, 12.9% of patients required reoperation because of sensing/pacing lead complications. Epicardial sensing lead systems and lead adapters are rarely used now, but this study made several important observations that have been subsequently repeatedly confirmed in the literature. First, the investigators reported that the most common clinical finding suggesting lead failure is oversensing, which frequently presents with inappropriate shocks. Second, sensing lead problems typically require reoperation to fix. Third, epicardial sensing tends to fail more frequently than transvenous systems only when adapters are included in the system. This observation highlights the importance of minimizing the number of adapters in an ICD system and keeping the connections to the ICD header as simple as possible. Finally, the investigators also noted that the enhanced diagnostic capabilities of ICDs allow for better surveillance of ICD lead systems during long-term follow-up.

In 1990 sensing and defibrillation function of ICD leads was combined onto a single transvenous lead and made clinically available. Initial ICD lead design was similar to pacemaker lead design, consisting of coaxial lead construction [4]. Coaxial lead design consists of a single coil defibrillation lead with either true or integrated bipolar sensing and pacing. The Medtronic Transvene™ (Medtronic, Minneapolis, MN) lead family and the St. Jude Medical/Ventritex TVL™ lead family (St. Jude Medical, Valley View Court, CA) was constructed with the coiled defibrillation conductor and the tip and ring pacing conductors separated by insulation layers between each of the conductor layers. Guidant's Endotak™ 60 series (Guidant, St. Paul, MN) lead design used integrated bipolar sensing (e.g. the device used the distal shocking electrode as the return electrode for rate sensing). This lead is constructed with a coaxial pace/sense branch, and with two high-voltage conductors in two additional lumens parallel to the pace sense conductor.

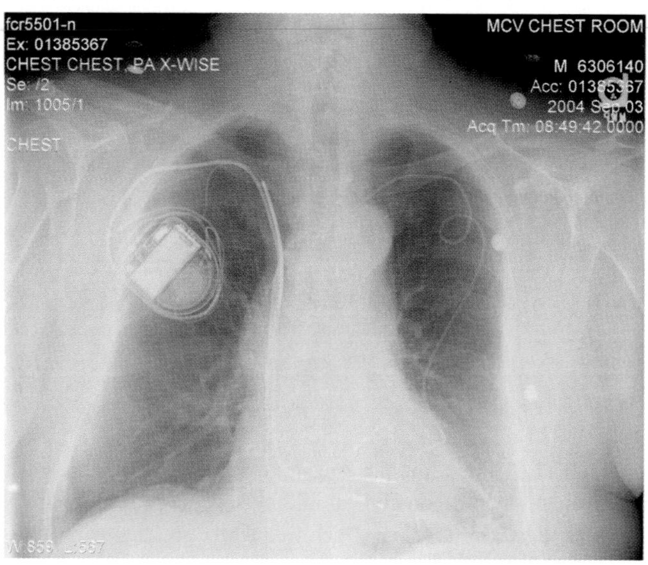

Figure 20.1 An elderly gentleman presented for routine ICD follow-up. At the time of single-chamber ICD generator change he was noted to have a lead failure during device testing. A new ICD lead was implanted. The patient now has three ICD leads, and no lead interactions were noted during testing.

The defibrillation conductor is made with braided strands instead of a coiled defibrillation conductor.

In contrast, more recent ICD lead design (Medtronic Sprint™, St. Jude Medical Riata™), and the Guidant leads of the Endotak™ 60 series and beyond (e.g. Endotak-DSP™, Endurance™, and Reliance™) consist of multilumen construction [4]. The Guidant leads have a coaxial pace/sense branch, with two high-voltage conductors in two additional lumens parallel to the pace/sense lumen (e.g. multilumen). In addition, they all have utilized integrated bipolar sensing (e.g. the distal shocking electrode is used as the return path for the rate sensing). With a multilumen design a wide variety of leads may be constructed including active/passive fixation, single- or dual-coil defibrillation, and integrated or true bipolar sensing. These leads all have in common the coiled and straight conductors running in parallel through a single insulating body with the conductors sheathed in an additional insulating layer. This design allows for the development of smaller more reliable leads that are more resistant to compression forces. Most current leads have silicone insulation between the conductors.

Reliability of ICD leads

A number of investigators reported a high incidence of transvenous ICD lead failures with early ICD leads [5–12]. A wide variety of different mechanisms has been reported as cause for transvenous lead failures. Different mechanisms have been noted to occur more commonly with specific leads from all the major manufacturers [5–12]. Some of the mechanisms of lead failure include (Table 20.1): macro-dislodgement, micro-dislodgement, conductor fracture at sites of stress or anchoring sutures, polyurethane insulation cracking due to metal ion oxidation, and lead fracture due to subclavian crush syndrome (Figures 20.2 and 20.3). Insulation stress or abrasion may result from transvenous leads tunneled down from the chest to an abdominal pocket (Figure 20.4). The mechanism of failure in an individual patient is often unknown. The most common clinical presentations of ICD lead failure are inappropriate shocks, followed by oversensing detected during routine ICD interrogation, and changes in pacing/sensing lead impedance (personal communication, H. Vlasak, Guidant). In one review of this subject, the overall rate of early transvenous ICD lead failure was 6.8% at the end of one year following implant (95% confidence interval: 5.8–7.8%) [5]. Finally, it is important to note the lead failure rate in clinical series is often higher than that reported by industry primarily due to incomplete ascertainment and follow-up of ICD leads in the manufacturers' databases.

A Multicenter Registry ICD lead database reported a specific lead associated with 54% of ICD

Table 20.1 Signs and causes of ICD lead failure.

Signs of ICD lead failure
Oversensing
Inappropriate shocks
Sensing of nonphysiologic signals
Marked changes in pacing/sensing thresholds
Marked changes in pacing/sensing lead impedance
Failure to defibrillate
Abnormal shocking impedance
Shock not delivered due to abnormal lead impedances
Visual abnormalities of lead body or insulation at the time of ICD generator change
Abnormal chest radiograph
Causes of ICD lead failure (most common)
Fracture of ICD pace/sense conductors
Abrasion of insulation, due to lead–lead interactions, lead–can interactions, fluid ingression, etc.
Terminal pin, terminal pin conductor, or terminal pin insulation damage
Fracture of ICD shocking coil
Failure of active fixation helix to extend/retract
Fluid ingression into lumen of lead
Macro- or micro-lead dislodgement
Fracture of lead extender or lead pin adapter

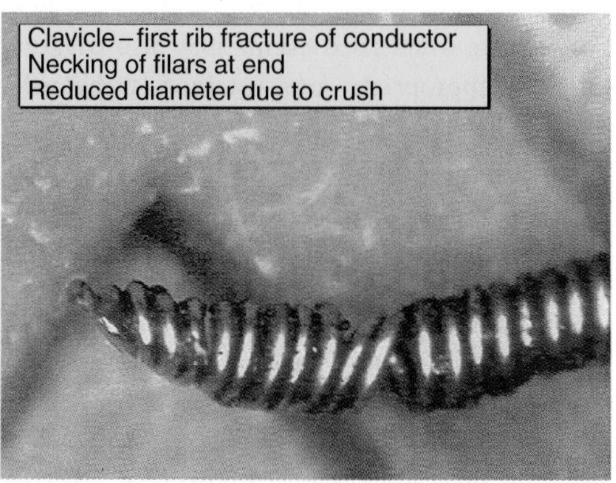

Figure 20.2 This patient presented with symptoms of inappropriate pacing and oversensing. The evaluation of the ICD lead revealed necking of the filar(s) in both the photographs (Figures 20.2 and 20.3). Reduction of overall coil diameter is seen indicating crush between the clavicle and first rib. (Reprinted with permission from Heidi Vlasek, Guidant Corporation.)

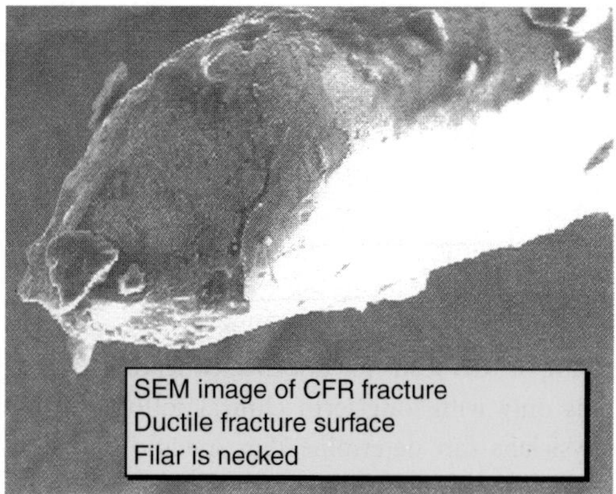

Figure 20.3 Scanning electron micrograph of the clavicle first rib fracture of the conductor coils shown above. (Reprinted with permission from Heidi Vlasek, Guidant Corporation.)

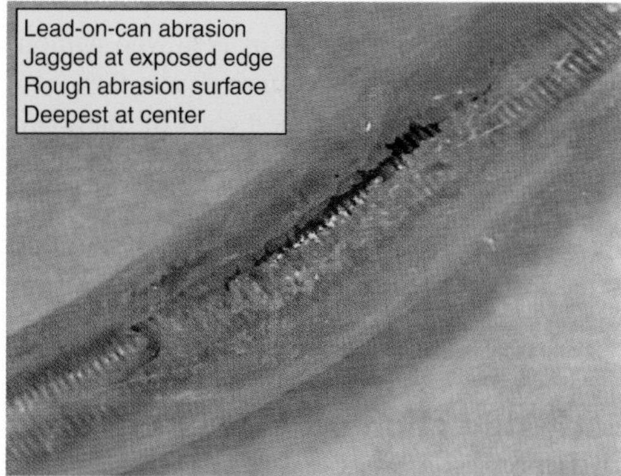

Figure 20.4 Insulation abrasion from rubbing of ICD pulse generator on lead.

lead failures in their registry [13]. Further investigation from a five center substudy estimated the survival probability of the coaxial polyurethane Medtronic Transvene™ model 6936/6966 to be 92% at 60 months and 80% at 84 months. The mean time to failure was 4.8 ± 2.1 years. The most common clinical presentation was oversensing (76%) with inappropriate shocks in 49% of the patients with ICD lead failure. Abnormalities of insulation were detected in 19 patients and of the pace/sense conductor were found in 15 patients. Other signs were found infrequently, including chest radiographic abnormalities in three patients, failure to capture in no patients, high defibrillation thresholds in one, visual abnormalities in two patients, and impedance changes in one patient. Management and follow-up strategies for patients with this lead or other lead problems were not studied. Based on their experience, however, the authors recommended device interrogation and threshold testing every 3–4 months with testing for oversensing by the use of provocative maneuvers, measurement of high-voltage coil and pace/sense lead impedance and periodic chest radiography to follow these patients. An accompanying editorial suggests that even with the careful preapproval lead testing process, the real-life function of an ICD lead can only be appreciated over years of follow-up [14]. The editorial further argues that manufacturers should not stop trying to improve leads, but rather focus on improving the postimplant monitoring of ICD leads for unexpected lead problems. It is only with long-term clinical follow-up that physicians can determine if a specific ICD lead functions within the predicted behavior based on animal and *in vitro* testing.

These findings are further supported by the experience of Dorwarth *et al.* [15]. This group reported a single center experience with follow-up of 261 consecutive patients with a 6936 lead after a mean follow-up of 4.0 ± 2.6 years. A lead-related sensing failure was observed in 12% who demonstrated oversensing. Lead survival was 98% at 4 years decreasing to 62% after 8 years of follow-up. Lead survival was not predicted by any clinical variable analyzed, including patient's age, implant access, or device implantation site. The authors argue for close follow-up of all patients with the 6936 lead.

Early detection of ICD lead failures

Analysis of the modes of failure with the Medtronic 6936 ICD lead was studied by our group [16]. We focused on trying to determine if early detection of ICD lead failure was possible. Pacing and sensing thresholds or changes in pacing lead impedance rarely changed from baseline or showed gross abnormalities in patients with lead failure. In a prospective evaluation of patients with the 6936 and no prior documented clinical malfunction, patients with an abnormally low, or a decrease in, ring to coil impedance or an increasing sensing integrity counter, which measured the number of nonphysiologic RR intervals, typically preceded ICD lead failures by at least several weeks to months. Additionally, we noted a unique presentation of 6936 ICD lead failure (i.e. oversensing of noise after an appropriate ICD shock). In patients without prior evidence of a lead problem, lead malfunction could be demonstrated by performing induction of ventricular tachycardia or ventricular fibrillation and then looking for oversensing after ICD shock delivery to terminate ventricular tachyarrhythmia (Figure 20.5). Dorwarth *et al.* also reported ICD interrogation showing rapid nonsustained ventricular tachycardia in 21 of 31 patients. In their study, this finding predicted ICD lead failure at an average of 40 ± 43 days before clinical presentation.

In a second study our group tested an algorithm that could identify ICD lead problems prior to clinical failure [17]. The algorithm that we tested used two measures of oversensing and one measure of abnormal lead impedance.

Oversensing due to lead failure typically results in sensed signals soon after the blanking period of the sensing amplifier. The sensing integrity counter quantifies oversensing by incrementing the counter for RR intervals <140 ms. A date/time stamp indicates when the counter first shows an increment since the last ICD interrogation. If the sensing integrity counter was ≥10 counts per day or >300 at the time of interrogation, the first component of the algorithm was satisfied. Consecutive oversensed events may also trigger a stored inappropriate nonsustained tachycardia episode. The ICD requires a minimum of five consecutive intervals in the tachycardia detection zone to store a nonsustained tachycardia episode. The nonsustained tachycardia log stores the 50 most recent episodes. Two nonsustained tachycardia episodes with RR intervals <200 ms within 1 week were required to satisfy the second component.

Impedance trends were stored in ICD memory for up to 1 year, including 14 daily and 52 minimum and maximum weekly measurements. An 8 week sliding window is used to create a baseline value to be compared with the most recent impedance value. The abnormal impedance criterion was satisfied when any of the following impedance algorithms were satisfied. First, three weekly maximum tip to ring impedances greater than 200% of the maximum baseline were required to indicate an abnormal impedance trend. Second, three weekly minimum tip to ring impedance measurements less than 50% of the minimum baseline were also required to satisfy the criterion of an abnormal impedance trend. The linear slope of a 5 beat

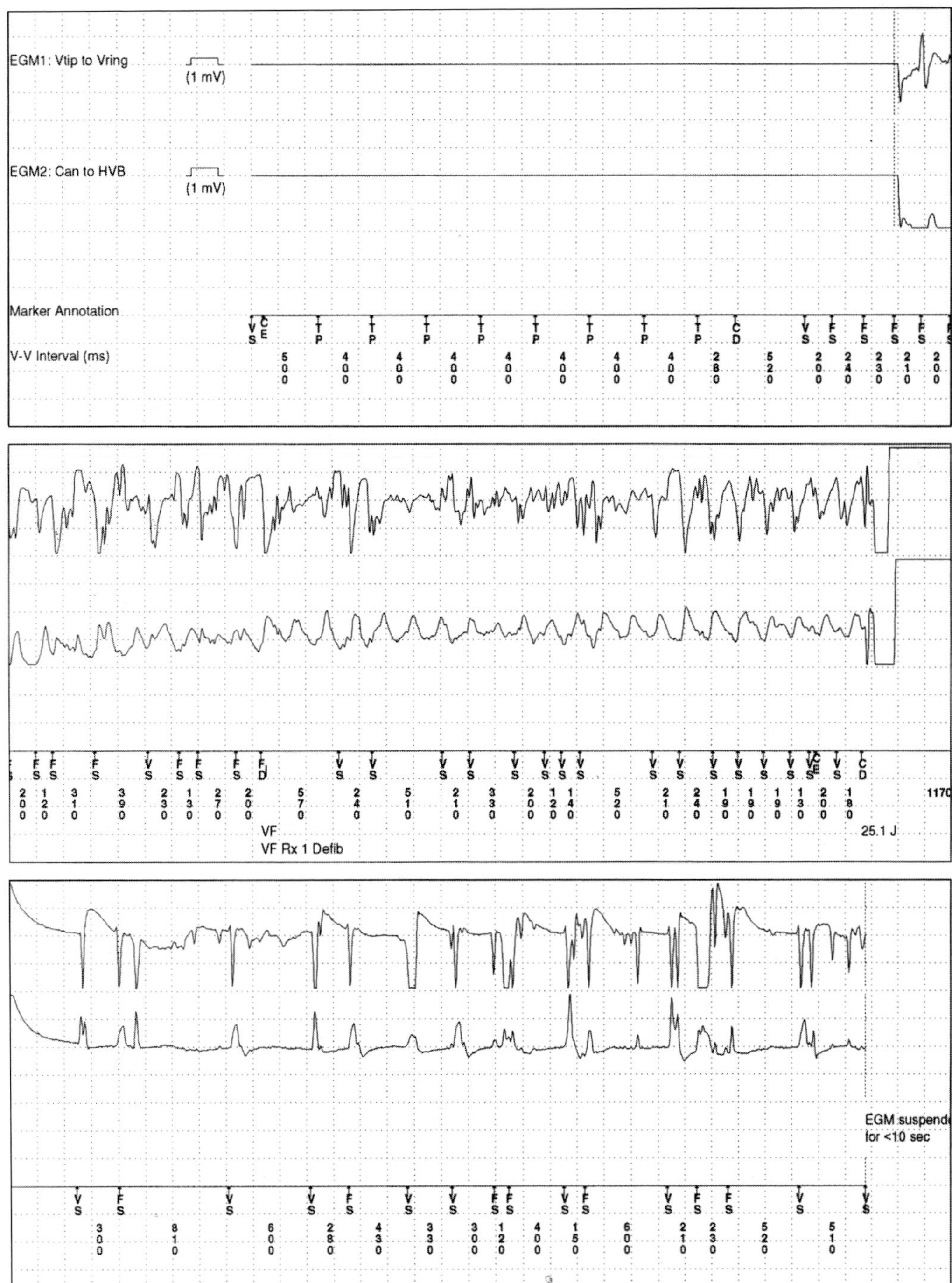

Figure 20.5 These are tracing from the patient shown in Figure 20.1. At the time of ICD pulse generator change, no abnormalities were noted until ventricular fibrillation was induced, after ICD discharge during testing, obvious noise is noted on sensing lead.

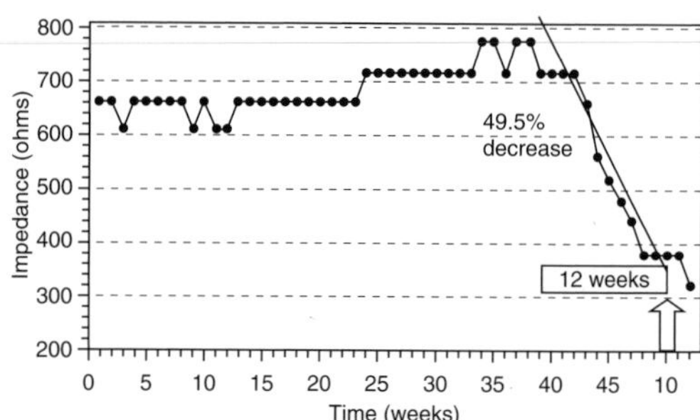

Figure 20.6 Example of abnormal lead impedance trend resulting in diagnosis of lead failure. On the *y*-axis is a plot of decreasing tip-ring impedances over time. The line shows the linear regression fit through the decreasing impedance values over 12 weeks. The arrow indicates the impedance criteria would have triggered 3 weeks before the inappropriate shock.

overlapping median window over 12 weeks was calculated. A third criterion was a 45% or greater decrease in the minimum tip to ring impedance (Figure 20.6). Finally, the algorithm was also satisfied when four of seven minimum ring to right ventricular coil impedances measured were less than 15 ohms.

The algorithm was designed using a database collected retrospectively from patients with and without ICD lead failures. The algorithm was then tested on a different preexisting database. The algorithm was tested on ICD stored information from 3848 patients at 13 centers. There were 1608 episodes of induced and spontaneous ventricular fibrillation, 62 patients with lead problems, 29 patients with evidence of noise or lead failure, and 6 patients with lead failures but no clinical adverse events yet. The average follow-up was 18.3 patient months. The ICD lead failures consisted of 12 patients with an ICD lead having a multilumen body design and 17 patients with an ICD lead having a coaxial body design. Patients were included in the normal group if they did not have any detected tachycardia episodes classified as inappropriate due to oversensing.

The ICD lead problem group averaged 11 ± 14 inappropriate detections per patient. The time to first inappropriate detection from lead implantation was 44 ± 6 27 months, with a range of 1–80 months and a median of 55 months. The sensitivity to identify a lead failure satisfying at least two of the three criteria was 82.8% (24/29). Three patients had only nonsustained tachycardia episodes with no abnormal impedance trend. One patient only satisfied the sensing integrity criteria and one patient did not satisfy any of the three criteria. Using the two oversensing criteria, the sensitivity was 72%. Using a combination of abnormal impedance and either of the two oversensing criteria, the sensitivity was 41%. All abnormal impedance trends also had at least one oversensing criteria satisfied. The nonsustained tachycardia had the highest individual sensitivity of 89%. There were no false positives in the normal group during 435 patient-years of follow-up resulting in a specificity of 100%. The impedance trend had the highest individual specificity of 99.7%.

The mean time from abnormal impedance to inappropriate detection was 8.1 ± 7.2 weeks, with a range of 1.4–22 weeks. The ICD was first interrogated 31 ± 39.7 days (median: 15 days, range: 0–158 days) after the first inappropriate detection. Of the 26 patients with nonsustained tachycardia, 16 patients had their logs overwritten with episodes occurring after the first inappropriate detection. The nonsustained tachycardia criterion was satisfied 20 ± 57 days (range: 0–181 days) before the first inappropriate detection for the 10 patients with all their nonsustained tachycardia episodes not overwritten prior to detection. We show that a 20 day average warning period is possible before an inappropriate ICD discharge. Additionally, we emphasized the importance of long-term continuous monitoring of ICD leads. Finally, although only Medtronic leads were studied, it is likely that leads from other companies would demonstrate similar findings.

Building on these observations, we have extended this approach to try to develop an algorithm that could discriminate between ICD lead failures and a variety of conditions that may simulate lead failure or malfunction [18]. The algorithm is outlined in Figure 20.7. Analysis of data not only includes RR intervals, but also the ventricular electrogram with 128 Hz sampling recorded between either the near-field tip and ring/coil sensing electrodes (NF-EGM) and the far field electrograms recorded from the coil or ICD can electrodes (FF-EGM). The morphology of the electrogram was also used in this analysis. Similar or different morphologies were

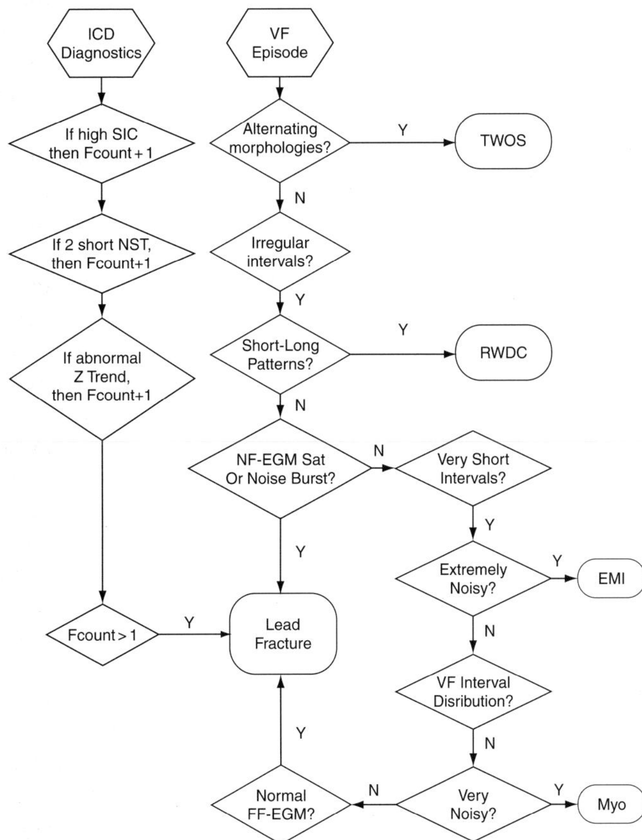

Figure 20.7 Design of algorithm tested in study. (Reproduced from *J Am Coll Cardiol* [17], with permission.)

determined using correlation waveform analysis. The algorithm used RR and electrogram data to identify oversensing coming from noncardiac sources (e.g. conductor fractures and electromagnetic interference) and cardiac oversensing (e.g. T-wave oversensing) from other detected episodes. The algorithm also incorporated information from special diagnostics: sensing integrity counter (e.g. RR intervals <140 ms), nonsustained episodes of tachycardia with a mean RR interval <200 ms, and impedance trends to identify lead failures. For example, successive voltages with a small difference between them made up a low-frequency unit. Continuous low-frequency units made up a low-frequency segment. An episode with noise bursts was defined as having irregular length low-frequency segments with a maximum noise segment of at least four units and <20% overall noise units. If an NF-EGM demonstrated maximum or minimum voltage or showed a noise burst, it was identified as a lead failure.

Ultimately, it would be desirable to have a series of algorithms and patient alerts that monitor pacing/sensing and defibrillator function included in the ICD. The device information would be interrogated on a daily or weekly basis by some sort of home telemetry system. The algorithms could be designed to take into account any differences between leads from different companies

Developments of new ICD lead technology

Several recent advances in ICD lead technology have been made over the last year. Recent commercial introduction of new multilumen leads with smaller French size and lubricious coatings makes it easier to pass more leads through the subclavian, axillary, or cephalic vein. A decade ago ICD leads generally required implantation through a 12 or 14 French introducer. Currently, all major US manufacturers have ICD leads that range in size from 7–9 French.

Manufacturers have employed a number of testing methods to ensure durability and improve reliability of the lead. As part of the design process, major and recurrent failure modes of previous lead generations were identified, studied, and subsequent leads were designed to decrease the chances of this failure mode recurring. For example, Guidant's Reliance™ leads have corrected problems with International Standard-1 (IS-1) terminal distal to the device header, elimination of yoke splice tube migration, and abrasion failures. Problems with lead abrasions were addressed by using a biopolymer of silicone that was more abrasion resistant, and thickening the wall of the conductors.

An interesting new development consists of the use of expanded polytetrafluoroethylene or ePTFE (WL Gore and Associates) to coat defibrillation coils [19]. This lead coating has acutely prevented tissue in-growth in sheep implanted with coated leads. In longer-term animal studies, the coating continues to prevent tissue in-growth at 6 months and in a smaller number of animals for up to 2 years. Importantly, the ePTFE coating is not associated with any change in the electrical properties of the ICD lead (e.g. either pacing or sensing thresholds or defibrillation thresholds). Long-term follow-up of this coating in animal and human studies will be anticipated.

Management of patients with ICD lead failure

Management of patients with ICD lead failure is a topic that has received relatively little examination. The increasing pool of younger and less ill patients undergoing ICD implantation leads to a large pool of patients who likely will live longer and be subject to ICD lead failure. Several different approaches to patient management are advocated. These include implantation of a new sensing lead for conductor or insulation fracture, or implantation of a new ICD lead. An alternative strategy is lead extraction, typically with laser sheaths and implantation of a new ICD lead. Without clinical trials comparing the different management strategies for ICD lead failure, specific recommendations cannot be given other than individualization of the risks and benefits of each approach for a given patient.

A significant body of literature already exists about the changes that occur at the electrode–myocardial interface in patients undergoing pacemaker lead implantation. Much less information exists about the pathologic changes that occur with implantation of nonthoracotomy ICD leads. Most of our information comes from a small study by Epstein *et al.* [20] of 8 patients whose hearts were examined at the time of heart transplantation or death. The electrode–myocardial interface in these patients was marked by intense fibrosis and these changes were remarkably consistent between patients. Each lead was encased by a ring of fibroelastic tissue and there was extensive fibrosis extending from the myocardium encapsulating the ICD lead. In some patients, fibrosis was also noted adjacent to the tricuspid valve. In this report, there is no mention of changes along the proximal defibrillator coil, which is particularly problematic for lead extraction.

A number of subsequent papers have reported on the feasibility and safety of ICD lead extraction. The number of patients studied in these series is small, but the literature emphasizes the considerable technical challenge involved with removal of ICD leads and especially the difficulty with fibrosis around the proximal coil. These early studies have used a variety of lead removal techniques, both superior and inferior approaches and primarily nonlaser sheaths [21, 22]. Later clinical series consist primarily of laser-assisted removal of ICD leads [23, 24]. A recent report about a series of children and young adults with congenital heart disease and ICD leads highlights these issues. Overall experience with laser lead extraction in experienced hands is typically associated with a 3.6% risk of serious or life threatening complications, and a 0.8% risk of mortality. The excimer laser sheath was used to extract ICD leads in this series, and was successful in 95% of patients. This group of young patients was characterized by exuberant lead fibrosis, primarily located in the region of venous entry, the high-voltage shocking coils, and the lead tip. One potential approach in these young patients advocated by the authors is implanting only single coil leads, thus avoiding the adhesion of the proximal coil to the heart and vessels as children experience further growth. Another approach as cited earlier would be using ICD leads with the ePTFE coating.

When an ICD lead fails because of oversensing and no apparent defibrillation problem is found, the clinician must weigh options carefully. Implantation of an additional sense/pace lead was advocated by our group in the mid-1990s as a safe approach for patients with ICD lead failures and either committed bipolar or integrated bipolar sensing [5, 6]. Extensive experience with Endotak™ leads shows that replacement of only the pace/sense portion of the lead is acceptable in many cases. Unpublished observations suggest that the pace/sense failures generally occur in the portion of the lead proximal to the yoke area, and hence do not affect the rest of the lead. Continued use of the defibrillation lead for high-voltage energy delivery is generally successful, only anecdotally has it been reported that defibrillation function is abnormal during additional follow-up. Leads with a defibrillation malfunction obviously need to be replaced. Additionally, any lead that has been replaced with a new sense/pace lead should be followed closely for evidence of malfunction of the defibrillation component. A concern often expressed as justification for ICD lead removal is the possibility of energy shunting between the two defibrillator coils. No reports of this phenomenon could be found in the literature. Another problem that can be avoided by judicious placement of ICD leads is oversensing due to creation of noise by electrodes from the two defibrillation leads making physical contact (see Figure 20.1).

A solution that has been advocated as an answer to concern about ICD lead malfunction is the "leadless" ICD. There is only limited published information. The concept of the "leadless" ICD is that it would be implanted easily by any physician subcutaneously. The device would be able to sense ventricular fibrillation and deliver a high enough energy shock to terminate the ventricular arrhythmia. It is unclear whether this device would be a "sentinel" device, and be replaced once it was clear the patient would likely receive additional shock or a fully functional device that would be left implanted in patients with recurrent ventricular tachyarrhythmias. Technical issues include size, shape, duration of battery life, maximal energy output, discrimination of electromagnetic interference, and myopotential discrimination from ventricular tachyarrhythmias (Table 20.2).

Table 20.2 Challenges associated with development of subcutaneous ICD.

General challenges
Shaped components will be expensive
Size will need to be larger because of higher defibrillation energy requirements
System must be relatively uniformly distributed but small enough to minimize implant difficulty, cosmetics, and patient discomfort
Technical challenges
Skeletal muscle artifacts may make arrhythmia detection more difficult
Motion artifacts may confound arrhythmia detection
EMI may lengthen ventricular arrhythmia detection
Subcutaneous signal amplitudes during ventricular arrhythmias will be much smaller than with transvenous sensing
DFTs expected to be higher (between 30 and 100 J)

Source:
Reprinted with permission from Paul A. Haefner, Guidant Corporation.

Ultimately, physicians must have access to complete and accurate information about lead survival and function that is similar in accuracy and completeness to the information collected in a randomized clinical trial. Physicians caring for or implanting ICDs, as well as engineers designing better ICD lead systems need accurate information in order to improve lead design. This information will only be collected by careful follow-up and evaluation of all ICD leads.

References

1 Gregoratos G, Abrams J, Epstein AE *et al.* ACC/AHA/NASPE 2002 guideline update for implantation of cardiac pacemakers and antiarrhythmia devices: summary article. *Circulation* 2002; **106**: 2145–2161.

2 Moss AJ, Zareba W, Hall WJ *et al.* (for the Multicenter Automatic Defibrillator Implantation Trial Investigators). Prophylactic implantation of a defibrillator in patients with myocardial infarction and a reduced ejection fraction. *N Engl J Med* 2002; **346**: 877–883.

3 Stambler BS, Wood MA, Damiano RJ *et al.* Sensing/pacing lead complications with a newer generation implantable cardioverter-defibrillator: worldwide experience from the guardian ATP 4210 clinical trial. *J Am Coll Cardiol* 1994; **23**: 123–132.

4 Gradaus R, Breithardt G, Böcker D *et al.* ICD leads: design and chronic dysfunctions. *PACE* 2003; **26**: 649–657.

5 Lawton JS, Wood MA, Gilligan DM *et al.* Implantable transvenous cardioverter defibrillator leads: the dark side. *PACE* 1996; **19**: 1273–1278.

6 Luria D, Glikson M, Brady PA *et al.* Predictors and mode of detection of transvenous lead malfunction in implantable defibrillators. *Am J Cardiol* 2001; **87**: 901–904.

7 Lawton JS, Ellenbogen KA, Wood MA *et al.* Sensing lead-related complications in patients with transvenous implantable cardioverter-defibrillators. *Am J Cardiol* 1996; **78**: 647–651.

8 Degeratu FT, Khalighi K, Peters RW *et al.* Sensing lead failure in implantable defibrillators: a comparison of two commonly used leads. *J Cardiovasc Electrophysiol* 2000; **11**: 21–24.

9 Reiter MJ, Mann DE *et al.* Sensing and tachyarrhythmia detection problems in implantable cardioverter defibrillators. *J Cardiovasc Electrophysiol* 1996; **7**: 542–558.

10 Mehta D, Nayak HM, Singson M *et al.* Late complications in patients with pectoral defibrillator implants with transvenous defibrillator lead systems: high incidence of insulation breakdown. *PACE* 1998; **21**: 1893–1900.

11 Gold MR, Peters RW, Johnson JW *et al.* Complications associated with pectoral implantation of cardioverter defibrillators. *PACE* 1997; **20**: 208–211.

12 Korte T, Jung W, Spehl S *et al.* Incidence of ICD lead related complications during long-term follow-up: comparison of epicardial and endocardial electrode systems. *PACE* 1995; **18**: 2053–2061.

13 Hauser RG, Cannom D, Hayes DL *et al.* Long-term structural failure of coaxial polyurethane implantable cardioverter defibrillator leads. *PACE* 2002; **25**: 879–882.

14 Maisel WH. Increased failure rate of a polyurethane implantable cardioverter defibrillator lead. *PACE* 2002; **25**: 877–878.

15 Dorwarth UWE, Frey B, Dugas M *et al.* Transvenous defibrillation leads: High incidence of failure during long-term follow-up. *J Cardiovasc Electrophysiol* 2003; **14**: 38–43.

16 Ellenbogen KA, Wood MA, Shepard RK *et al.* Detection and management of an implantable cardioverter defibrillator lead failure. *J Am Coll Cardiol* 2003; **41**: 73–80.

17 Gunderson BD, Patel AS, Bounds CA, Shepard RK, Wood MA, Ellenbogen KA. An algorithm to predict implantable cardioverter-defibrillator lead failure. *J Am Coll Cardiol* 2004; **44**: 1898–1902.

18 Gunderson BD, Patel AS, Bounds CA, Ellenbogen KA. Automatic identification of clinical lead problems. *Pacing Clin Electrophysiol* 2005; **28**: 563–567.

19 Rosenthal L, Zagrodzky J, Johnson T *et al.* Initial Results of a new defibrillation lead with expanded polytetrafluoroethylene coated shocking coils. *PACE* 2003; **26**: 1123.

20 Epstein AE, Kay N, Plumb VJ *et al.* Gross and microscopic pathological changes associated with nonthoracotomy implantable defibrillator leads. *Circulation* 1998; **98**: 1517–1524.

21 Franc PL, Klug D, Jarwe M *et al.* Extraction of endocardial implantable cardioverter-defibrillator leads. *Am J Cardiol* 1999; **84**: 187–191.

22 Kantharia BK, Padder FA, Pennington III JC *et al.* Feasibility, safety, and determinants of extraction time of percutaneous extraction of endocardial implantable cardioverter defibrillator leads by intravascular countertraction method. *Am J Cardiol* 2000; **85**: 593–597.

23 Wilkoff BL, Byrd CL, Love CJ *et al.* Pacemaker lead extraction with the laser sheath: results of the pacing lead extraction with the excimer sheath (PLEXES) trial. *J Am Coll Cardiol* 1999; **33**: 1671–1676.

24 Cooper JM, Stephenson EA, Berul CI *et al.* Implantable cardioverter defibrillator lead complications and laser extraction in children and young adults with congenital heart disease: implications for implantation and management. *J Cardiovasc Electrophysiol* 2003; **14**: 344–349.

21

CHAPTER 21
Optimization of defibrillation function

Michael R. Gold, MD, PhD *& Paul J. DeGroot,* MS

Introduction

Over the 20 years since initial Food and Drug Administration (FDA) approval in 1985, the implantable cardioverter defibrillator (ICD) has undergone a remarkable transformation as a treatment of life threatening ventricular arrhythmias. Initially, this device was used in the 1980s as salvage therapy for the few patients who survived multiple aborted sudden death episodes. Today, in the United States most devices are implanted for primary prevention of sudden death, often with little or no specific arrhythmia risk stratification. After more than two decades of study, the ICD is established as the best prevention of sudden cardiac death.

The rapid increase and acceptance of the ICD has been paralleled by an equally rapid evolution of technology. Initially, these pulse generators were large devices implanted in the abdomen, and a thoracotomy was required for the placement of defibrillation patches. The earliest versions of the ICD only delivered high-energy shocks to treat tachyarrhythmias and had simple counters to document activity. Patients typically spent about a week in the hospital recovering from surgery. Now, pectoral transvenous implantation is routine and can often be performed as an outpatient procedure. All ICD systems have pacing capabilities and widely programmable detection criteria in addition to enhanced diagnostics and electrogram storage to facilitate therapy interpretation. Lead systems have been developed to allow for dual-chamber defibrillators with pacing and shock capability in the right atrium as well as ventricle, and multichamber ICDs with left ventricular pacing via the coronary sinus, as adjunctive therapy for the treatment of congestive heart failure. Despite these advances in technology, the fundamental and distinguishing aspect of an ICD is the ability to deliver high-energy shock automatically to treat ventricular tachyarrhythmias. It is this shock therapy that is responsible for the mortality reductions observed with these devices. This chapter will summarize the recent data available for optimization of defibrillation therapy.

Defibrillation shocks can be divided into two groups: truncated exponential waveforms and other waveforms. ICDs have historically used truncated exponential waveform because the electrical components used to generate them require little space, an obvious benefit for an implantable device. The defibrillation output circuit for such a waveform is essentially a capacitor and a switch, allowing for either monophasic or biphasic shocks (Figure 21.1). After charging the capacitor with energy from the battery, a switch between the capacitor

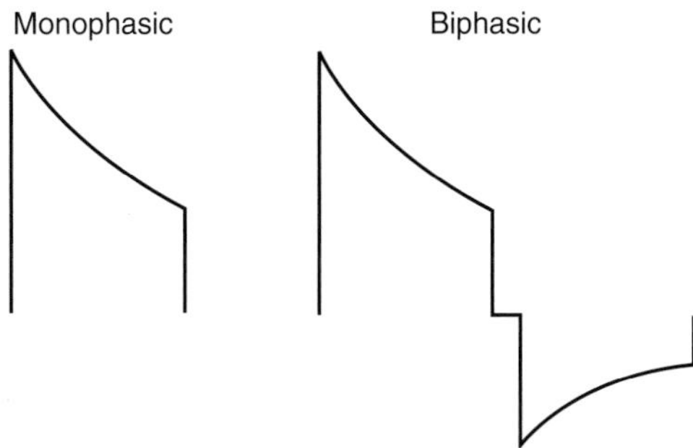

Figure 21.1 Truncated exponential waveforms. Monophasic and biphasic shock waveforms are shown. The amplitude of the pulse represents the voltage on the capacitor.

and electrodes in the patient's body is closed, discharging the energy across the heart. This results in an exponentially declining voltage between the electrodes. Until the energy required for defibrillation is reduced by an order of magnitude or new battery technologies are discovered, a capacitor will remain an integral part of ICD designs.

Measuring defibrillation efficacy

A necessary aspect of all defibrillation research protocols is measurement of the defibrillation threshold, or DFT. While "threshold" implies an all-or-none phenomenon, defibrillation is in fact a highly probabilistic outcome and is best represented by a success curve which transitions from low to high probability of success over a range of several joules rather than at one distinct energy. While a single number is often used to describe the DFT of a patient with a given lead system and waveform, studies on patients [1] and animals [2] have shown that even consecutive DFT measurements can vary dramatically (Figure 21.2). Traditionally, human studies have expressed the DFT in joules, or the amount of energy needed to defibrillate. However, peak voltage or current can also be used. In fact, some early studies of transthoracic defibrillation indicted that current was the critical factor needed to achieve defibrillation [3].

A variety of DFT protocols have been used to compare the performance of different defibrillation configurations. Historically, a step-down DFT protocol was the method of choice (Figure 21.3). After ventricular fibrillation (VF) induction, the first shock is delivered at a relatively high energy. If successful, subsequent shocks are delivered at progressively lower energy until defibrillation fails. Theoretically, this identifies on average the energy that successfully defibrillates about 70% of the time (DFT_{70}). Another popular method to measure DFT has been the binary search DFT protocol (Figure 21.4). In this method, an energy at about the predicted 50% success for defibrillation (DFT_{50}) is used for the first shock. Using higher energy following a failure and less energy following a success, subsequent shocks are delivered midway between previously tested energies (or the range minimum or maximum) until the desired resolution of the DFT is achieved. This method offers the advantage of having a predetermined number of shocks in the protocol, whereas the step-down method requires more episodes/shocks for patients with lower DFTs.

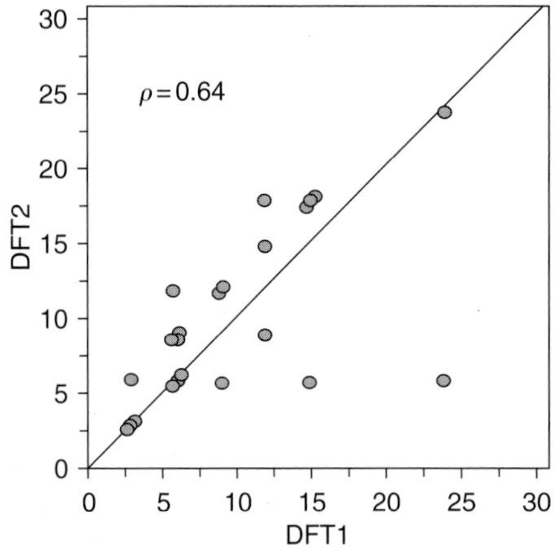

Figure 21.2 Reproducibility of DFTs. Two consecutive DFT measurements were made (DFT1 and DFT2) and are plotted on this graph. r = correlation with black unity line. (Data are from Reference 1.)

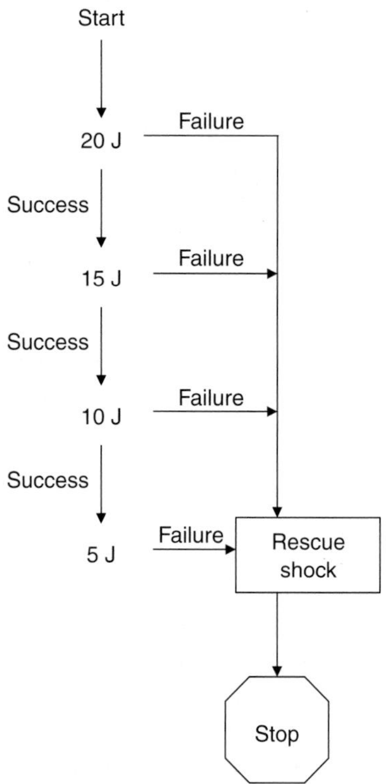

Figure 21.3 Schematic diagram of a step-down DFT protocol. Usually, the initial shock energy for the first trial is either 20 J, as shown, or 15 J.

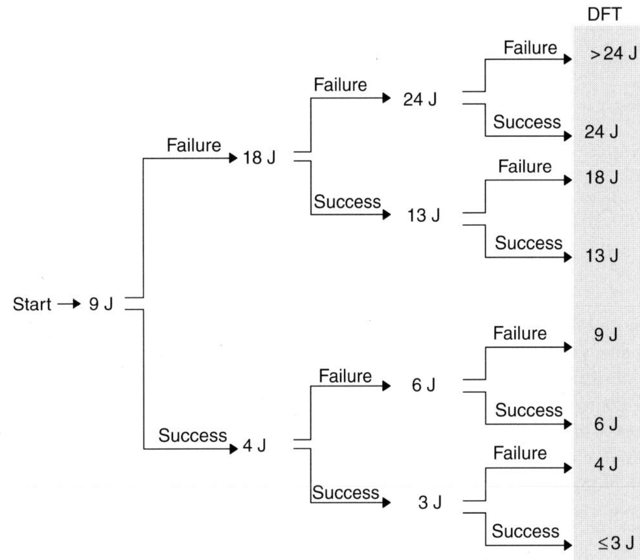

Figure 21. 4 Schematic diagram of a binary search DFT protocol. Note that the first shock energies for successive VF inductions are dependent on the success or failure of the preceding induction.

Though theoretical differences exist between the DFTs estimated using these two methods, we have shown a statistically and clinically insignificant difference between DFTs measured by each method [4]. Finally, another DFT method used in clinical investigation is a step-up DFT. In this protocol, the first shock energy is delivered using the lowest energy of interest with subsequent shocks delivered at progressively higher energies. Unlike the first two methods, shocks are delivered into the same episode of induced VF until defibrillation is successful. Like the step-down method, the number of shocks depends on the DFT. However, with this method, duration of VF also depends on the DFT, with the potential for long VF episodes coming with high DFTs being a significant drawback. However, a comparison of step-up and binary search protocols has also shown no difference in DFT, with the average total time in VF actually less for the step-up method [5].

Though important for defibrillation research, a true DFT is measured in <10% of ICD implants at present. Rather, shocks are most often given at a single energy level to assess the patient's safety margin. Based on empiric observation that patients with epicardial patch electrodes and monophasic waveform ICDs who had at least a 10 J safety margin were served adequately by their ICD [6, 7], modern day implants still are most often implanted after observing success using two shocks at 10 J below the maximum output of the ICD. A 5 J safety margin may be adequate if three successive terminations of VF are demonstrated [8]. This is because the more successive successful shocks for VF termination that are obtained, the more likely that this energy is at the higher part of the DFT probability curve. This is shown graphically in Figure 21.5. However, given the desire for less testing at implant, we have recently demonstrated that a single shock given ~20 J below maximum output may also be a viable criterion [9, 10]. While these practices are supported by long-standing practice, statistical models provide evidence that the sensitivity and specificity of implant test protocols are significantly less than perceived, bringing into question the value of basing implant decisions on such limited testing [11, 12]. It is not uncommon for patients with limited defibrillation success at implant and apparently high DFTs to exhibit adequate defibrillation efficacy during testing on another day. It is not well understood if this is merely an unlucky probabilistic phenomenon or a transient period when the patient has higher defibrillation energy requirements. Either way, it brings into question the role of extensive lead revision or subcutaneous array placement at ICD implant. Rather, retesting several days later or adding a Class III antiarrhythmic drug such as Dofetilide may be a simpler strategy [13].

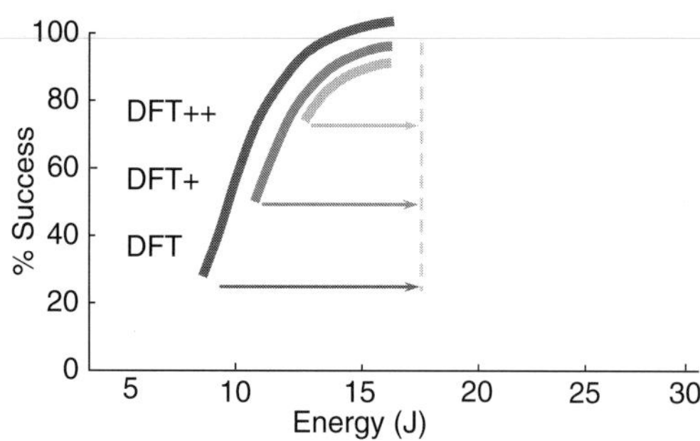

Figure 21.5 More rigorous DFT testing should allow for smaller safety margins. Theoretic curves are shown for defibrillation efficacy for a step-down protocol (DFT), one where two successive shocks at the DFT are required (DFT+) and one where three successive shocks are required (DFT++). Note that as testing is more rigorous, the probability of still being relatively low on the efficacy curve is reduced. (Arrow = safety margin).

Defibrillation waveforms

In the 1980s, the first implantable defibrillators used a monophasic truncated exponential waveform, wherein a capacitor was discharged once across the defibrillation electrodes. The energy required to defibrillate, or DFT, was shown to be less when not all the energy was discharged from the capacitor [14]. It was believed that refibrillation occurred at low voltages, which was prevented by truncating the waveform. Hence, the exponentially decaying waveform used in ICDs is truncated at some point during delivery. Initially, the duration was set at about 1 time constant of decay or truncated at about 35% residual voltage (i.e. 65% tilt, see below). Subsequent models and animal experiments suggested that this was close to the optimal monophasic duration. However, human studies failed to demonstrate an optimal duration, with DFTs increasing only with very short duration pulses (≤2 ms). Pulses of 18–20 ms in duration had no deleterious effects on defibrillation [15].

While a single discharge was most common, sequential pulses from two capacitors were sometimes used in order to spatially distribute energy more evenly across the heart, thereby reducing the energy requirement [16]. In the 1990s, undoubtedly the most significant advance in shock waveform was the advent of the biphasic waveform. As the name implies, the biphasic waveform consists of two truncated exponential waveforms. As implemented in ICDs, the second phase is delivered in the opposite polarity using energy remaining on the capacitor after the truncation of the first phase. The biphasic waveform resulted in a dramatic reduction in the DFT, making successful ICD shock therapy nearly certain with the epicardial patch electrodes in use at the time and paving the way for routine use of simple transvenous lead systems. By simply reversing the polarity of the shock, the peak or leading edge voltage of the second phase cannot be greater than the minimal or trailing edge voltage of the first phase of the pulse. Studies comparing different biphasic waveforms demonstrated that keeping the leading edge voltage of the second phase equal to the trailing edge voltage of the first phase is superior to diminishing the second phase voltage further [17]. Furthermore, defibrillation efficacy is relatively insensitive to second phase duration. DFTs only increase with very short second phase durations (1–2 ms). Contrary to predictions from animal experiments, human studies showed that second phase durations up to 3 times as long as first phase durations had no deleterious effects on DFTs [18].

One waveform variable programmable in some ICDs is the waveform tilt. Tilt, related to waveform duration, is a measure of the percent of voltage dropped from beginning to end of the truncated exponential waveform. For example, a 65% tilt waveform has a trailing edge voltage equal to 35% of the starting voltage, and would have less voltage at the end (and have shorter duration) than the same waveform but with 50% tilt. As noted above, studies of human defibrillation showed no effect of tilt for monophasic waveforms over a large range of tilts (40–95%), implying that this is not an important factor [15].

The effect of tilt on biphasic waveforms is more complex, although all devices employ tilts in the range of 50–65%. Using three-electrode/two-pathway configurations, studies have shown that waveforms with lower tilt have lower DFTs than those with higher tilt [17, 19, 20], though this finding has not always been observed [21]. However, two-electrode/one-pathway systems, which have higher resistance and hence longer time constants ($\tau = RC$, where R is the resistance and C is the capacitance) do not show significant effect of tilt on DFT [21–23]. Based on these data, commercial pulse generators use either 50% tilt for each phase (Medtronic), 60% tilt for the first phase and 50% tilt for the second (Guidant), or offer programmable tilt, with 65% tilt recommended for both phases (St. Jude). Despite several studies showing a statistically lower DFT (or at worse no difference) with a shorter tilt, it is unclear whether programming individual patients to longer tilts has true benefit or if the apparent difference is simply a reflection of the probabilistic nature of defibrillation. Given the limitations of DFT testing, it is possible that programmable tilt may only appear to improve defibrillation efficacy. For that reason, we believe an ICD with a low, fixed tilt to be preferable and that other options be explored when faced with difficulty meeting implant criterion.

Another variable known to affect DFT is the defibrillation waveform time constant, τ, which reflects the rate of exponential decay of the voltage waveform. This is usually modified experimentally by changing capacitance, although phase duration is longer for either higher capacitance or resistance. In the defibrillation studies on tilt referred above, note that the optimal tilt is dependent on the number of current pathways – a major determinant of overall resistance, and therefore determines τ. As further evidence of the importance of τ, Swerdlow *et al.* [24] showed that for a fixed tilt waveform, the lowest DFT for a given ICD capacitance was dependent on the resistance. When capacitance was 60 μF, the higher resistance configurations had the lower DFT, and when $C = 120$ μF the lower resistance configurations had the lower DFT. Additional studies on the effect of capacitance and tilt using conventional transvenous electrode systems indicate that the ideal waveform time constant is likely between 3.5 and 4.0 ms [25–27], though one study has shown little or no difference in DFT using waveforms with τ between 3.5 and 4 ms [28]. It is interesting that this is close to the cardiac membrane time constant for defibrillation [29].

Assuming an ideal $\tau = 3.6$ ms and a resistance of 40 ohms, typical of present day dual-coil, pectoral shock configuration (Can + SVC → RV), the ideal ICD capacitance would be 90 μF. Connected to a single-coil lead, a Can → RV configuration has a resistance of ~60 ohms and an ideal capacitance of 60 μF. In contrast to these ideal capacitances, present day ICDs utilize capacitances ranging from 90 to 150 μF. The reason lies in capacitor technology.

Implantable cardioverter defibrillator capacitors use a technology developed for flash photography. This technology, aluminum electrolytic, provided a relatively lightweight, high-energy density capacitor. The maximum voltage that an aluminum electrolytic capacitor can hold is nominally 375 V, and stacking two components together yields a peak voltage of 750 V. Determination of the energy stored by the capacitor (StE) is made using the equation $\text{StE} = \frac{1}{2}CV^2$. With this a 90 μF device only offers a maximum energy of 25 J – on the low end of output necessary to reliably defibrillate most patients. Higher output ICDs are achieved by employing a higher capacitance with a minor compromise in the defibrillation waveform time constant. Recently, wet tantalum capacitors have been developed for ICDs. This technology offers a higher energy density than aluminum electrolytic and therefore the potential for a smaller ICD. Besides having a noticeably higher mass, another downside is a lower peak voltage, meaning even higher capacitance to achieve the desired energy and the potential for further compromise in defibrillation efficacy.

Shock polarity and lead configuration

With the goal of improving efficacy and/or decreasing device size, significant research has aimed at optimizing defibrillation efficacy with transvenous lead system using truncated exponential waveforms. As noted above, these parameters include capacitance and tilt/duration. In addition, shock polarity and lead configuration can affect the shock vector and have important effects on DFTs. Some of these parameters can be fixed into the design of the ICD with the implanting physician having no control, or can be provided as programmable parameters that can be tested during implant.

Polarity is one parameter often changed through programming at implant or follow-up when faced with a patient with marginal or no defibrillation success. Though research has shown that monophasic waveform DFTs are lower when the RV coil is the anode for the first phase [30], the effect of polarity on the DFT with a biphasic waveform remains unclear. While several studies seem to corroborate the results using a monophasic waveform [31–34], there are a number of trials that found no significant difference [35, 36]. Curiously, none of the studies that found a difference favor starting with the RV as cathode. We have found that patients with DFT > 15 J show lower DFT with RV anode while patients with DFT < 15 J exhibit no difference based on polarity [34]. Thus, the ability of any study to show a difference may simply be the baseline DFT of the patients enrolled. Another potential theory is that polarity in fact has no effect on DFT but rather allows a second chance for success when encountering an occasional probabilistic failure to defibrillate with an otherwise adequate configuration. Narasimhan *et al.* [37] showed that the polarity associated with the lower DFT is not reproducible in DFT measurements conducted at implant and at the prehospital discharge. While there is no definitive study, most agree that both polarities should be tested at implant before resorting to more complicated alternatives in order to meet ICD implant criteria. Furthermore, since any difference seems to favor RV anode, it seems prudent to start testing with that polarity.

A major advance in the development of reliable transvenous defibrillation lead systems was the active pectoral pulse generator, or "active can." Initially, energy was only applied between transvenous electrodes or epicardial patches. However, Bardy *et al.* [38] showed that the pulse generator could act as an electrode in the left pectoral area producing a favorable defibrillation vector from the right ventricle to the left shoulder. They coined this the unipolar defibrillation configuration and showed that it helped to reduce DFTs compared with a two-coil shocking vector. Subsequently, we showed that adding an active can to a dual-coil transvenous lead creating three electrodes, which we termed the triad lead configuration, was even more effective for reducing DFTs [39]. Moreover, the benefit of an active can was greatest for those patients with the highest DFTs, thus eliminating virtually all outliers with an unacceptable defibrillation safety margin. The primary benefit of the triad lead configuration is to reduce shock impedance, since peak current is not reduced. Subsequent studies have shown that the position of the proximal or SVC coil is not critical in the presence of an active can, so a single pass dual-coil lead provides the simplest implantation approach [40]. An active can in the right pectoral space does not reduce DFTs [41], so a left sided approach is preferred. The dual-coil, active left pectoral lead configuration has become the standard for transvenous defibrillation. It is only in unusual circumstances, such as a pediatric patient, when a single-coil lead is preferred, or when a left sided system is contraindicated (e.g. AV fistula, infection, mastectomy, persistent left SVC, etc.) that a right sided approach is favored.

Alternative waveforms

In addition to biphasic waveforms, other capacitor discharge waveforms have been tested attempting to improve defibrillation efficacy. Recently, research has been performed using an "auxiliary" pulse delivered using an electrode on the left ventricle. As with sequential pulses employed in ICDs in the early 1990s, it is hypothesized that the extra discharge will distribute current to areas not reached with a single discharge. While animal studies showed dramatic reduction [42], results in patients did not show a statistically significant reduction in DFT using RV → SVC + Can followed by LV → SVC + Can shock pathways compared with a conventional RV → Can + SVC configuration [43]. Although patients with a more apical lead placement appeared to have some benefit, the lack of universally positive results plus the difficulty of positioning a lead in a coronary vein need to be overcome before this approach becomes a viable alternative.

Another approach to lower DFTs is to use additional pulses to optimize depolarization of the cardiac tissue. Triphasic waveforms have been explored in several studies but they do not appear to reduce DFTs further. A recent study by Huang *et al.* [44] demonstrated that factors such as triphasic waveform polarity and tilt could affect DFT, but no statistical difference was observed comparing them to biphasic waveform DFTs.

Others have proposed using additional discharges without switching polarity. Predictions using mathematical models treating the cardiac cell membrane as a capacitor show that membrane voltage rises with the onset of a truncated exponential shock. But as the shock voltage decays, the membrane voltage itself reaches a peak and also begins to fall [45–46]. By timing another shock to begin near the peak, the membrane voltage can further increase achieving a voltage sufficient to generate an action potential. One version of this waveform is generated starting with two capacitors electrically tied in parallel for the first part of the delivery and then switching them in series at the appropriate time. This switching doubles the applied voltage and decreases τ to 25% of the original discharge. Yamanouchi *et al.* [47] reported results showing a significant reduction in stored energy DFT with this "parallel–series" waveform compared with 135 and 90 μF biphasic waveforms. More recently, Seidl *et al.* [48] showed a statistically nonsignificant 19% decrease using a "stepped defibrillation waveform" compared with a 110 μF biphasic waveform in 21 patients.

As described above, capacitive discharge waveforms are employed in ICDs because they are easy to generate. However, they are far from ideal from the standpoint of maximizing the efficiency of stimulating the myocardium. In 1972, Klafter [49] described the theoretically optimal waveform for charging a capacitive membrane. In contradistinction to a capacitive discharge waveform, which has a sudden onset and then decreasing voltage, the Klafter waveform has a small step at onset and then ascends until delivery is stopped. Inspired by this prediction, we compared DFTs using an ascending ramp waveform to a conventional biphasic waveform [50, 51]. In two studies, comparison was made between a 125 μF, 50%/50% tilt biphasic (control) waveform with an ascending ramp biphasic waveform (Figure 21.6). The ramp waveform had either 12 ms or 7 ms ramp waveform for phase 1 transitioning to a short exponentially decaying segment followed by a reverse polarity truncated exponential waveform for phase 2. In both studies, the ramp waveform required significantly lower voltage at DFT than the control waveform. The 7 ms ramp showed a 17% reduction in delivered energy threshold while the 12 ms waveform yielded no significant difference. Of interest, Bardy *et al.* [53] previously showed lower transvenous DFTs using a damped sinusoid, another slow rise waveform popular in external defibrillators, again hoping to find a superior alternative to a truncated exponential. These findings confirmed the potential for a lower energy device, but the complex circuitry required to deliver an ascending waveform would consume any size reduction achieved by reducing the ICD maximum output. These waveforms may hold potential for the future as technology advances high-frequency switching circuits.

Summary and future directions

Implantation of ICD and defibrillation testing has become routine with modern lead systems and waveforms. With almost uniform defibrillation success of dual-coil, active left pectoral shocking configurations, the need for any defibrillation testing at all has been questioned. Moreover,

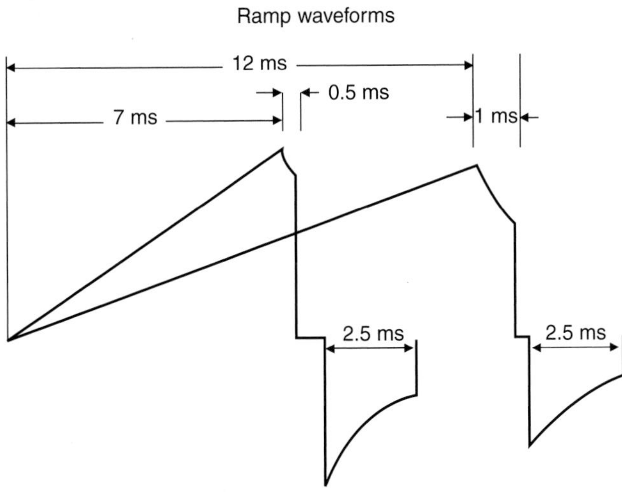

Figure 21.6 Ascending ramp waveform. A schematic diagram of the voltage contour of this waveform is shown.

defibrillation research has decreased markedly given the success of current ICD systems. One area of interest has been the evaluation of "leadless" ICD systems, in which defibrillation is achieved by shocking between an active pectoral can and a subcutaneous electrode, thus obviating the need for any transvenous leads [52]. Other simple prophylactic "shock boxes" have been proposed with limited programmability and no pacing capabilities as a way to reduce costs and further disseminated this technology. Whether either of these strategies becomes mainstream therapy is unclear, as a majority of ventricular tachyarrhythmias can be painlessly pace terminated, avoiding the need for shocks [54]. Thus, these simple systems may not be well accepted by patients or clinicians if they result in frequent unnecessary although appropriate shocks.

References

1 Swerdlow C, Davie S, Ahern T *et al.* Comparative reproducibility of defibrillation threshold and upper limit of vulnerability. *PACE* 1996; **19:** 2103–2111.

2 Jones D, Fujimura O, Klein G. Minimum replications to estimate average threshold energy for defibrillation. *Me Inst* 1988; **22:** 298–303.

3 Lerman B, DiMarco J, Haines D. Current-based versus energy-based ventricular defibrillation: a prospective study. *JACC* 1988; **12:** 1259–1264.

4 Shorofsky SR, Peters RW, Rashba EJ *et al.* Comparison of step-down and binary search algorithms for determination of defibrillation threshold in humans. *PACE* 2004; **27:** 218–220.

5 Annamraju S, Lieberman R, Meissner M *et al.* ICD defibrillation threshold determination via single VF induction. *PACE* 2002; **25:** 618 (abstract).

6 Marchlinski F, Flores B, Miller J *et al.* Relation between the intraoperative defibrillation threshold to successful postoperative defibrillation with an automatic implantable cardioverter defibrillator. *Am J Cardiol* 1988; **62:** 393–398.

7 Epstein A, Ellenbogen K, Kirk K, Kay N, Dailey S, Plumb V. Clinical characteristics and outcomes of patients with high defibrillation thresholds: a multicenter study. *Circulation* 1992; **86:** 1206–1216.

8 Gold MR, Higgins S, Klein R *et al.* Efficacy and temporal stability of reduced safety margins for ventricular defibrillation: primary results from the Low Energy Safety Study (LESS). *Circulation* 2002; **105:** 2043–2048.

9 Gold MR, Breiter D, Leman R *et al.* Safety of a single successful conversion of ventricular fibrillation before the implantation of cardioverter defibrillators. *PACE* 2003; **26:** 483–486.

10 Higgins S, Mann D, Calkins H *et al.* One VF induction is adequate for ICD implant: a subanalysis from the Low Energy Safety Trial (LESS). *PACE* 2002; **24:** 549 (abstract).

11 DeGroot P, DeSouza C, Wang W. Is testing defibrillation efficacy during defibrillator implant worth it? *PACE* 1999; **22:** 723 (abstract).

12 Smits K, DeGroot P. A bayesian approach to reduced implant testing of a ventricular defibrillator: a computer simulation. *Europace Suppl* 2004; **6:** 97 (abstract).

13 Simon RD, Sturdivant JL, Leman R *et al.* The role of dofetilide to reduce defibrillation thresholds in patients with an inadequate defibrillation safety margin. *Heart Rhythm* 2004; **1:** S42 (abstract).

14 Schuder JC, Gold JH, Stoeckle H *et al.* Tansthoracic ventricular defibrillation in the 100 kg calf with untruncated and truncated exponential stimuli. *IEEE Trans Biomed Eng* 1980; **27:** 37–43.

15 Shorofsky SR, Foster AH, Gold MR. Effect of waveform tilt on defibrillation thresholds in humans. *J Cardiovasc Electrophysiol* 1997; **8:** 496–501.

16 Bardy G, Stewart R, Ivey T *et al.* Intraoperative comparison of Medtronic sequential pulse and CPI/Intec single pulse defibrillation methods. *Circulation* 1986; **74:** 184 (abstract).

17 Natale A, Sra J, Dhala A *et al.* Effects of initial polarity on defibrillation threshold with biphasic pulses. *PACE* 1995; **18:** 1889–1893.

18 Shorofsky SR, Gold MR. Effect of second-phase duration on the strength–duration relation for human transvenous defibrillation. *Circulation* 2002; **2:** 2239–2242.

19 Swartz J, Fletcher R, Karasik P. Optimization of biphasic waveforms for human nonthoracotomy defibrillation. *Circulation* 1993; **88:** 2646–2654.

20 Sweeney MO, Natale A, Volosin KJ *et al.* Prospective randomized comparison of 50%/50% versus 65%/65% tilt biphasic waveform on defibrillation in humans. *PACE* 2001; **24:** 60–65.

21 Shepard RK, DeGroot P, Pacifico A *et al.* Prospective randomized comparison of 65%/65% versus 42%/42% tilt biphasic waveform on defibrillation thresholds in humans. *J Interv Card Electrophysiol* 2003; **8:** 221–225.

22 Li H, Yee R, Mehra R *et al.* The effect of biphasic shock waveform tilt upon defibrillation efficacy. *Circulation* 1993; **88:** I113 (abstract).

23 Poole J, Bardy G, Kudenchuk P *et al.* Prospective randomized comparison of biphasic waveform tilt using a unipolar defibrillation system. *PACE* 1995; **18:** 1369–1373.

24 Swerdlow C, Kass R, Chen P *et al.* Effect of capacitor size and pathway resistance on defibrillation threshold for implantable defibrillators. *Circulation* 1994; **90:** 1840–1846.

25 DeGroot P, Norenberg M, Mehra R. Effect of capacitance on defibrillation thresholds in dogs. *Am Heart J* 1994; **128:** 640 (abstract).

26 Lin J, Stotts L, Rosborough J *et al.* Comparison of defibrillation efficacy using biphasic waveforms delivered from various capacitances/pulse widths. *PACE* 1997; **20:** 158–162.

27 Yamanouchi Y, Brewer JE, Mowrey K *et al.* The strength–duration relationship of monophasic waveforms with varying capacitance sizes in external defibrillation. *PACE*, 2003; **26:** 2213–2218.

28 Brugada J, Herse B, Sandstedt B *et al.* Clinical evaluation of defibrillation efficacy with a new single-capacitor biphasic waveform in patients undergoing implantation of an implantable cardioverter defibrillator. *Europace* 2001; **3:** 278–284.

29 Shorofsky S, Rashba E, DeGroot P *et al.* Is the membrane time constant for defibrillation independent of the shock waveform? *PACE* 2003; **25:** 620 (abstract).

30 Strickberger S, Hummel J, Horwood L *et al.* Effect of shock polarity on ventricular defibrillation threshold using a transvenous lead system. *JACC* 1993; **24:** 1069–1072.

31 Natale A, Sra J, Krum D *et al.* Comparison of biphasic and monophasic pulses: does the advantage of biphasic shocks depend on the waveshape? *PACE* 1995; **18:** 1354–1361.

32 Keelan E, Sra J, Axtell K *et al.* The effect of polarity on the initial phase of a biphasic shock waveform on the defibrillation threshold of pectorally implanted defibrillators. *PACE* 1997; **20:** 337–342.

33 Olsovsky MR, Shorofsky SR, Gold MR. Effect of shock polarity on biphasic defibrillation thresholds using an active pectoral lead system. *J Cardiovasc Electrophysiol* 1998; **9:** 350–354.

34 Rashba EJ, Shorofsky SR, Peters RW *et al.* Effect of shock polarity on defibrillation thresholds with a hybrid patch-coil lead system. *J Interv Card Electrophysiol* 2003; **9:** 391–396.

35 Strickberger SA, Man KC, Daoud EG *et al.* Effect of first-phase polarity of biphasic shocks on defibrillation threshold with a single transvenous lead system. *J Am Coll Cardiol* 1995; **25:** 1605–1608.

36 Neuzner J, Pitschner H, Schwarz T *et al.* Effects of electrode polarity on defibrillation thresholds in biphasic endocardial defibrillation. *Am J Cardiol* 1996; **78:** 96–97.

37 Narasimhan C, Panotopoulos P, Deshpande S *et al.* Reversing the initial phase polarity in biphasic shocks: the polarity benefit reproducible? *PACE* 1999; **22:** 60–64.

38 Bardy G, Johnson G, Poole J *et al.* A simplified single-lead unipolar transvenous cardioversion-defibrillation system. *Circulation* 1993; **88:** 543–547.

39 Gold M, Foster A, Shorofsky S. Effects of an active pectoral-pulse generator shell on defibrillation efficacy with a transvenous lead system. *Am J Cardiol* 1996; **78:** 540–543.

40 Gold MR, Olsovsky MR, DeGroot P *et al.* Optimization of transvenous coil position for active can defibrillation thresholds. *J Cardiovasc Electrophysiol* 2000; **11:** 25–29.

41 Kirk M, Shorofsky S, Gold M. Right sided active pectoral pulse generators do not reduce defibrillation thresholds. *Am J Cardiol* 2001; **88:** 1308–1311.

42 Kenknight BH, Walker RG, Ideker RE. Marked reduction of ventricular defibrillation threshold by application of an auxiliary shock to a catheter electrode in the left posterior coronary vein of dogs. *J Cardiovasc Electrophysiol* 2000; **11:** 900–906.

43 Butter C, Meisel E, Engelmann L *et al.* Human experience with transvenous biventricular defibrillation using an electrode in a left ventricular vein. *PACE* 2002; **25:** 324–331.

44 Huang J, KenKnight BH, Rollins DL *et al.* Ventricular defibrillation with triphasic waveforms. *Circulation* 2000; **101:** 1324–1328.

45 Blair HA. On the intensity–time relations for stimulation by electric currents. II. *J Gen Physiol* 1932; **15:** 731–755.

46 Walcott G, Walker R, Cates A *et al.* Choosing the optimal monophasic and biphasic waveforms for ventricular defibrillation. *J Cardiovasc Electrophysiol* 1995; **6:** 737–750.

47 Yamanouchi Y, Brewer JE, Mowrey KA *et al.* Sawtooth first phase biphasic defibrillation waveform: a comparison with standard waveform in clinical devices. *J Cardiovasc Electrophysiol* 1997; **8:** 517–528.

48 Seidl K, Molder C, Mouchawar G *et al.* Stepped defibrillation waveform is more efficient than the biphasic waveform. *Europace Supplements* 2004; **6:** 144 (abstract).

49 Klafter RD. An optimally energized cardiac pacemaker. *IEEE Trans BME* 1973; **20:** 350–356.

50 Gold M, Shorofsky S, Rashba E *et al.* A modified ramp waveform reduces defibrillation voltage, but an energy, in humans. *PACE* 2002; **25:** 686 (abstract).

51 Shorofsky S, Rashba E, Havel W, *et al.* Improved defibrillation efficacy with an ascending ramp waveform in humans. *Heart Rhythm* 2005; **2:** 388–394.

52 Bardy G, Zagho H, Gartman D *et al.* A prospective randomized comparison of defibrillation efficacy of truncated pulses and damped sine wave pulses in humans. *J Cardiovasc Electrophysiol* 1994; **5:** 725–730.

53 Bardy G, Cappato R, Smith W *et al.* The totally subcutaneous ICD system (The S-ICD). *PACE* 2002; **25:** 578 (abstract).

54 Wathen M, DeGroot P, Sweeney MO *et al.* Prospective randomized multicenter trial of empirical antitachycardia pacing versus shocks for spontaneous rapid ventricular tachycardia in patients with implantable cardioverter-defibrillators. *Circulation* 2004; **110:** 2591–2596.

22

CHAPTER 22

Remote web-based device monitoring

Edmund Keung, MD *&* *Yang Xue,* BS

Background of remote device monitoring

Transtelephonic pacemaker monitoring (TTM) is probably one of the earliest forms of remote device monitoring and telemedicine with its beginning dated back to 1970 [1, 2]. The objectives of TTM include the following: (1) to detect pacing system malfunctions that occur between clinic visits and before patients become symptomatic, (2) to detect battery depletion before voltage output ceases, (3) to provide monitoring and pacing expertise for facilities without pacemaker follow-up expertise, (4) to provide minimum monitoring for patients who cannot travel or who have to travel long distance to a medical facility for regular visit. The patient is given a transmitter and a magnet. A typical arrangement is showed in Figure 22.1. The patient places one electrode band on each wrist and the transmission of ECG tracing is accomplished by placing the phone on the transmitter. The test has to be performed with a land-based, analog phone line (however, cordless phones have provided successful transmissions). Pacemaker checks can either be initiated by telephone calls from the patient or from medical staff at a clinic or by a commercial monitoring service. The protocol includes transmission of at least 30 s of nonmagnet, or presenting or free-running tracing. This is followed by placing a magnet over the pulse generator to initiate transmission of 30 s or more of magnet tracing. The tracings are evaluated by qualified professional personnel for presence of pacing outputs, capture and sensing, and battery elective replacement indicator (ERI) from the magnet response rate and reports sent to referring physicians. The transmitted tracings may reveal the presence of atrial and ventricular tachyarrhythmias.

Home monitoring of pacemaker with TTM has proven to be very safe provided that some guidelines are strictly followed. Magnet tests should be avoided if the heart rate is above 100 beats per minute (bpm), frequent ventricular premature complexes or atrial and ventricular tachyarrhythmias are present, and while the patient is having chest pain. Magnet tests should not be performed on patients with an internal cardioverter defibrillator, for application of the magnet would "blind" the device to tachycardia detection and may even inactivate the device. Very rarely, application of the magnet has resulted in supraventricular tachycardia (SVT) and pacemaker-mediated tachycardia.

The functionalities of TTM remain very limited. Sensing and pacing can only be evaluated with a 30–60 s ECG snapshot of pacemaker actions obtained during each test, and there have only been a few studies examining its effectiveness in recent years [3, 4]. Although major advances in pacing technology have occurred in recent years, very few of these were transferred to TTM. There are some well-known technical inadequacies in TTM, some of which result from new developments in pacing since 1970. Bipolar pacing configuration frequently prevents stimulus artifacts from being recorded because of the small signal amplitude. Introduction of a special TTM feature by Medtronic greatly enhanced recording of the stimulus artifacts. When the TTM is programmed ON,

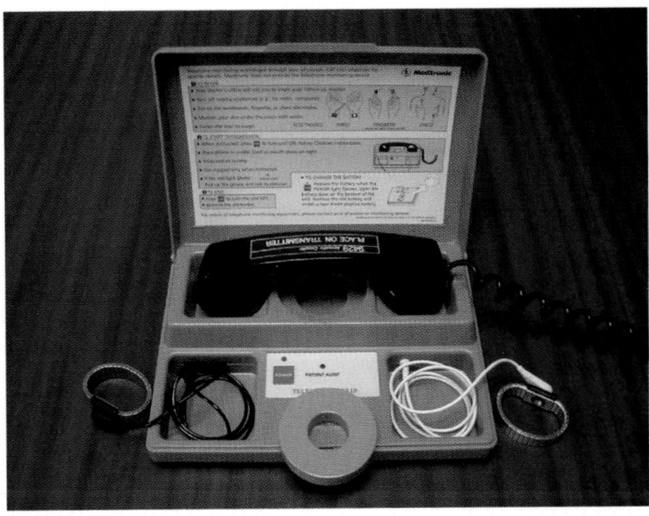

Figure 22.1 A typical transmitter used for TTM.

application of the magnet temporarily set the pacing polarity from bipolar to unipolar to provide improved ECG artifact detection and thus one has to make sure that the pacemaker is pacing properly in the unipolar configuration. In patients with both an implantable defibrillator and a pacemaker, unipolar pacing can cause a double counting of the heart rate that may result in inappropriate therapy. Another often-encountered TTM technological inadequacy is failure to document atrial capture and sensing (Figure 22.2). When TTM was first introduced in 1970, single-chamber ventricular pacemakers provided pacing in most of the patients. Documentation of sensing and pacing was easily accomplished. With the introduction of the dual-chamber pacemaker, evaluation of atrial pacing function by TTM has often become an exercise of inference. Because the small P-wave signal is often not well represented on TTM tracings, atrial sensing abnormality frequently has to be inferred from circumstantial evidence. For example, the presence of frequent safety pacing provides strong evidence for P-wave undersensing, while irregularly irregular atrial synchronous pacing may be due to atrial fibrillation.

Since the inception of TTM, manufacturers have added a small number of functionalities. Shortening of atrioventricular delay (AVD) during magnet test in a dual-chamber pacemaker maximizes documentation of ventricular capture in patients whose AVD delay is programmed to longer duration to ensure intrinsic AV conduction. Several tests for threshold safety margin (Threshold Margin Test, TMT) have been introduced. For Medtronic pacemakers, application of a magnet initiated 3 cycles at 100 ppm with AVD of 100 ms. The output voltage of the fourth stimulus was reduced by 20%. Intermedics pacemakers TMT consisted of 4 cycles at 90 ppm with magnet test. The pulse width of the fifth stimulus was reduced by 50%. A more detailed measurement of pacing threshold was introduced by Siemens (named Vario) and Ela Medical. Application of magnet initiates a train of pacing outputs that are successively decreased to zero. The pacing threshold can be calculated to <0.5 V accuracy. One significant problem with this approach is that in patients with high pacing threshold, prolonged asystole, and subsequent adverse clinical event could result as the pacing output continued to be decremented to zero during the test. In this group of patients, this feature is usually programmed off.

The next enhancement of functionalities of TTM was the Fully Automated Self-Test (FAST) introduced with Medtronic's Kappa series pacemakers. If this feature is enabled, a specific pattern of pacing occurs during magnet application if out-of-range pacing impedance is recorded or Capture Management measures unusually high ventricular thresholds (resulting in 5 V and 1 ms pacing output). This feature represents the first expansion of TTM functionalities to include historical event data.

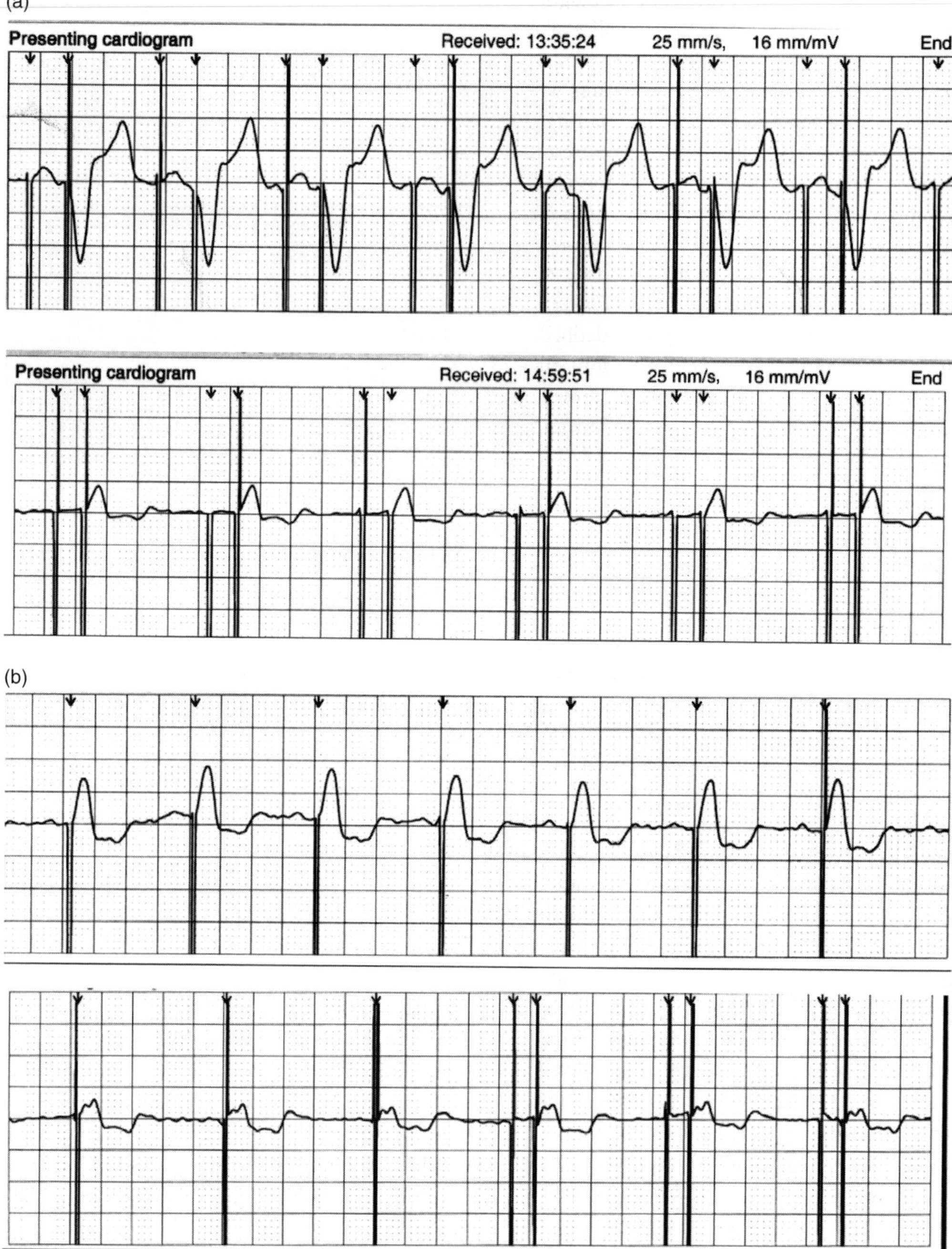

Figure 22.2 Technical inadequacies of TTM: atrial capture often cannot be documented. (a) In the upper tracing, atrial capture is clearly demonstrated by distinct atrial depolarizations in response to the output stimuli. However, as often the case, as shown in the lower tracing, no recognizable atrial deflections are present on the TTM tracings to confirm capture. (b) In the upper TTM tracing, P-waves can clearly be identified. In the lower TTM tracing, there are no recognizable P-waves in the first three complexes. The presence of P can only be inferred from the suppression of atrial pacing spikes.

Recognition of battery ERI from the magnet rate remains the most important functionality of TTM. Remote home surveillance allows close monitoring of the battery status of older pacemakers without increasing the burden of traveling, waiting time, and utilization of clinic or office resources. However, after more than 30 years of service, TTM is approaching its own replacement time. This is brought on by advancement in three areas: development and incorporation of diagnostic clinical data and automaticity features in pacemaker, introduction of implantable cardioverter defibrillators (ICD) and cardiac resynchronization therapy (CRT) devices, and the exponential growth and adoption of Internet, telecommunication, and web applications.

Development of extended telemetry and automaticity features in devices

In the past few years, a number of self-diagnostic and monitoring functionalities have been incorporated into pacemakers and defibrillators [5]. The automaticity features include automatic programmed setting adjustments, such as polarity switch and sensitivity adjustment, as well as self-adjustment of pacing output based on device-initiated atrial and ventricular pacing threshold testing. These features not only detect changes in device performance but also make corrections as soon as they happen. They also take any guesswork out of atrial and ventricular capture and sensing evaluation in TTM. Telemetry capability has also been greatly expanded. Historical device data (such as P- and R-wave amplitude trends, atrial and ventricular impedance monitoring) and clinician-selected diagnostic clinical events (e.g. high atrial and ventricular rate events, mode-switching episodes, heart rate trends, mode of pacing) are now stored and can be retrieved with a programmer. The rapidly widening information and functionality gap between device and TTM creates an impetus for the medical community and device manufacturers to develop and adopt a new generation of remote monitoring system and reevaluate the objectives of device monitoring.

A new generation of remote device monitoring

Recently technology has been developed to enable remote transmission of comprehensive data on pacemaker and ICD performance and therapy history (equivalent to interrogation with a programmer) to a network server. It is quite apparent that a full-feature download of data is far superior to TTM. With automaticity functionalities and extensive telemetry device data, healthcare professionals can provide a comprehensive and more accurate evaluation of the performance of the device. For ICD, ability to transmit EGM tracing recorded during a tachycardia episode will allow a physician to remotely evaluate the appropriateness and effectiveness of detection and therapy. Figure 22.3 shows the EGM of a "ventricular fibrillation" (VF) episode transmitted during a periodic remote transmission scheduled between office visits. Examination of the tracing showed that frequent extrinsic noise was detected, resulting in false identification of VF. The patient underwent lead revision to correct the problem. Because of early detection, inappropriate shock was avoided. Furthermore, diagnostic event history will assist physicians in managing the patient's disease condition. For example, presence of frequent and prolonged episodes of mode-switching, atrial tachycardia response, and high atrial rate events strongly suggest atrial tachyarrhythmias and raise the question of atrial fibrillation and its associated complications. Retrieved telemetry data will take on even more significant clinical relevance when more diagnostic functionalities are incorporated into CRT devices in patients with heart failure.

Three device manufacturers are now marketing remote monitoring system in the United States. Medtronic and St. Jude Medical have adopted this full-disclosure model for their remote monitoring system. The retrieval, just as performed during office visit, is achieved by magnetically coupling the device to a transmitter using an antenna or wand that is physically linked to the transmitter. The notable difference is that the patient performs the transmission at home. Like TTM, the retrieved data are transmitted by land-based phone line to a receiving center, or to a central computer server, for

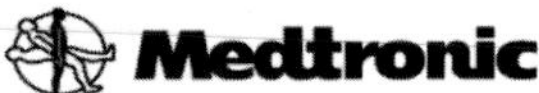

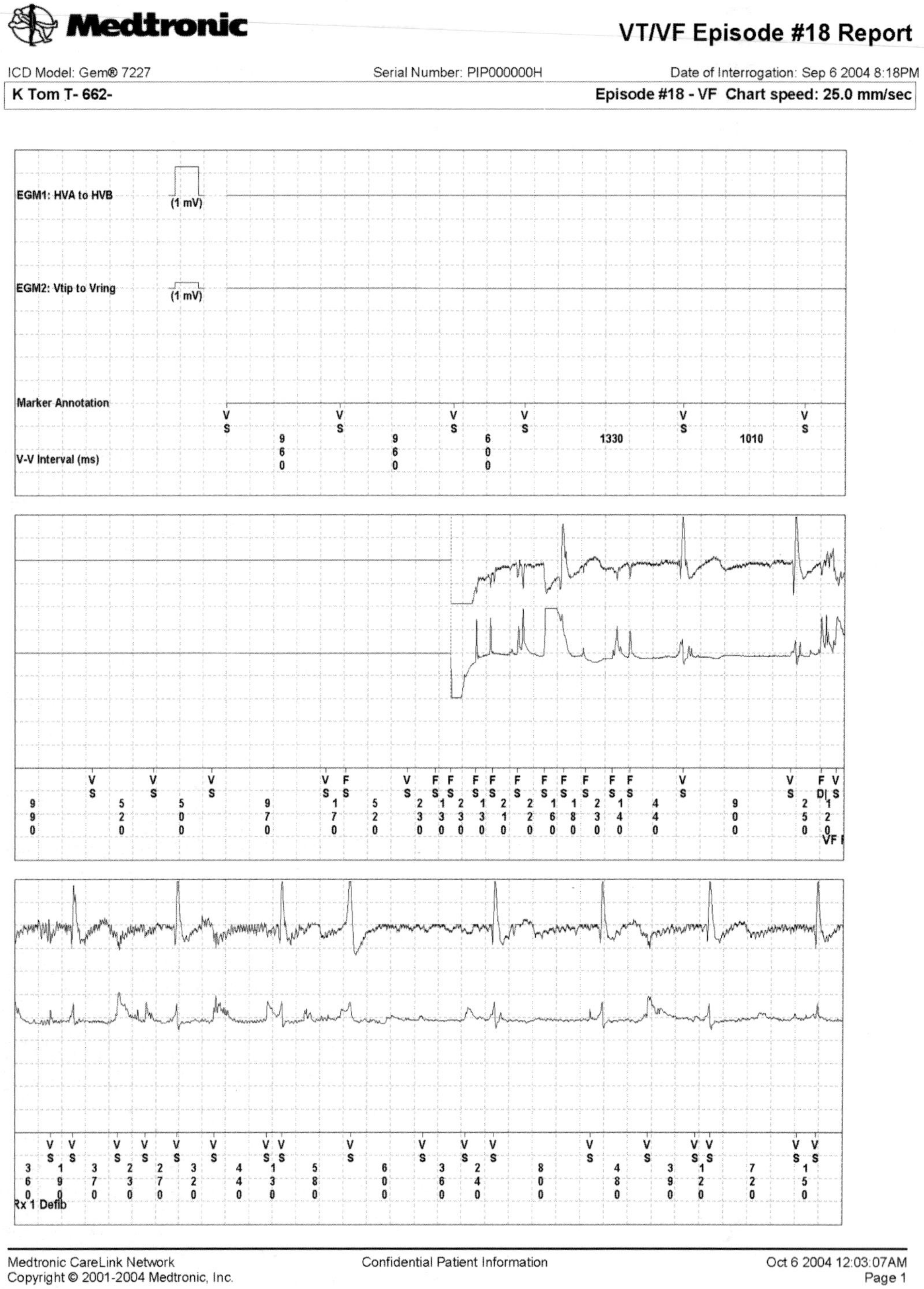
VT/VF Episode #18 Report
ICD Model: Gem® 7227
Serial Number: PIP000000H
Date of Interrogation: Sep 6 2004 8:18PM
K Tom T- 662-
Episode #18 - VF Chart speed: 25.0 mm/sec
EGM1: HVA to HVB
(1 mV)
EGM2: Vtip to Vring
(1 mV)
Marker Annotation
V-V Interval (ms)
1330
1010
VF
Rx 1 Defib
Medtronic CareLink Network
Copyright © 2001-2004 Medtronic, Inc.
Confidential Patient Information
Oct 6 2004 12:03:07AM
Page 1

Figure 22.3 A VT/VF episode report from the Medtronic CareLink® Network System. Inclusion of EGM from the episode allowed the physician to recognize false identification of a VF episode resulting from a malfunctioning lead.

processing and review. Because data retrieval has to be done with an antenna or wand placed over the device, the transmission session has to be initiated by the patient. In the Medtronic Carelink® Network for Medtronic pacemaker and ICD, at the scheduled time the patient connects the CareLink® monitor (Figure 22.4) to a standard analog phone line, powers on the monitor, and places the antenna over the implanted device. The monitor will retrieve the data and then automatically dial a toll-free, preprogrammed telephone number and upload the data to a secure server. The entire process takes 2–12 min, depending on the volume of data being transmitted. The device continues to perform its regular function during the transmission. There is no human interaction and feedback of the transmission session is limited to lights on the monitor confirming proper antenna placement and completion of data transmission. The St. Jude Medical Housecall Plus™ Remote Follow-Up System adopts the basic features of the standard TTM approach. It is limited to St. Jude Medical ICD only. A transmission session can be initiated by a phone call either from the patient to the receiving center or by a healthcare professional to the patient. The transmitter (Figure 22.5) is connected to a phone jack and to the patient's regular telephone. Wristband electrodes allow transmission of

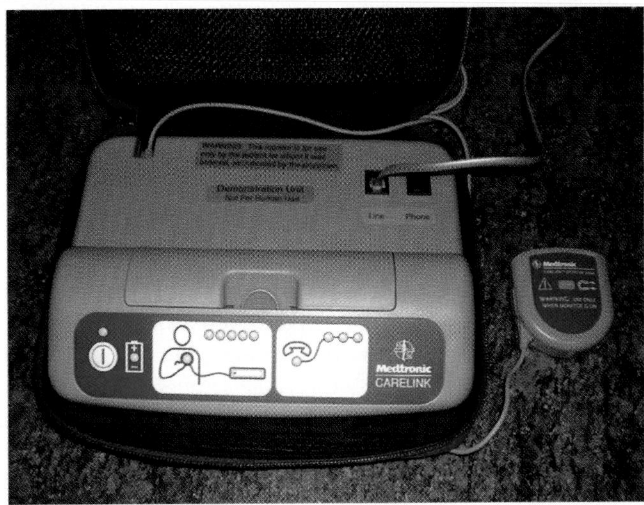

Figure 22.4 A Medtronic CareLink® monitor. The monitor automatically dials a toll-free, preprogrammed telephone number over a land-based phone line and sends the retrieved data to a secure computer.

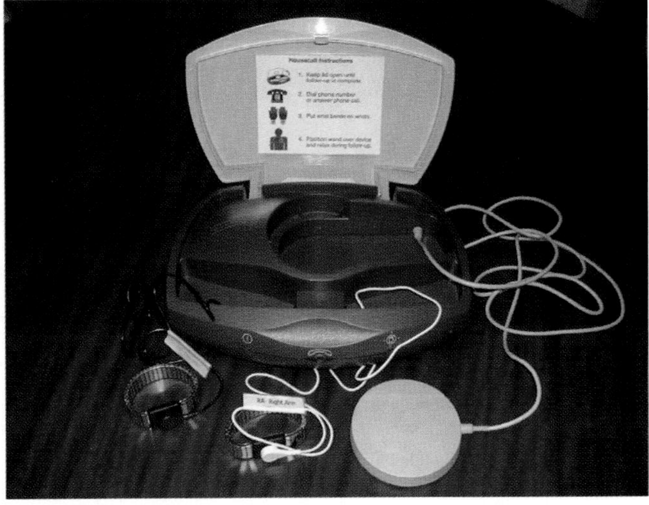

Figure 22.5 A St. Jude Medical HouseCall Plus™ transmitter (model 3180-T). The patient dials or answers phone call from his or her monitoring facility to initiate a transmission session. Inclusion of wristbands allows transmission of TTM-type ECG tracings to the monitoring facility during the session.

real-time TTM-type ECG tracing to the receiving center during the session. The wand is placed over the implanted device, and the person at the receiving center remotely controls collection and transmission of data over the telephone line. Similar to TTM, voice communication between the caller and the patient is available during the session except when data are being transmitted.

Biotronik adopted a different philosophy in remote monitoring. It employs a sentinel approach. Instead of performing scheduled full-disclosure data transmissions, its Home Monitoring System emphasizes continuous surveillance and immediate (real-time) communication of changes (alert) to healthcare professionals (http://www.earlydetection.net). Although scheduled and patient initiated transmissions of selected data are also part of their protocol, the salient characteristic is that transmissions are event-triggered, alert triggered, or need based. The report (Figure 22.6) consists of information on the occurrence of therapy events and selected functional status of the device. It also includes line graphs depicting VF/VT (ventricular tachycardia) instances, intrinsic rhythm (with pacing mode), and pacing and shock lead impedance trend. Transmitted data (and triggered events) from its Lexos® DR-T ICD include the following: (1) detection of VT, VF, and SVT; (2) ATP counter (started, successful); (3) shock counter (started, successful, aborted); (4) 30 J shock counter (unsuccessful); (5) information about the intrinsic rhythm; (6) voltage and status of battery with date of measurement; (7) atrial and ventricular pace impedances with date of measurement; and (8) shock impedance with date of measurement. No EGM tracings are included. With the Philos® DR-T pacemaker, automatic transmission is triggered by one of the following events: (1) atrial or ventricular lead impedance out of range (<300 and >3000 ohms), (2) low P- or R-wave amplitude (<50% safety margin), (3) ventricular runs (4–8 beats) and ventricular events (VT > 8 beats), and (4) ERI. Because it is not a full-disclosure data transmission system, Biotronik does not recommend extending intervals between regular office visit for device interrogation. The advantage of the Home Monitoring System is that it does not require the patient's active participation. Hence, there are no missed appointments (transmissions) and no burden on patients to keep track of their transmission schedule. To accomplish this, Biotronik employs a cell-phone-like transceiver, CardioMessenger®, that performs wireless retrieval of data from the implanted device using the Medical Implant Communications Service (MICS) band and transmission of data to a receiving center in Germany using the Global System for Mobile (GSM) Communications digital wireless phone system (Figure 22.7).

Medical implant communications service and wireless remote monitoring

Until 1999, the only means to retrieve data from a pacemaker or ICD, whether it was done remotely at home or during an office visit, was by magnetically coupling the device to an external programmer or a transmitter. This magnetic coupling required that the device be physically linked to a programmer or transmitter, usually with a wand. Because of this requirement, the patient or the healthcare professional has to initiate the communication of data. In addition, such communication sessions operate with very slow data rates, sometimes requiring up to several minutes for the required data. We learned from our experience, with remote monitoring of 1600 patients at the VA National ICD Surveillance Center that the patient-triggered transmission approach often results in a high non-compliance rate. An ideal remote monitoring system should allow wireless retrieval of data from implanted devices and communication of data to a receiving center for viewing and analysis. Automated communication of information from an implant to a home receiver will greatly improve the compliance rate. The patients' quality of life will improve because the burden and worry of keeping track of their transmission schedule is removed. Moreover, preprogrammed home monitoring can automatically trigger communication sessions. Physicians can then be notified of potential problems with minimal delay, instead of waiting for the next scheduled follow-up office visit. While the benefits are clear, there are several important technical factors to be considered in wireless transmission. The amplitude of the radio signals emitted from an implanted device must be large enough to overcome

CARDIO REPORT

BIOTRONIK

Hotline Tel.: 800–284–6689
Fax: 888–387–2681

To attending physician	**Fax:**

Patient ID	Patient Device No.	Last Message received at Patient Device	**07–08–2003 at 08:40:17**
		Last Message received at Service Center	**07–08–2003 at 08:40:01**
		Consecutive Report No.	**7**
	Implant / Serial No.	Consecutive Report: Date / Time	**07–08–2003 at 08:49:26**
	Belos DR–T /	Date of Preceding Cardio Report	**06–17–2003 at 06:04:08**

Event Report – VF Detected

	Since last Follow Up **04–16–2003**	Since Implantation
DETECTION		
Episodes in VT1 Zone	0	0
Episodes in VT2 Zone	0	0
Episodes in VF Zone	6	11
SVT	0	0
THERAPY		
ATPs started	0	0
ATPs successful	0	
Shocks started	7	12
Shocks successful	1	
Shocks aborted	6	7
30 J Shock without Success	0	

INTRINSIC RHYTHM* *Detection also during SVT	**Since restart statistics**	**Since last Reporting Interval**
Atrial senses (As/Ax) [%]	92	–––––
Ventricular senses (Vs/Vx) [%]	92	–––––

BATTERY		
Status	BOL 83 %	
Voltage measured on	6.24 V	07–08–2003

LEADS	**Atrial**	**Ventricular**
Pace Impedance measured on	695 Ohm 07–08–2003	493 Ohm 07–08–2003
Shock Impedance measured on		50 Ohm 05–27–2003

DEVICE STATUS SUMMARY / REMARK	
Status	OK
Remark	

• VT1 Episodes cumulative since Follow-up ▼ SVT

• VF Episodes cumulative since Follow-up ▼ VT2

Intrinsic Rhythm (%) ▼As / Ax •Vs / Vx

▼Shock Imp. (Ohm) Pacing Imp. (Ohm) •Ventricular ◆Atrial

prev. Follow-up 04/20 05/18 06/15

Monitoring Mode Settings	Monitoring Interval (periodic message from implant):	24 hours
	Reporting Interval between Follow Up (interval of periodic reports):	4 weeks

Figure 22.6 A Cardio Report from the Biotronik Home Monitoring System. Reproduced with permission from Biotronik USA.

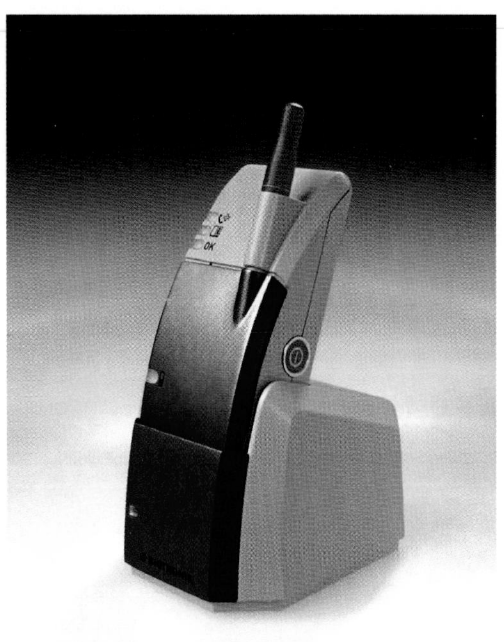

Figure 22.7 A CardioMessenger® wireless transceiver for the Biotronik Home Monitoring System. The effective range is 6 ft. Data are transmitted from the implant device to the transceiver using the MICS band of 401–406 MHz. The data are then sent to a receiving center in Germany using the GSM Communications digital wireless phone system. Reproduced with permission from Biotronik USA.

body tissue propagation losses without prematurely depleting the battery. A frequency band for medical telemetry must be relatively free of interference from external transmitters such as those found in the broadcast (600 kHz to 1.6 MHz for AM radio and 88–108 MHz for FM radio) cellular phone (800–900 MHz) and two-way frequency bands. Additionally, a suitable frequency band must be sufficiently separated in frequency from these bands in order to avoid disruption to communication sessions.

In 1998, the International Telecommunications Union (a worldwide regulatory authority) recommended sharing of the MICS with Meteorological Aids in the 401–406 MHz band on a worldwide basis in ITU-R SA 1346. (ITU-R Recommendation SA 1346: "Sharing between the meterological aids service and medical implant communication systems (MICS) operating in the mobile service in the frequency band 401–406 MHz.") At the urging of the medical community and device manufacturers, the Federal Communications Commission (FCC) adopted the ITU-R recommendation and established the MICS in 1999 (http://wireless.fcc.gov/services/personal/medicalimplant/) for the 402–405 MHz band. Other countries, including the European Union, have also adopted the 402–405 MHz band for MICS. The FCC defined the MICS as an ultra-low power, unlicensed, mobile radio service for transmitting data in support of diagnostic or therapeutic functions associated with implanted medical devices. The goal is to establish high-speed, dependable, short-range wireless links (within 6 ft) from implantable devices, such as pacemaker and defibrillator to programmers and receivers, without causing interference to other users of the electromagnetic radio spectrum. The FCC made the 402–405 MHz frequency band available for MICS operations on a shared, secondary basis. The use of the 402–405 MHz frequency band for the MICS does not pose a significant risk of interference to other radio operations with primary status in that band, which include the Meteorological Aids, Meteorological Satellite, or Earth Exploration Satellite Services operating in the same or adjacent frequencies. The 402–405 MHz frequencies have propagation characteristics that allow engineers to design MICS system to optimize the transmission of radio signals from devices within the human body without sacrificing size, antenna performance, and power usage.

The MICS rules took effect on January 14, 2000. While a license is not required to operate MICS equipment, it must be operated by a duly authorized healthcare professional, which is defined by the FCC as a physician or other individual authorized under state or federal law to provide healthcare services using medical implant devices. MICS transmitters must select channels to avoid interference with other MICS transmissions via a "listen-before-talk" access protocol. In the listen-before-talk protocol, external device programmer and MICS transmitters must incorporate a mechanism for monitoring the channel or channels that the MICS system devices intend to occupy. One FCC rule that has a significant effect on the development of home wireless transmission of pacemaker and ICD data is that except in response to a medical implant event (e.g. alerts triggered by changes in measured values or device functions that may adversely affect the safety or well-being of the patients), devices are not permitted to initiate transmission sessions on their own. Accordingly, regularly scheduled device-initiated surveillance transmissions do not qualify as medical implant events and are not permitted by the FCC. At present, a waiver has to be obtained from the FCC for permission to perform wireless, periodic, scheduled transmissions of device data.

The adoption of the MICS was a major milestone in the development of wireless remote monitoring of pacemakers and defibrillators. The listen-before-talk protocol complies with the ITU-R recommendation for frequency agility in order to avoid other MICS users in the band and ambient interference sources. This protocol preserves the safety and integrity of the band for patients and their physicians and forms the foundation for the future development of wireless transmission.

Banking and distribution of transmitted data: web-based monitoring

One obvious result from the new remote monitoring systems is accumulation of voluminous amounts of data, especially from full-disclosure systems. This presents several immediate problems to the healthcare professionals. The data will need to be stored electronically in an easily accessible and retrievable location and in formats that are scalable and portable. St. Jude Medical's HouseCall Plus™ system basically consists of a personal computer (PC) with proprietary software that functions essentially as a programmer (but without programming capability) operated remotely by a healthcare professional to perform full interrogation of the patient's device via a transmitter by telephone. The data are transmitted and stored as individual files in proprietary format in the hard drive of the operator's PC, and data from each interrogation can be printed and stored as paper files. Limited amount of text data can be transferred via a serial cable or by a removal disk to a Medtronic Paceart® System for electronic filing. This limitation is partly due to Paceart® System's ICD modules not having been updated to accommodate diagnostic and therapy event data, which are now available in newer ICDs, and there is no transfer mechanism for EGM tracings. Taking advantage of the exponential growth and adoption of the Internet, broadband connectivity, and the popularity of web applications, both Medtronic CareLink® Network and Biotronik Home Monitoring System created web-based remote monitoring of device data. The transmitted data are uploaded to a secure server. They are then processed and displayed in HTML (Hypertext Markup Language) in web pages on their websites. The Medtronic CareLink® Network System web application (http://medtroniccarelink.net) has limited dynamic functions. It basically serves as a data-viewing site where EGM tracings can be viewed in reports packaged in Portable Document Format (PDF). There is no notification of instances of transmission to patient's healthcare provider. The Biotronik Home Monitoring System does not transmit EGM tracing and reports are limited to text and line graphs mainly because its primarily goal is to serve as a trip-wire for events (http://www.earlydetect.com). The physician will be notified of an instance of transmission by a predefined method of his or her choice: fax, email, or short message system (SMS). Based on the information in the transmitted report, a decision will then be made by the provider on whether a full in-office interrogation of the device is warranted.

The World Wide Web

A healthcare professional will not need to understand what a web-based system is to appreciate its remarkable convenience and multiple functionalities. However, some understanding of this powerful application will help us appreciate the potential benefits of web-based device monitoring and, eventually, patient monitoring and management. Furthermore, our increased awareness and knowledge will help us to work with and lobby the industry to adopt, expand, and define future directions in web-based monitoring. Web-based device monitoring is a web application. A healthcare professional uses a web browser (e.g. Internet Explorer, Netscape) in a computer that is connected to the Internet (a client computer) to access a web application stored at a server computer. The latter runs special software called web server to send web pages to the web browsers. The client and server computers communicate with each other using the ubiquitous Hypertext Transfer Protocol (http). A web application is a set of web pages that are generated in response to user requests. When a web page contains so-called web controls (text boxes, drop-down lists, submit buttons) it becomes a web form. A dynamic web page is a document generated by a web application in response to information sent from a web browser (Figure 22.8). We are utilizing dynamic web pages when we use search engines such as Yahoo and Google, shop at online stores or eBay, manage our account using online banking service, and express our opinions in discussion groups or forum. It is very obvious that dynamic web pages have significant potential applications to healthcare providers. They allow service providers to offer interactive and customized services using customized web pages to healthcare professionals and patients. Dynamic web applications and relational database management system (RDBMS) such as Microsoft Access, Microsoft SQL Server 2000, and Oracle can be integrated to provide a more interactive and comprehensive remote monitoring program with central data banking of device and clinical data that is readily accessible by patients and healthcare providers [6]. The data can easily be ported and queried by users to retrieve information pertinent to their needs and practice. For example, heart failure physicians and electrophysiologists who now often co-manage patients with CRT devices can both review their patient data on a customized personal web page and receive reports they personally designed to provide data pertinent to their area of practice (Figure 22.9). At the Veterans Affairs National ICD Surveillance Center, we are working to realize these ideas by constructing a secure, password protected remote monitoring web application that is hosted in a central server located behind the VA's own firewall and is accessible by all VA facilities using the VA intranet. At present, the Medtronic Paceart® System, which is built on Microsoft SQL Server 2000, is the application software and RDBMS that drives the monitoring operation. Central data banking service is provided through interactive dynamic web pages that offer online registration and update of patient data (demographic, clinical, and device) and referring medical center data, and viewing of customized reports on scheduled or unscheduled transmitted data after they are reviewed by the National Center staff. The referring centers can also access the website to find out their patients' transmission schedule as determined by

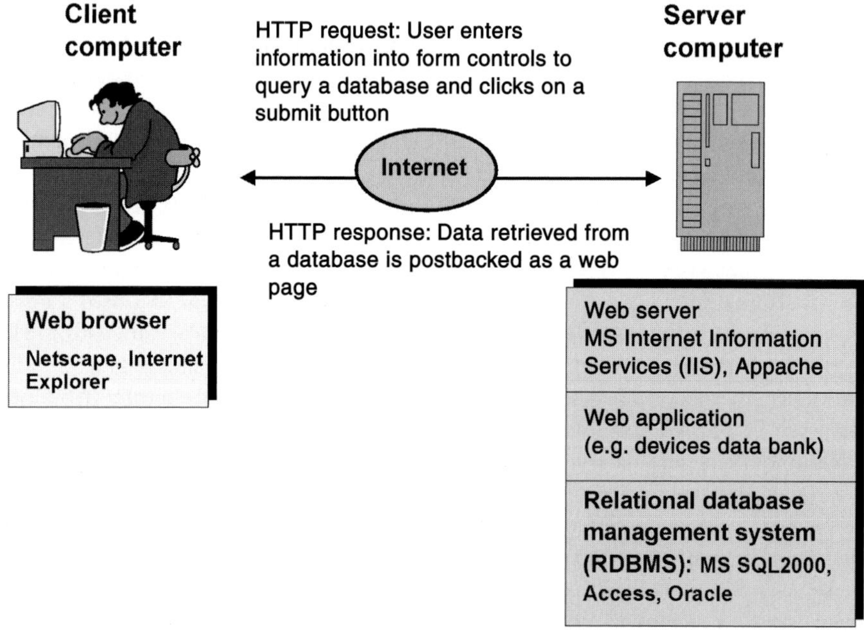

Figure 22.8 Basic components of a web application and processing of dynamic web pages by a web server.

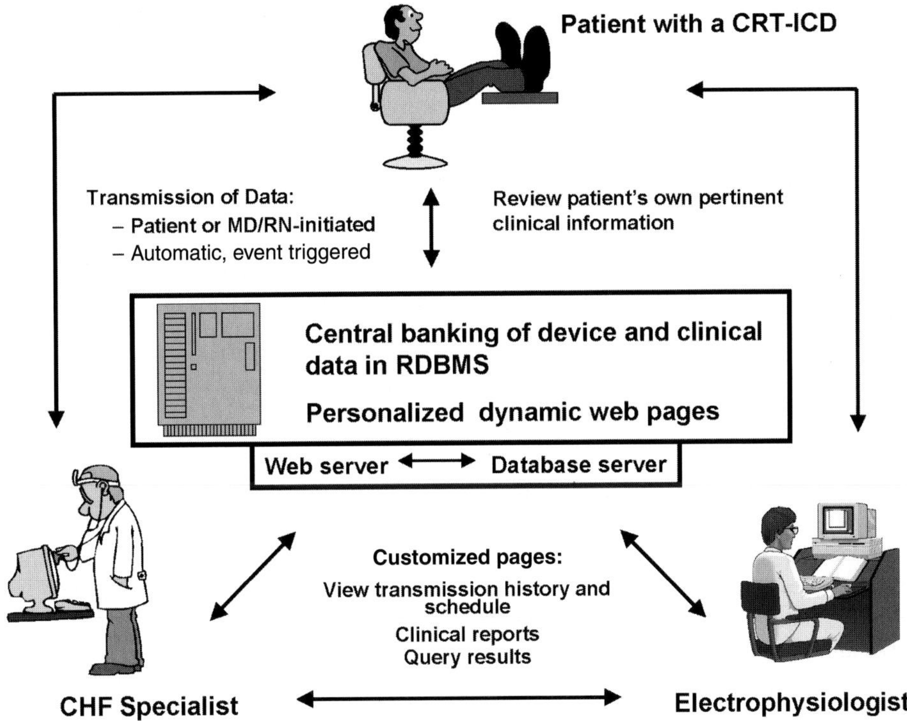

Figure 22.9 Usefulness of central banking of clinical data for patients with CRT devices. Data are shared between the heart failure specialist and the electrophysiologist.

the National Center or to change schedule or even takeover the scheduling themselves. They will also be able to query the database using some built-in selective filters.

Future work and problems of web-based remote device monitoring

Device manufacturers are spending a considerable amount of effort and resources to advance device remote monitoring beyond TTM. We are already witnessing several different approaches to accomplish this task. The ideal system is a combination of full data disclosure and event-triggered transmissions using wireless connectivity. Full interrogation and transmission of device data can be performed on a regularly scheduled basis. These are supplemented with event-triggered instances so that a healthcare professional can respond immediately to potentially damaging adverse events. A major potential problem is that each manufacturer is independently creating its own web-based operation. It may be centralized banking for device data from each manufacturer; healthcare professionals are forced to visit several "central" banks to view patient data because their patient panel will likely contain devices from more than one manufacturer. This creates a burden on the healthcare professionals because they will have to track each patient's device manufacturer, history of transmissions, transmission schedules, and the different operation protocol of reporting and notification (if included) used by different manufacturers. This problem is compounded by the lack of data export functionality in the Medtronic CareLink® Network System and the St. Jude Medical HouseCall™ Plus System. The remotely uploaded device data cannot be exported to any RDBMS. Even with some form of built-in export function (The Biotronik Home Monitoring data can be exported in CSV, comma separated value, file format) there is no available application software that can accommodate all the transmitted data from all the different manufacturers and manage device follow-up. We have reached a juncture in the development of remote monitoring at which it is imperative that the manufacturers begin to work together to adopt some standard of reporting and a standard transfer protocol to allow sharing or easy transfer of data among data banking websites. There is a need for independent device management application software that is designed to work with the new remote monitoring systems. Once a standard is accomplished, the inevitable task of migrating the remote device data into electronic medical record system will be less daunting. Finally, we still have to deal with pages of data printed from regular programmers from different manufacturers during clinic visit. For years, we have been dutifully filing them in paper folders and hand transcribed the information into the patients' medical records. If these printed data can be uploaded from the programmer and integrated with web-based monitoring (a concept that is being developed in the Guidant Latitude® System) from which they can also be transferred to a device management software application, we will be taking a giant step in dismantling the Tower of Babel that is being built in device monitoring and truly enjoy the convenience provided by the new technology.

There is no doubt that the new remote monitoring system will offer unprecedented convenience and comfort to our patients and the healthcare providers. Several recent small studies have demonstrated safety and convenience in remote ICD monitoring [7–11]. The patients no longer will feel the need to seek unscheduled office or clinic appointment with their healthcare provider after an ICD shock therapy is delivered. Visit to device clinic will be reduced as will long distance travel and waiting at the doctor's office. On the other hand, there will be a need to design studies to examine if this new monitoring system, with its ever expanding, on-demand, online data available to healthcare professionals, will improve management of our patients and result in better clinical outcomes. Faced with voluminous amount of transmitted data, healthcare providers will undoubtedly appreciate some form of algorithm to automate interpretation of pacemaker and ICD data, at least for screening purpose. Once we address the above issues, the new generation of web-based remote monitoring will truly be embraced and appreciated by physicians and allied professionals and become an indispensable part of our practice.

References

1 Furman S, Parker B, Escher DJ. Transtelephone pacemaker clinic. *J Thorac Cardiovasc Surg* 1971; **61:** 827–834.

2 Furman S, Escher DJ. Transtelephone pacemaker monitoring: five years later. *Ann Thorac Surg* 1975; **20:** 326–338.

3 VonFeldt L, Neubauer S, Hayes DL. Is transtelephonic monitoring a useful method to detect pacing system abnormalities? *PACE* 1992; **15:** 544.

4 Keung E, Massie B, Gajewski A. What are current pacemaker failure rates? Experience from a large trans-telephonic monitoring program. *Circulation* 1999; **100:** I-569.

5 Neuzner J, Schwarz T, Sperzel J. Pacemaker automaticity. *Am J Cardiol* 2000; **86**(Suppl. 1): K104–K110.

6 Syverson B. (2003) *Murach's SQL for SQL Server.* Mike Murach & Assoc, Fresno.

7 Joseph GK, Wilkoff BL, Dressing T *et al.* Remote interrogation and monitoring of implantable cardioverter defibrillators. *J Interv Card Electrophysiol* 2004; **2:** 161–166.

8 Fauchier L, Kouakam C, Briand F *et al.* Benefit of telemedicine in implantable cardioverter defibrillator recipients related to distance from institution. *Heart Rhythm* 2004; **1**(Suppl.): S57.

9 Sauberman RB, Hsu W, Machado CB *et al.* Technical performance and clinical benefits of remote wireless monitoring of implantable cardioverter defibrillators. *Heart Rhythm* 2004; **1**(Suppl.): S215.

10 Dorszewski A, Kottkamp H, Schirdewahn P *et al.* Long term follow-up of patients with implantable defibrillators using telemetric homemonitoring. *Heart Rhythm* 2004; **1**(Suppl.): S273.

11 Schoenfeld MH, Compton SJ, Mead RH *et al.* Remote monitoring of implantable cardioverter defibrillators: a prospective analysis. *PACE* 2004; **27:** 757–763.

23

CHAPTER 23
New ICD indications

Erik Sirulnick, MD, *Amin Al-Ahmad*, MD, & *Paul J. Wang*, MD

Evolution of indications for ICD implantation

Antiarrhythmic drug therapy for ventricular arrhythmias

The treatment of ventricular tachyarrhythmias has evolved dramatically since the initial approval of the implantable cardioverter defibrillator (ICD) by the Food and Drug Administration (FDA) in the United States of America in 1985 [1, 2]. Prior to the introduction of the implantable defibrillator, antiarrhythmic drug therapy, primarily with Class Ia agents and subsequently amiodarone, was the primary treatment of ventricular arrhythmias and was relied upon to decrease the risk of sudden death in these patients. Patients were routinely started on antiarrhythmic drug therapy and underwent repeat electrophysiologic testing on the antiarrhythmic drug. If the patient became noninducible, the patient was discharged on these medications [3]. The role of serial electrophysiological testing in guiding antiarrhythmic therapy came under question with the results of the Cardiac Arrest in Seattle: Conventional versus Amiodarone Drug Evaluation (CASCADE) trial [4], which demonstrated a superiority of empiric amiodarone therapy compared with Class Ia antiarrhythmic therapy, altering the standard of care of patients surviving cardiac arrest.

Introduction of the implantable defibrillator

From the time of FDA approval of the implantable defibrillator, there was considerable optimism about the effectiveness of the implantable defibrillator in preventing sudden cardiac death with recognized limitations of antiarrhythmic drug therapy in preventing cardiac arrest. Initially, prior to randomized clinical trials of ICDs, ICDs were indicated for patients surviving two cardiac arrests. ICDs were quickly adopted in many electrophysiology centers in such patients. Nevertheless, rather than implanting an ICD in all such patients, it was still routine for patients to undergo three or more antiarrhythmic drug trials prior to receiving an implantable defibrillator, often requiring 2 or more weeks of in-hospital monitoring. Because of recurrences of ventricular tachycardia or cardiac arrest on antiarrhythmic therapy, implantable defibrillators became increasingly accepted in the treatment of ventricular arrhythmias. ICDs gradually were introduced earlier and earlier in the treatment algorithm. The ICD became accepted therapy for patients with inducible ventricular tachyarrhythmias on Class I antiarrhythmic drug therapy.

Randomized data supporting ICD use in ventricular arrhythmias

Despite the FDA approval for implantable defibrillators, there were no randomized data supporting the use of these devices. The landmark study called the Antiarrhythmics Versus Implantable Defibrillators (AVID) trial (Table 23.1) demonstrated a statistically significant increase in survival with ICD implantation compared with antiarrhythmic drug treatment in patients surviving cardiac arrest or hemodynamically significant sustained ventricular tachycardia [16]. Two additional randomized trials, the Cardiac Arrest Study Hamburg (CASH) [6], and the Canadian Implantable Defibrillator Study (CIDS) in similar patient groups also demonstrated the superiority of ICD therapy over any conventional medical therapy [7, 17, 18]. Hence, by the time the 1998 guidelines were released, the evidence for

Table 23.1 Pivotal trials leading to evolution of ICD indications.

Trial name	*Year published*	*Inclusion criteria*	*Summary of results*
ICD versus antiarrhythmic drugs			
Antiarrhythmics Versus Implantable Defibrillator AVID trial [5]	1997	Patients with cardiac arrest or hemodynamically significant sustained VT	1016 patients randomized to ICD or antiarrhythmic therapy. Survival was greater in the ICD arm: 75.4% versus 64.1% at 3 years, a 31% reduction in mortality
Cardiac Arrest Study Hamburg (CASH) [6]	2000	Patients surviving cardiac arrest	ICD versus antiarrhythmic drug (amiodarone, propafenone, or metoprolol; propafenone was discontinued in 1992). ICD arm exhibited trend toward decreased mortality
Canadian Implantable Defibrillator Study (CIDS) [7]	2000	Patients with VT or VF or unmonitored syncope	659 patients randomized to ICD versus amiodarone. 20% relative risk reduction by ICD that was not statistically significant
Primary prevention trials			
Multicenter Automatic Implantable Defibrillator Trial (MADIT)	1996	Patients with coronary artery disease, nonsustained VT EF $\leq$ 35%, inducible VT not suppressed by Class Ia antiarrhythmic drug	196 patients randomized to ICD versus no ICD. ICD arm had hazard ratio of 0.46 for overall mortality, $p = .009$
Multicenter Unsustained Tachycardia Trial (MUSTT) [8]	1999	Patients with coronary artery disease, EF $\leq$40%	704 patients randomized to receive no antiarrhythmic therapy or electrophysiological study guided antiarrhythmic drug or ICD therapy. Risk of cardiac arrest significantly lower in patients receiving ICD
Multicenter Automatic Implantable Defibrillator Trial II (MADIT II) [9]	2002	Patients with coronary artery disease, EF $\leq$30%, more than 1 month after myocardial infarction and 3 months after revascularization	1232 patients randomized to ICD versus no ICD. At 20 months mortality in 19.8% in conventional arm and 14.2% in ICD arm (hazard ratio 0.69, $p = .016$)
Cardiomyopathy Arrhythmia Trial (CAT) [10]	2002	Patients having nonischemic cardiomyopathy of $\leq$ 9 months and EF $\leq$ 30%	104 patients randomized to ICD versus no ICD. No difference in mortality
Amiodarone versus Implantable cardioverter Defibrillator Trial (AMIOVERT) [11]	2003	Patients having nonischemic cardiomyopathy, nonsustained VT, EF $\leq$ 35%	103 patient randomized to ICD versus amiodarone. No difference in mortality
Defibrillators in Nonischemic Cardiomyopathy Trial (DEFINITE) [12]	2004	Patients had nonischemic cardiomyopathy, EF $<$ 36%, premature ventricular beats or nonsustained VT	458 patients randomized to ICD versus no ICD. After mean of 29 months, 35% lower risk death with ICD compared with no ICD ($p = .08$). Significant decrease in sudden death rate in ICD arm
Defibrillator in Acute Myocardial Infarction Trial (DINAMIT) [13]	2004	Patients 6–40 days after acute myocardial infarction, EF $\leq$ 35%, impaired heart rate variability or elevated mean heart rate	674 patients were randomized to ICD versus no ICD. No difference in mortality

Continued

Table 23.1 (*Continued*)

Trial name	*Year published*	*Inclusion criteria*	*Summary of results*
Sudden Cardiac Death in Heart Failure Trail (SCD-HeFT) [14]	Pending	Patients with EF≤ 35%, NYHA Class II or III	2521 patients randomized to ICD versus amiodarone versus no ICD. ICD arm had mortality of 28.9% versus 35.8% in control arm
COMPANION [15]	2004	Patients with Class III/IV heart failure, EF ≤ 35%, QRS width ≥ 120 ms, PR≥ 150 ms, 1 heart failure hospitalization in 1–12 months	1520 patients were randomized to optimal medical therapy, biventricular pacing, biventricular ICD. Primary endpoint of mortality and hospitalization was decreased in both treatment arms. Mortality decreased in biventricular ICD by 36%.

EF, ejection fraction; VT, ventricular tachycardia; VF, ventricular fibrillation; and NYHA, New York Heart Association.

ICDs as first line treatment for sudden death survivors became irrefutable [19].

Introduction of the prophylactic use of implantable defibrillators

More than a decade after the FDA approval of the ICD, the Multicenter Automatic Implantable Defibrillator Trial (MADIT) I in 1996 provided the first evidence that the ICD decreased all-cause mortality in a patient population without prior cardiac arrest or sustained ventricular tachycardia [20] (Table 23.1). The patients randomized in the MADIT I study had coronary artery disease, ejection fraction ≤35%, inducible ventricular tachycardia not suppressed by intravenous antiarrhythmic medications. The Multicenter Unsustained Tachycardia Trial (MUSTT) demonstrated that patients undergoing electrophysiologic testing-guided therapy including ICD implantation had a greater survival compared with antiarrhythmic drug therapy alone [8]. The 1998 guidelines incorporated the findings of the AVID trial for sudden death survivors and the MADIT trial for primary prevention (Table 23.2).

2002 Revision of guidelines for implantable defibrillators

Additional clinical trials

Of the major trials leading to expanded indications for the ICD in the 2002 revision of the guidelines, the MADIT II [9] study had the greatest impact. In this study, patients with prior myocardial infarction and ejection fraction of 30% or less were randomized to receive ICD therapy or no ICD therapy. In this study, 1232 patients were followed for an average of 20 months. The all-cause mortality rate of 19.8% in the conventional therapy arm was statistically significantly greater compared with the 14.2% all-cause mortality rate in the ICD arm ($p = .016$), thus demonstrating a significant role of ICDs in decreasing mortality in this patient population.

Changes in 2002 guidelines

As a result of the MADIT II study, the 2002 ACC/AHA guidelines for the indications appropriate for ICD implantation were amended to include a Class IIa indication for ICD implantation for patients with left ventricular dysfunction and coronary artery disease. Changes in the 2002 guidelines are highlighted in the published version to assist in readily identifying these revisions [21, 22].

In addition to the MADIT II-based changes, three major differences should be mentioned in the 2002 guidelines compared with the 1998 guidelines. The 2002 guidelines recognize that patients who benefit the most from ICDs are those with structural heart disease. Hence, patients with ventricular arrhythmias without the presence of structural heart disease are usually better candidates for ablation procedures and such. Syncope in a patient with

Table 23.2 Classification of indications in guidelines for ICD therapy.

Degrees of agreement	
Class I	Conditions for which there is evidence and/or general agreement that a given procedure or treatment is beneficial, useful, and effective
Class II	Conditions for which there is conflicting evidence and/or divergence of opinion about the usefulness/ efficacy of a procedure or treatment
Class IIa	Weight of evidence/opinion is in favor of usefulness/efficacy
Class IIb	Usefulness/efficacy is less well established by evidence/opinion
Class III	Conditions for which there is evidence and/or general agreement that a procedure/treatment is not useful/effective and in some cases may be harmful
Levels of evidence	
Level A	If the data were derived from multiple randomized clinical trials involving a large number of individuals
Level B	When data were derived from a limited number of trials involving comparatively small numbers of patients or from nonrandomized studies or observational data registries
Level C	When consensus of expert opinion was the primary source of recommendation

electrocardiographic evidence of Brugada syndrome is designated as a Class IIb indication for ICD implantation based on the high incidence of ventricular tachycardia in this patient population. At the time the guidelines were published, there were only limited data demonstrating risk in this population of patients [23–25]. Subsequently, additional studies have demonstrated significant incidence of sudden death in this patient population. In addition, a randomized study called the defibrillator versus beta-blockers for unexplained death in Thailand [26] provided further clinical data supporting this aggressive approach.

The 2002 guidelines also contained a new recommendation supporting the role of ICD implantation in patients with advanced structural heart disease presenting with syncope without a clear cause despite thorough invasive and noninvasive investigation. This patient population is felt to be at a high risk despite a negative evaluation.

Future revisions of the ICD guidelines

Clinical trials

New clinical trials, which completed the 2002 guidelines will likely form the basis for new indications in future revisions [27]. Of these trials the Sudden Cardiac Death-Heart Failure Trial (SCD-HeFT) [28–30], the DEFINITE trial, and the COMPANION trial will have the greatest impact on new ICD indications. While these studies have important differences in their study populations, they both expand the indications for patients with heart failure and severe left ventricular dysfunction of both ischemic and nonischemic causes. In the SCD-HeFT trial, 2521 patients were enrolled from September 1997 through July 2001 and followed until October, 2003. The patients in the study had Class I, II, or III with an ejection fraction <35% on optimal medical regimens. Of the patients, 52% had ischemic cardiomyopathy. The patients were randomized to (1) conventional therapy for heart failure plus placebo, (2) conventional therapy plus amiodarone, or (3) conventional therapy plus an ICD. The median ejection fraction was 25%. The average follow-up was 2.5 years. The 3 year mortality rate was 22% in the placebo arm, 24% in the amiodarone arm, and 17% in the ICD arm.

The defibrillators in nonischemic cardiomyopathy treatment evaluation study (DEFINITE) [12, 31], was a randomized prospective clinical trial evaluating ICD therapy in exclusively nonischemic cardiomyopathy patients. A total of 458 patients at 48 centers from July 1998 to June 2002, were followed with a mean follow-up of 29.0 months. Patients had nonischemic cardiomyopathy, an ejection fraction ≤35%, a history of at least Class II congestive heart failure (CHF), and at least 10 or more premature-ventricular contractions (PVCs) per hour on an ambulatory ECG monitor. All-cause mortality was 7.9% in the ICD arm versus 14.1% in the medical therapy arm, $p = .08$. The sudden death mortality was significantly reduced.

The comparison of medical therapy, pacing and defibrillation in chronic heart failure (COMPANION) [15]trial was a randomized controlled trial conducted at 128 medical centers in the United States comparing medical treatment, biventricular pacing, or biventricular pacing, with ICD in patients with ischemic or nonischemic cardiomyopathy, Baseline characteristics revealed an average ejection fraction 22% and mean QRS duration 160 ms, with 55% of patients having ischemic cardiomyopathy. For the primary endpoint of mortality and all-cause hospitalization, both the biventricular pacing (0.81 RR) and biventricular ICD (0.80 RR) arms had a statistically lower event rate than optimal medical therapy alone. For all-cause mortality, the biventricular pacing arm showed a trend toward benefit while the biventricular pacing-ICD arm decreased mortality by 36%.

Clinical trials that did not reveal benefit of the ICD may also be used to modify the indications for ICDs. The Defibrillator IN Acute Myocardial Infarction Trial (DINAMIT) [13] examined a particularly high-risk patient population 6–40 days after a myocardial infarction and with ejection fraction <35% and decreased heart rate variability or elevated heart rate. A total of 676 patients were randomized to ICD versus medical therapy. The mean follow-up time was 30 months. A significant number of patients required hemodynamic support for cardiogenic shock. The ICD reduced arrhythmic death significantly, but had no impact on all-cause mortality, probably due to increased nonarrhythmic mortality in this high-risk population. It is unknown whether future indications will exclude such high-risk patients with decreased heart rate variability and history of a need for hemodynamic support.

Syncope

Nonrandomized studies have shown that the ICD is effective in preventing sudden death in patients with syncope and inducible arrhythmias [32]. The current guidelines refer to syncope in several different locations and contexts (Table 23.3). As shown in Table 23.4, a Class I indication for ICD implantation (Table 23.3) includes syncope and inducible ventricular tachycardia or fibrillation when drug therapy is not effective or preferred. Class IIb indication is listed as essentially the same indication but without the requirement for drug therapy to be ineffective or not preferred. Similarly, ICD is accepted as a Class IIb indication for an ICD if the patients have advanced structural heart disease and a thorough investigation has not revealed other potential cause of syncope. Future guidelines may consolidate and simplify these indications, particularly removing the generally outdated approach of using drug therapy of patients with inducible ventricular tachycardia and syncope. Also incorporation of the new indications for patients with severely diminished left ventricular function may simply result in the ICD being indicated in these patients with or without syncope.

Role of the electrophysiological test and antiarrhythmic drug suppression of inducibility

Current and past guidelines continue to discuss the role of electrophysiological testing and the role of antiarrhythmic drug suppression of inducibility. Syncope with inducibility of a hemodynamically significant ventricular tachycardia will undoubtedly and appropriately remain an indication for ICD implantation. However, the role of drug therapy should be eliminated in this setting.

The guidelines state that "cardiac arrest presumed to be due to VF when electrophysiological testing is precluded by other medical conditions, is an indication for ICD implantation according to the guidelines." This implies that the results of electrophysiological testing should determine the decision to implant an ICD. The role of electrophysiological testing remains controversial. However, some clinicians have argued that electrophysiological testing remains valuable since it may identify other important causes of cardiac arrest [33, 34].

Possible areas of investigation for new indications

Refinement of prophylactic indications for ICD

Many clinicians and healthcare policymakers have asked for a further definition of the patient populations that would benefit from the ICD. Underlying this request is a belief that there exists a population of patients for whom the ICD presents the greatest

Table 23.3 Guidelines for ICD therapy.

Class I

- Cardiac arrest due to VF or VT not due to a transient or reversible cause
- Spontaneous sustained VT in association with structural heart disease
- Syncope of undetermined origin with clinically relevant, hemodynamically significant sustained VT or VF induced at electrophysiologic study when drug therapy is ineffective, not tolerated, or not preferred
- Nonsustained VT in patients with coronary disease, prior MI, LV dysfunction, and inducible VF or sustained VT at electrophysiological study that is not suppressible by a Class I antiarrhythmic drug
- Spontaneous sustained VT in patients without structural heart disease not amenable to other treatments

Class IIa

- Patients with LV ejection fraction of ≤ 30% at least 1 month post-MI and 3 months postcoronary artery revascularization surgery

Class IIb

- Cardiac arrest presumed to be due to VF when electrophysiologic testing is precluded by other medical conditions
- Severe symptoms (e.g. syncope) attributable to ventricular tachyarrhythmias in patients awaiting cardiac transplantation
- Familial or inherited conditions with a high-risk for life-threatening ventricular tachyarrhythmias such as long-QT syndrome or hypertrophic cardiomyopathy
- Nonsustained VT with coronary artery disease, prior MI, and LV dysfunction, and inducible sustained VT or VF at electrophysiologic study
- Recurrent syncope of undetermined origin in the presence of ventricular dysfunction and inducible ventricular arrhythmias at electrophysiologic study when other causes of syncope have been excluded
- Syncope of unexplained origin or family history of unexplained sudden cardiac death in association with typical or atypical right bundle-branch block and ST-segment elevation (Brugada syndrome)
- Syncope in patients with advanced structural heart disease in whom thorough invasive and noninvasive investigations have failed to define a cause

Class III

- Syncope of undetermined cause in a patient without inducible ventricular tachyarrhythmias and without structural heart disease
- Incessant VT or VF
- VF or VT resulting from arrhythmias amenable to surgical or catheter ablation; for example, atrial arrhythmias associated with the Wolff–Parkinson–White syndrome, RV outflow tract VT, idiopathic LV tachycardia, or fascicular VT
- Ventricular tachyarrhythmias due to a transient or reversible disorder (e.g. AMI, electrolyte imbalance, drugs, or trauma) when correction of the disorder is considered feasible and likely to substantially reduce the risk of recurrent arrhythmia
- Significant psychiatric illnesses that may be aggravated by device implantation or may preclude systematic follow-up
- Terminal illnesses with projected life expectancy < 6 months
- Patients with coronary artery disease with LV dysfunction and prolonged QRS duration in the absence of spontaneous or inducible sustained or nonsustained VT who are undergoing coronary bypass surgery
- NYHA Class IV drug-refractory CHF in patients who are not candidates for cardiac transplantation

NYHA, New York Heart Association; VF, ventricular fibrillation; VT, ventricular tachycardia; LV, left ventricular; RV, right ventricular; and MI, myocardial infarction.

benefit in terms of survival and a population of patients for whom the ICD presents a minimal benefit in terms of survival. Some clinical analyses using techniques such as T-wave alternans have provided data regarding groups that may receive greater or lesser benefit from ICD therapy [35]. However, there are randomized data demonstrating in such a patient population that ICD therapy does or does not provide a survival benefit. There are two major issues preventing such randomized data from occurring. Many clinicians argue that it is no longer ethical to randomize patients meeting currently MADIT II criteria to ICD versus no ICD, even if a test such as T-wave alternans is used. On the other hand, others feel that it is so important to further define subgroups that benefit the most from the ICD that such a strategy is justified. The DINAMIT study suggests that heart rate variability

Table 23.4 Syncope in 2002 guidelines.

Class I

- Syncope of undetermined origin with clinically relevant, hemodynamically significant sustained VT or VF induced at electrophysiological study when drug therapy is ineffective, not tolerated, or not preferred

Class IIb

- Severe symptoms (e.g. syncope) attributable to sustained ventricular tachyarrhythmias while awaiting cardiac transplantation
- Recurrent syncope of undetermined etiology in the presence of ventricular dysfunction and inducible ventricular arrhythmias at electrophysiological study when other causes of syncope have been excluded
- Syncope of unexplained etiology or family history of unexplained sudden cardiac death in association with typical or atypical right bundle-branch block and ST-segment elevations (Brugada syndrome)
- Syncope in patients with advanced structural heart disease in which thorough invasive and noninvasive investigation has failed to define a cause

Class III

- Syncope of undetermined cause in a patient without inducible ventricular tachyarrhythmias and without structural heart disease

VF, ventricular fibrillation; VT, ventricular tachycardia.

may not be the appropriate marker [13]. Since heart rate variability may have a relationship with heart turbulence, heart rate turbulence also may not be appropriate. Instead, T-wave alternans may be a more desirable screening test [35].

Patients with less severe left ventricular dysfunction after myocardial infarction

While patients with severe left ventricular dysfunction have the highest incidence of sudden death, patients with less severe left ventricular dysfunction make up the greatest proportion of patients having a cardiac arrest. Identifying a subgroup of these patients who are at a risk comparable to patients with more severe left ventricular dysfunction is the next major challenge facing the field. If such a subgroup could be identified using as a diagnostic test such as T-wave alternans, a randomized study might be conducted [36]. Assuming a 2 year recruitment and 3 year follow-up period, power of 0.8 and α of 0.05, a reduction in survival in the ICD from 0.91 to 0.99 would require a sample size of ~300 patients in each group.

Hypertrophic cardiomyopathy

Data to date has demonstrated a significant ability of the ICD to prevent sudden cardiac death in this population [37, 38]. However, despite a prevalence of 1 out of 500 individuals patients having hypertrophic cardiomyopathy, many high-risk individuals do not receive ICD therapy. It may be possible to establish the clinical utility of ICDs in high-risk individuals with a randomized clinical trial [39]. If one can identify a subgroup at increased risk, for example, 5% per year and to reduce the risk to 2.5% per year, a total number of 546 patients would be needed with a 3 year follow-up.

Cardiac arrest in the setting of acute myocardial infarction

For decades, it has been believed that patients experiencing a cardiac arrest in the setting of an acute myocardial infarction are not at increased risk of having a future event compared to patients without a cardiac arrest. However, some retrospective analyses of patients having cardiac arrest in this setting suggest that these patients may have an increased risk despite correction for the degree of left ventricular dysfunction. The initial cardiac arrest may signify an increased propensity to having a cardiac arrest that may make a future cardiac arrest more likely. On the other hand, the arrhythmogenic events in the acute myocardial infarction may make it unlikely that the patient will again have a cardiac arrest.

First month post-myocardial infarction

Recent studies such as the MADIT II study excluded patients within 1 month of an acute myocardial infarction. While DINAMIT trial did not show benefit of an ICD, this is likely because of identification of a patient population at high risk for nonarrhythmic death based on the abnormal heart rate variability. Indices predicting absence of significant recovery of ejection fraction will be invaluable in stratifying patients following acute myocardial infarction. Viability scans using radionuclide or MRI techniques show promise in predicting early recovery of heart function. Since the first month following myocardial infarction carries with it the highest risk of sudden death, it is likely that the benefit of an ICD can be demonstrated in patients predicted to have little or no recovery of systolic function.

Genetic markers as predictors of sudden death

With the recognition of the limitations of clinical parameters other than ejection fraction to predict arrhythmic death rather than overall cardiac mortality, some investigators have proposed using genomic analysis to identify individuals at increased risk of sudden death. The use of SNP analysis has been proposed as a method of identifying such a genetic risk profile [40].

Cost-effectiveness of ICD therapy

Societal acceptance of any therapy implies a recognition of its cost-effectiveness. However, to differing extents, therapies such as ICDs have been examined using cost-effectiveness analysis as each new indication has emerged. In some cases, the cost-effectiveness has been analyzed after initial regulatory and reimbursement approvals have been completed. Nevertheless, cost-effectiveness analysis has played an important role in understanding the appropriate use of ICDs within the healthcare system [41–43]. Even when cost-effectiveness has been demonstrated, there are extensive concerns that the healthcare system is able to afford these costs [44–47]. The cost-effectiveness in some populations has been questioned and will undoubtedly be the subject of future analyses [48].

Early implantation after revascularization

Recent clinical trials included largely excluded patients early after revascularization. This exclusion from clinical studies has led to the clinical practice of depriving such individuals of early ICD therapy in a potentially high-risk period. In a 10 year retrospective analysis, Bolad *et al.* [49] have demonstrated a high event rate early following revascularization. Further studies are needed to justify the exclusion of these patients from receiving early ICD therapy.

Guideline evolution and development

Evolution of indications and barriers to implementation

Indications for ICD implantation have followed a step-by-step evolutionary pattern from technological development (Figure 23.1) to clinical studies and regulatory approval, eventually leading to reimbursement approval and adoption and implementation. There are numerous barriers to implementation (Table 23.2). There is an educational and information gap that initially prevents implementation or adoption of new indications. Implementation requires a range of physicians from primary care physicians to specialists to be familiar with the new indications and the strength of the data demonstrating the importance of the ICD indications. Adoption of the new ICD indications requires that these range of physicians have a thorough understanding of the indications and the need for referring to an electrophysiologist or implanting physician. Keys to this adoption of the new ICD indications are a multipronged educational effort that includes incorporation into professional organization's symposia, direct mailing to healthcare providers, CME and other educational programs, dissemination from professional organizations, and written materials.

There are major issues of familiarity with the technology and comfort with the technology. There are frequent perceptions that ICD therapy is an extreme therapy that should be reserved for a small subset of patients who are perceived to derive the greatest benefit. There is also a strong perception that ICD therapy has a significant negative impact on the quality of a patient's life [50–55]. There is often a familiarity with psychological stress and device malfunction rather than the overall significant freedom from complications and abnormalities.

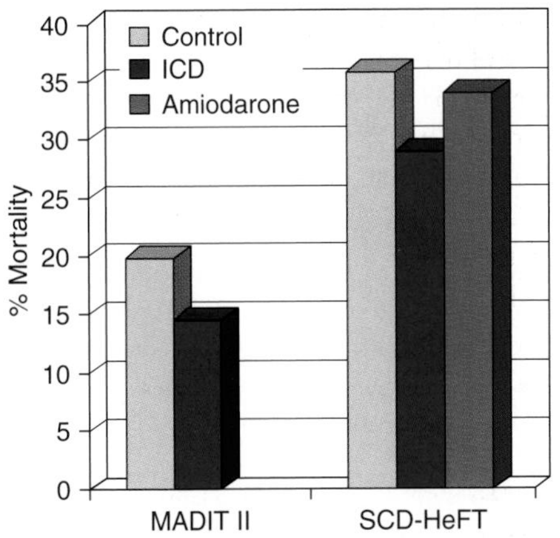

Figure 23.1 Percent mortality in MADIT II and SCD-HeFT trials.

Because of the unit cost of the devices, a common barrier to adoption of the ICD indications has been the perception of the impact of the ICD implementation [56]. Strong data regarding the cost-effectiveness of ICD therapies for each new indication must be disseminated and presented in a clear manner for these technologies to be accepted.

Ultimately, physicians must understand the benefit of patients who have had life-saving therapy from ICDs. Physicians should be notified when a patient has received successful therapy. Finally, for widespread adoption there must be easy access and availability of ICDs and implanting physicians.

Process of guideline development

The guidelines developed by the American College of Cardiology, American Heart Association, and the Heart Rhythm Society play an important role in guiding physician practice as well as providing acceptance of new ICD indications. They reflect the evolving body of knowledge and provide a critical examination of the published literature and consensus among experts. The most recent guideline was published in 2002 as the Guideline Update for Implantation of Cardiac Pacemakers and Antiarrhythmia Devices: A Report of the American College of Cardiology/American Heart Association Task Force on Practice Guidelines. The classification of degrees of agreement and the level of evidence is shown in Table 23.2.

There is currently no mechanism to provide an interim update of the guidelines as new information emerges and as indications evolve. Thus, it is frequent that the guidelines are not coordinated with the results of clinical trials, regulatory approvals, and reimbursement approvals. The guideline process must balance the advantages of a comprehensive revision of the guidelines with up-to-date modifications of the guidelines.

Conclusions

The indications for implantable defibrillators continue to increase based on carefully performed randomized clinical trials. Future studies will likely identify new patient groups that will benefit from ICD therapy.

References

1 Cannom DS, Prystowsky EN. Evolution of the implantable cardioverter defibrillator. *J Cardiovasc Electrophysiol* 2004; **15**(3): 375–385.

2 DiMarco JP. Implantable cardioverter-defibrillators. *N Engl J Med* 2003; **349**(19): 1836–1847.

3 Reiffel JA. Prolonging survival by reducing arrhythmic death: pharmacologic therapy of ventricular tachycardia and fibrillation. *Am J Cardiol* 1997; **80**(8A): 45G–55G.

4 The CASCADE Investigators. Randomized antiarrhythmic drug therapy in survivors of cardiac arrest (the CASCADE Study). *Am J Cardiol* 1993; **72**(3): 280–287.

5 Investigators TAVIDA. A comparison of antiarrhythmic-drug therapy with implantable defibrillators in patients resuscitated from near-fatal ventricular arrhythmias. *N Engl J Med* 1997; **337**(22): 1576–1583.

6 Kuck KH, Cappato R, Siebels J, Ruppel R. Randomized comparison of antiarrhythmic drug therapy with implantable defibrillators in patients resuscitated from cardiac arrest: the Cardiac Arrest Study Hamburg (CASH). *Circulation* 2000; **102**(7): 748–754.

7 Connolly SJ, Gent M, Roberts RS *et al.* Canadian implantable defibrillator study (CIDS): a randomized trial of the implantable cardioverter defibrillator against amiodarone. *Circulation* 2000; **101**(11): 1297–1302.

8 Buxton AE, Lee KL, Fisher JD, Josephson ME, Prystowsky EN, Hafley G. A randomized study of the prevention of sudden death in patients with coronary artery disease. Multicenter unsustained tachycardia trial investigators. [Erratum appears in N Engl J Med 2000; **342**(17): 1300]. *N Engl J Med* 1999; **341**(25): 1882–1890.

9 Moss AJ, Zareba W, Hall WJ *et al.* Prophylactic implantation of a defibrillator in patients with myocardial infarction and reduced ejection fraction. *N Engl J Med* 2002; **346**(12): 877–883.

10 Bansch D, Antz M, Boczor S *et al.* Primary prevention of sudden cardiac death in idiopathic dilated cardiomyopathy: the Cardiomyopathy Trial (CAT). *Circulation* 2002; **105**(12): 1453–1458.

11 Strickberger SA, Hummel JD, Bartlett TG *et al.* Amiodarone versus implantable cardioverter-defibrillator: randomized trial in patients with nonischemic dilated cardiomyopathy and asymptomatic nonsustained ventricular tachycardia – AMIOVIRT. *J Am Coll Cardiol* 2003; **41**(10): 1707–1712.

12 Kadish A, Dyer A, Daubert JP *et al.* Prophylactic defibrillator implantation in patients with nonischemic dilated cardiomyopathy. *N Engl J Med* 2004; **350**(21): 2151–2158.

13 Hohnloser SH, Kuck KH, Dorian P *et al.* Prophylactic use of an implantable cardioverter-defibrillator after acute myocardial infarction. *N Engl J Med* 2004; **351**(24): 2481–2488.

14 Cleland JG, Coletta AP, Nikitin N, Louis A, Clark A. Update of clinical trials from the American College of Cardiology 2003. EPHESUS, SPORTIF-III, ASCOT, COMPANION, UK-PACE and T-wave alternans. *Eur J Heart Fail* 2003; **5**(3): 391–398.

15 Bristow MR, Saxon LA, Boehmer J *et al.* Cardiac-resynchronization therapy with or without an implantable defibrillator in advanced chronic heart failure. *N Engl J Med* 2004; **350**(21): 2140–2150.

16 The AVID Investigators. A comparison of antiarrhythmic-drug therapy with implantable defibrillators in patients resuscitated from near-fatal ventricular arrhythmias. *N Engl J Med* 1997; **337**(22): 1576–1583.

17 Connolly SJ, Hallstrom AP, Cappato R *et al.* Meta-analysis of the implantable cardioverter defibrillator secondary prevention trials. AVID, CASH and CIDS studies. Antiarrhythmics vs implantable defibrillator study. Cardiac Arrest Study Hamburg. Canadian Implantable Defibrillator Study. *Eur Heart J* 2000; **21**(24): 2071–2078.

18 Oseroff O, Retyk E, Bochoeyer A. Subanalyses of secondary prevention implantable cardioverter-defibrillator trials: Antiarrhythmics Versus Implantable Defibrillators (AVID), Canadian Implantable Defibrillator Study (CIDS), and Cardiac Arrest Study Hamburg (CASH). *Curr Opin Cardiol* 2004; **19**(1): 26–30.

19 Gregoratos G, Cheitlin MD, Conill A *et al.* ACC/AHA guidelines for implantation of cardiac pacemakers and antiarrhythmia devices: executive summary – a report of the American College of Cardiology/American Heart Association Task Force on practice guidelines (Committee on Pacemaker Implantation). *Circulation* 1998; **97**(13): 1325–1335.

20 Moss AJ, Hall WJ, Cannom DS *et al.* Improved survival with an implanted defibrillator in patients with coronary disease at high risk for ventricular arrhythmia. Multicenter automatic defibrillator implantation trial investigators. *N Eng J Med* 1996; **335**(26): 1933–1940.

21 Epstein AE. An update on implantable cardioverter-defibrillator guidelines. *Curr Opin Cardiol* 2004; **19**(1): 23–25.

22 Gregoratos G, Abrams J, Epstein AE *et al.* ACC/AHA/NASPE 2002 guideline update for implantation of cardiac pacemakers and antiarrhythmia devices; summary article: a report of the American College of Cardiology/American Heart Association Task Force on practice guidelines (ACC/AHA/NASPE Committee to update the 1998 pacemaker guidelines). *Circulation* 2002; **106**(16): 2145–2161.

23 Brugada P, Brugada R, Mont L, Rivero M, Geelen P, Brugada J. Natural history of Brugada syndrome: the prognostic value of programmed electrical stimulation of the heart. *J Cardiovasc Electrophysiol* 2003; **14**(5): 455–457.

24 Brugada P, Brugada R, Brugada J, Geelen P. Use of the prophylactic implantable cardioverter defibrillator for patients with normal hearts. *Am J Cardiol* 1999; **83**(5B): 98D–100D.

25 Brugada J, Brugada P, Brugada R. The syndrome of right bundle branch block ST segment elevation in V1 to V3 and sudden death – the Brugada syndrome. *Europace* 1999; **1**(3): 156–66.

26 Nademanee K, Veerakul G, Mower M *et al.* Defibrillator Versus beta-Blockers for Unexplained death in Thailand (DEBUT): a randomized clinical trial. *Circulation* 2003; **107**(17): 2221–2226.

27 Prystowsky EN. Primary prevention of sudden cardiac death: the time of your life. *Circulation* 2004; **109**(9): 1073–1075.

28 Grimm W, Alter P, Maisch B. Arrhythmia risk stratification with regard to prophylactic implantable defibrillator therapy in patients with dilated cardiomyopathy. Results of MACAS, DEFINITE, and SCD-HeFT. *Herz* 2004; **29**(3): 348–352.

29 Grimm W. Clinical trials of prophylactic implantable defibrillator therapy in patients with nonischemic cardiomyopathy: what have we learned and what can we expect from future trials? *Card Electrophysiol Rev* 2003; **7**(4): 463–467.

30 Cleland JG, Ghosh J, Freemantle N *et al.* Clinical trials update and cumulative meta-analyses from the American College of Cardiology: WATCH, SCD-HeFT, DINAMIT, CASINO, INSPIRE, STRATUS-US, RIO-Lipids and cardiac resynchronisation therapy in heart failure. *Eur J Heart Fail* 2004; **6**(4): 501–508.

31 Schaechter A, Kadish AH, Evaluation DEIN-ICT. DEFibrillators in non-ischemic cardiomyopathy Treatment Evaluation (DEFINITE). *Card Electrophysiol Rev* 2003; **7**(4): 457–462.

32 Steinberg JS, Beckman K, Greene HL *et al.* Follow-up of patients with unexplained syncope and inducible ventricular tachyarrhythmias: analysis of the AVID registry and an AVID substudy. Antiarrhythmics Versus Implantable Defibrillators. *J Cardiovasc Electrophysiol* 2001; **12**(9): 996–1001.

33 Becker R, Melkumov M, Senges-Becker JC *et al.* Are electrophysiological studies needed prior to defibrillator implantation? *PACE* 2003; **26**(8): 1715–1721.

34 Brembilla-Perrot B, Miljoen H, Houriez P *et al.* Causes and prognosis of cardiac arrest in a population admitted to a general hospital: a diagnostic and therapeutic problem. *Resuscitation* 2003; **58**(3): 319–327.

35 Pruvot EJ, Rosenbaum DS. T-wave alternans for risk stratification and prevention of sudden cardiac death. *Curr Cardiol Rep* 2003; **5**(5): 350–357.

36 Hohnloser SH, Ikeda T, Bloomfield DM, Dabbous OH, Cohen RJICRJ. T-wave alternans negative coronary patients with low ejection and benefit from defibrillator implantation. *Lancet* 2003; **362**(9378): 125–126.

37 Jayatilleke I, Doolan A, Ingles J *et al.* Long-term follow-up of implantable cardioverter defibrillator therapy for hypertrophic cardiomyopathy. *Am J Cardiol* 2004; **93**(9): 1192–1194.

38 Maron BJ, Shen WK, Link MS *et al.* Efficacy of implantable cardioverter-defibrillators for the prevention of sudden death in patients with hypertrophic cardiomyopathy. *N Engl J Med* 2000; **342**(6): 365–373.

39 Maron BJ, Estes NA III, Maron MS, Almquist AK, Link MS, Udelson JE. Primary prevention of sudden death as a novel treatment strategy in hypertrophic cardiomyopathy. *Circulation* 2003; **107**(23): 2872–2875.

40 Arking DE, Chugh SS, Chakravarti A, Spooner PM. Genomics in sudden cardiac death. *Circulat Res* 2004; **94**(6): 712–723.

41 Hlatky MA. Evidence-based use of cardiac procedures and devices. *N Eng J Med* 2004; **350**(21): 2126–2128.

42 Hlatky MA, Sanders GD, Owens DK. Cost-effectiveness of the implantable cardioverter defibrillator. *Card Electrophysiol Rev* 2003; **7**(4): 479–482.

43 Larsen G, Hallstrom A, McAnulty J *et al.* Cost-effectiveness of the implantable cardioverter-defibrillator versus antiarrhythmic drugs in survivors of serious ventricular tachyarrhythmias: results of the Antiarrhythmics Versus Implantable Defibrillators (AVID) economic analysis substudy. *Circulation* 2002; **105**(17): 2049–2057.

44 Armstrong PW, Bogaty P, Buller CE, Dorian P, O'Neill BJ, Canadian Cardiovascular Society Working Group. The 2004 ACC/AHA guidelines: a perspective and adaptation for Canada by the Canadian Cardiovascular Society Working Group. *Can J Cardiol* 2004; **20**(11): 1075–1079.

45 Barold HS. Using the MADIT II criteria for implantable cardioverter defibrillators – what is the role of the Food and Drug Administration approval? *Card Electrophysiol Rev* 2003; **7**(4):443–446.

46 Boriani G, Biffi M, Martignani C *et al.* Cardioverter-defibrillators after MADIT-II: the balance between weight of evidence and treatment costs. *Eur J Heart Fail* 2003; **5**(4): 419–425.

47 Camm AJ, Nisam S. The utilization of the implantable defibrillator – a European enigma. *Eur Heart J* 2000; **21**(24): 1998–2004.

48 Chen L, Hay JW. Cost-effectiveness of primary implanted cardioverter defibrillator for sudden death prevention in congestive heart failure. *Cardiovasc Drug Therapy* 2004; **18**(2): 161–170.

49 Bolad I, MacLellan C, Karanam S *et al.* Effectiveness of early implantation of cardioverter defibrillator for postoperative ventricular tachyarrhythmia. *Am J Cardiol* 2004; **94**(3): 376–378.

50 Dougherty CM, Pyper GP, Benoliel JQ. Domains of concern of intimate partners of sudden cardiac arrest survivors after ICD implantation. *J Cardiovasc Nurs* 2004; **19**(1): 21–31.

51 Dougherty CM. Psychological reactions and family adjustment in shock versus no shock groups after implantation of internal cardioverter defibrillator. *Heart Lung: J Acute Crit Care* 1995; **24**(4): 281–291.

52 Dougherty CM, Pyper GP, Frasz HA. Description of a nursing intervention program after an implantable cardioverter defibrillator. *Heart Lung* 2004; **33**(3): 183–190.

53 Edelman S, Lemon J, Kidman A. Psychological therapies for recipients of implantable cardioverter defibrillators. *Heart Lung* 2003; **32**(4): 234–240.

54 McCready MJ, Exner DV. Quality of life and psychological impact of implantable cardioverter defibrillators: focus on randomized controlled trial data. *Card Electrophysiol Rev* 2003; **7**(1): 63–70.

55 Sears SF, Jr., Conti JB. Quality of life and psychological functioning of icd patients. *Heart (Brit Card Soc)* 2002; **87**(5): 488–493.

56 Reynolds MR, Josephson ME. MADIT II (Second Multicenter Automated Defibrillator Implantation Trial) debate: risk stratification, costs, and public policy. *Circulation* 2003; **108**(15): 1779–1783.

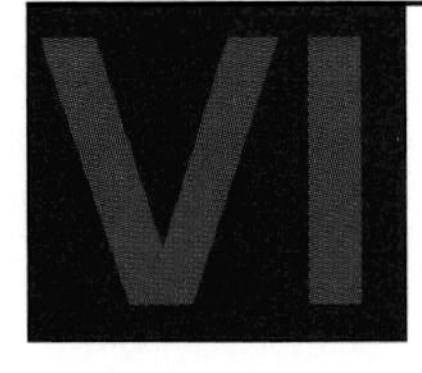

PART VI

Advances in catheter surgical ablation

24

CHAPTER 24

Advances in surgical ablation devices for atrial fibrillation

Spencer J. Melby, MD, *Anson M. Lee*, BS, *& Ralph J. Damiano, Jr.*, MD

Introduction

The Cox–Maze procedure was introduced by Dr James Cox at Barnes-Jewish Hospital in St. Louis in 1987. The operation involved creating a myriad of incisions across both the right and left atria. It was designed to block the multiple macro-reentrant circuits that were felt at the time to be the mechanism responsible for atrial fibrillation (AF). Over the next decade, this operation became the gold standard for the surgical treatment of AF [1]. The 10 year freedom from AF in our series has been 96%. These excellent results have been reproduced by other groups around the world [2–4]. Despite its efficacy, this procedure has not been widely performed. This has been attributed to its complexity and technical difficulty. Few surgeons were willing to add the Cox–Maze procedure to a valve or coronary operation.

Recently, the introduction of new ablation technology has significantly changed this attitude. In order to simplify the operation and make it easier to perform, the incisions of the traditional cut-and-sew Maze procedure were replaced with linear lines of ablation. Various energy sources have been used, including cryoablation, radiofrequency (RF) energy, microwave, laser, and high-frequency ultrasound. This chapter will review the present state-of-the-art in surgical ablation therapy.

Requirements for surgical ablation

For ablation technology to reliably replace an incision in AF surgery, it must meet several important criteria. First of all, it must produce bidirectional conduction block. This is the mechanism by which incisions prevent AF. They either block macro- or micro-reentrant circuits or isolate trigger foci. There continues to be a debate concerning the necessity to produce fully transmural lesions in order to achieve this goal. It has been demonstrated that nontransmural lesions, which leave only a thin rim of viable tissue, can cause conduction block during AF [5]. However, it is difficult, if not impossible, to discern the adequate depth of a lesion required to create conduction block in the operating room. Therefore, the only guarantee of effectiveness is a fully transmural lesion. This always results in complete conduction block. A device must be able to make transmural lesions on the arrested heart from either the epicardial or endocardial surface for ablation performed during valve or coronary surgery.

The second important attribute of the technology is that it must be safe. This requires a precise definition of dose–response curves to limit excessive or inadequate ablation. The surgeon also requires knowledge of the effect of the specific ablation technology on surrounding vital structures, such as the coronary sinus, coronary arteries, and heart valves.

Third, a device should make AF surgery easier and quicker to perform. This would require features such as rapidity of lesion formation, simplicity of use, and adequate length and flexibility.

Finally, the device optimally would have to be adaptable to a minimally invasive approach. This would require the ability to insert the device through minimal access or ports. It would also require the device to be capable of creating epicardial transmural lesions on the beating heart. In the chapter below, we will discuss each ablation technology and its potential advantages and disadvantages. We will review the evidence available that each of the ablation devices can fulfill the abovementioned goals.

Cryoablation

Device characteristics

There are two commercially available sources of cryothermal energy that are being used in cardiac surgery. The older technology utilizes nitrous oxide and is manufactured by Cooper Surgical (Trumbull, Connecticut). The nitrous oxide devices use rigid reusable electrodes. More recently, CryoCath Technologies (Montreal, Quebec, Canada) has developed a device using argon (Figure 24.1). This device uses a flexible catheter that has a 10 cm ablation electrode. At one atmosphere of pressure, nitrous oxide is capable of cooling tissue to −89.5°C, while argon has a minimum temperature of −185.7°C.

Cryothermal energy is delivered to myocardial tissue by using a cryoprobe. This probe consists of a hollow shaft, an electrode tip, and an integrated thermocouple for distal temperature recording. A console houses the tank containing the liquid refrigerant. This liquid is pumped under high pressure to the electrode through an inner lumen. Once the fluid reaches the electrode, it converts from a liquid to a gas phase, absorbing energy and resulting in rapid cooling of the tissue. The gas is then aspirated by vacuum through a separate return lumen to the console. At the tissue–electrode interface, there is a well-demarcated line of frozen tissue, termed an "ice ball."

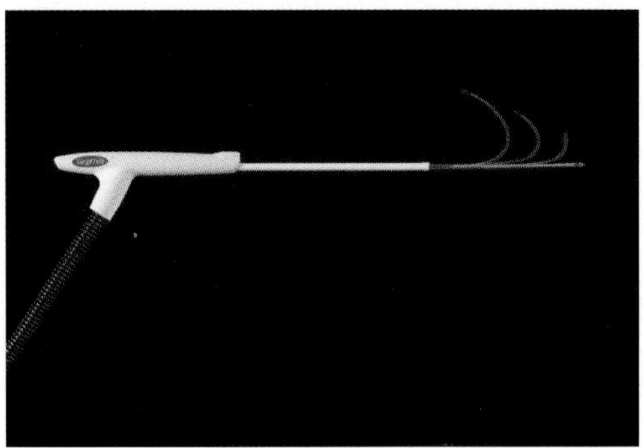

Figure 24.1 CryoCath Surgifrost™ flexible catheter with a 10 cm electrode.

Mechanism and histology of tissue injury

Cryothermal energy destroys tissue through the formation of intracellular and extracellular ice crystals. This disrupts the cell membrane and the cytoplasmic organelles. Following the cryoablation, there is development of hemorrhage, edema, and inflammation over the first 48 h. Irreversible injury is usually evident within this early time period. There is also evidence of apoptosis, the induction of which may expand the area of initial cell death [6].

Healing is characterized by extensive fibrosis, which begins approximately 1 week after lesion formation. Cryoablation is the only currently available energy source that does not alter tissue collagen; it preserves normal tissue architecture. This makes it an excellent energy source for ablation close to valvular tissue or the fibrous skeleton of the heart. Histologically, lesions exhibit dense homogenous scar formation. There is a distinct absence of cicatrization and a lack of thrombus formation over the lesions. The homogenous scar has been shown to have a low arrhythmogenic potential [7–9].

In a human study, specimens that underwent endocardial cryoablation on the arrested heart were examined. The histology revealed extensive myocellular damage and transmural lesions. Morphologic features included sarcoplasmic vacuolization, increased cell roundness with indistinct membranes, and loss of contraction bands [10].

Ability to create transmural lesions

The size and depth of cryolesions are determined by numerous factors, including probe temperature, tissue temperature, probe size, the duration and number of ablations, and the particular liquid used as the cooling agent [9]. With conventional nitrous oxide, 2–3 min ablations have been shown to reliably create transmural lesions on both the right and left atrium. Because of the heat sink provided by circulating endocardial blood, epicardial cryolesions on the beating heart with nitrous oxide have not been transmural.

There is little available data for argon cryoablation. There has been one published study on epicardial cryoablation using the argon device in a sheep model and one study of safe use on a single patient [11, 12]. In the animal study, they examined epicardial cryoablation for 2 min at −160° C. They were able to get transmural lesions 62% of the time around the pulmonary veins. Five out of six lesions on the right atrial appendage were transmural, but only two out of eight (25%) on the left atrial appendage were transmural. Thus, this device appears to be capable of creating transmural epicardial lesions, but not in a reliable fashion.

Safety profile

Cryoablation has the benefit of preserving the fibrous skeleton of the heart and thus is one of the safest of all the technologies available. Nitrous oxide cryoablation has extensive clinical use and has an excellent safety profile. While experience has shown that cryothermal energy appears to have no permanent effects on valvular tissue or the coronary sinus, experimental studies have shown late minimal hyperplasia of coronary arteries and these should be avoided [10, 13–15]. In the report by Doll *et al.* [11], they were able to create mild esophageal lesions in seven of the eight cases with epicardial cryoablation. Indiscriminate use of freezing has certain potential of esophageal destruction that could lead to esophageal perforation and possible atrio-esophageal fistula. There is no published data regarding the safety profile of the argon device.

Summary

Cryoablation is unique among the presently available technologies in that it destroys tissue by freezing instead of heating. The biggest advantage of this technology is its ability to preserve tissue architecture. The nitrous oxide technology has a well-defined dose curve and safety profile and is generally safe except around coronary arteries.

The potential disadvantages of this technology include the relatively long time necessary to create an ablation (2–3 min). There also is difficulty in creating lesions in the beating heart because of the heat sink of the circulating blood volume. The CryoCath device may overcome this problem. However, if blood is frozen, it coagulates, and this may be another potential risk to epicardial cryoablation on the beating heart.

Radiofrequency energy

Radiofrequency (RF) energy has been used for cardiac ablation for many years in the electrophysiology laboratory [16]. It was one of the first energy sources to be used in the operating room for AF ablation. RF energy can be delivered by either unipolar or bipolar electrodes. The electrodes can be either dry or irrigated.

Device characteristics

There are a number of unipolar RF devices available for surgical ablation. Boston Scientific has marketed a Cobra™ catheter (Figure 24.2). This is a dry unipolar catheter that is a segmented, flexible device with variable lesion lengths of 10–95 mm. It has seven electrodes, which can be individually selected and temperature controlled. It has been used widely around the world. The newer Cobra Cooled™ surgical probe is the same size catheter but has a cooled tip for better heat transfer.

Medtronic has developed the Cardioblate™ catheter (Figure 24.3). It is an irrigated unipolar RF catheter. It is a pen-like device used to make point-by-point ablations by dragging it across tissue to make a linear lesion.

Bipolar RF is similar to unipolar energy except that two electrodes, instead of one, are used to focus the path of energy. This allows for faster ablation, usually <10 s, while limiting destruction to tissue that is in close proximity to the electrodes.

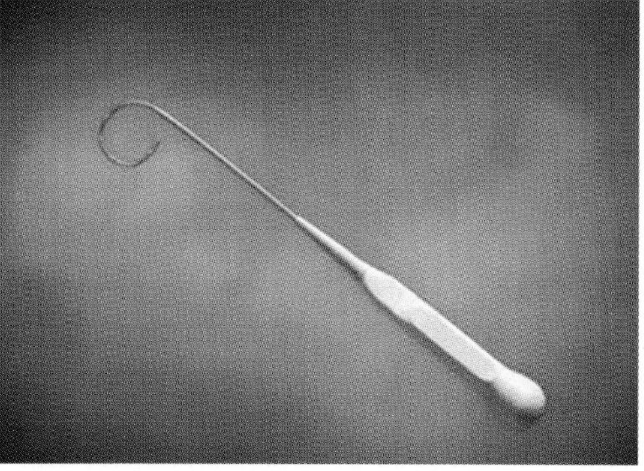

Figure 24.2 Cobra™ dry unipolar segmented, flexible device with variable lesion lengths of 10–95 mm.

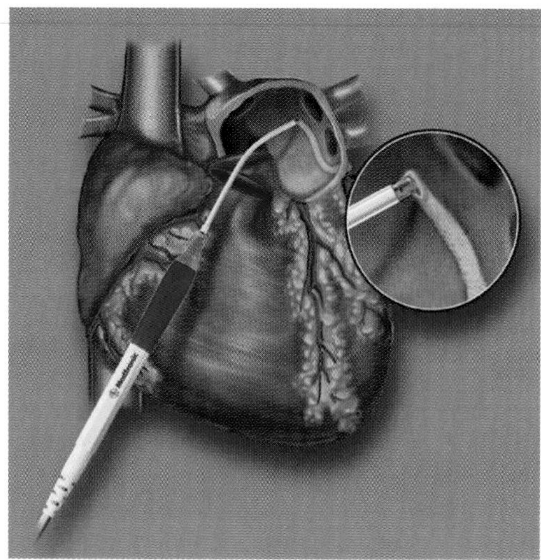

Figure 24.3 Medtronic Cardioblate™ pen irrigated unipolar RF catheter.

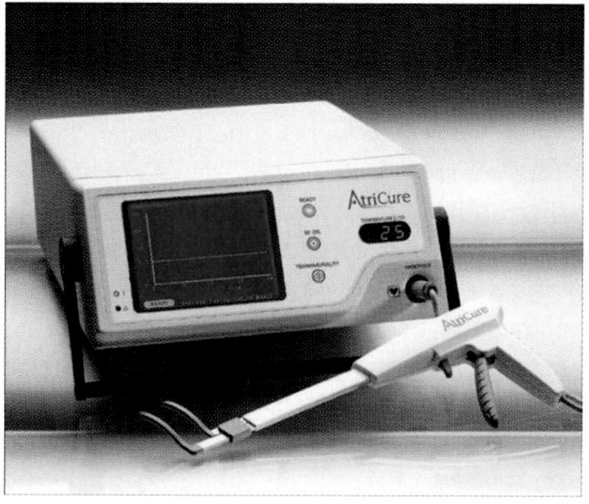

Figure 24.4 Atricure Isolator™ bipolar RF clamp.

For bipolar RF, the electrodes are clamped over the targeted atrial tissue. The first bipolar RF device was introduced by Atricure, Inc. (Figure 24.4). The Isolator™ is a specially designed clamp with 1 mm wide, 5 cm long electrodes embedded in the jaws. The newer Isolator™ long has 6.1 cm long electrodes and a longer handle. The device was the first on the market to have an online measurement of lesion transmurality. The conductance between the electrodes is measured during ablation. When the conductance drops to a stable minimum level, this correlates well both experimentally and clinically to histologically transmural lesions [17]. This allows for total energy delivery to be customized to the individual tissue characteristics. Two other bipolar ablation devices have since been released by Medtronic and Boston Scientific [18, 19]. The Medtronic bipolar device, the Cardioblate™ BP, has an irrigated, flexible jaw along with an articulating head. The electrodes are 5 cm long.

Mechanism and histology of tissue injury

Radiofrequency energy uses an alternating current in the range of 100–1000 kHz. This frequency is high enough to prevent rapid myocardial depolarization and the induction of ventricular fibrillation, yet low enough to prevent tissue vaporization and perforation. Resistive heating occurs only within a narrow rim of tissue in direct contact with the electrode, usually less than 1 mm. The deeper tissue heating occurs via passive conduction. With unipolar catheters, the energy is dispersed between the electrode tip and an indifferent electrode, usually the grounding pad applied to the patient. In the bipolar clamp devices, alternating current is generated between two closely approximated electrodes. This results in a more focused ablation. The lesion size depends on electrode–tissue contact area, the interface temperature, the current and voltage (power), and the duration of delivery. The depth of the lesion can be limited by char formation at the tissue–electrode interface. To resolve this problem, irrigated catheters were developed; this reduces char formation by keeping temperatures cooler at the tissue interface. These irrigated catheters have been shown to create larger volume lesions than dry RF devices [20, 21].

On histologic evaluation of radiofrequency lesions, a focal coagulation necrosis predominates acutely. This correlates with the irreversible nature of the injury, which occurs at high temperatures. There is destruction of myocardial/collagen matrix and replacement with fibrin and collagen in chronic studies. In chronic models, contraction and scarring occurs with large lesions. At very high temperatures (>100°C), char formation predominates. Char presents as an impediment to heat transduction and has been associated with asymmetrical ablations. Bipolar RF ablation results in discrete, transmural lesions with no evidence of contraction or scarring. In a chronic animal study from our laboratory, the atria, vena cava, and pulmonary veins were examined 30 days following ablation and revealed no evidence of thrombus or stricture formation. By microscopic examination, all lesions were transmural, continuous, and discrete with a single ablation using the conductance algorithm. Lesion width varied depending on tissue depth and the duration of ablation; the measured lesions were typically 2–3 mm but up to 5 mm in width on the thickest parts of the atrium [17, 22]. This study and others have suggested that the bipolar technology produces consistent transmural lesions.

Ability to create transmural lesions

The dose–response curves for unipolar RF have been described [23–25]. While in animals, unipolar RF has been shown to create transmural lesions on the arrested heart with sufficiently long ablation times (60–120 s), there have been problems in humans. After 2 min endocardial ablations during mitral valve surgery, only 20% of the *in vivo* lesions were transmural [24]. Epicardial ablation has been even more difficult. Animal studies have consistently shown that unipolar RF is incapable of creating epicardial transmural lesions on the beating heart [25, 26]. A recent clinical study has confirmed this problem. Epicardial RF ablation in humans resulted in only 7% of the lesions being transmural despite electrode temperatures of up to 90°C [27].

Bipolar RF ablation has been shown to be capable of creating transmural lesions without difficulty on the beating heart. This has been shown both in animals and in humans with average ablation times between 5 and 10 s [17, 22, 28].

Safety profile

Because RF ablation is a well-developed technology, much is known about its safety profile. The complications of unipolar RF devices have been described after extensive clinical use and include coronary artery injuries, cerebrovascular accidents, and the devastating creation of esophageal perforation leading to atrio-esophageal fistula [29–32]. Use of the bipolar RF devices has eliminated most of the collateral damage that is created with the unipolar devices. The energy is focused between the two electrodes of the device, eliminating the diffuse radiation of heat. There have been no described clinical injuries with this device.

Summary

Unipolar RF ablation has been shown to be able to create endocardial transmural lesions most of the time, but is incapable of creating epicardial transmural lesions on the beating heart. As with all unipolar energy sources, it radiates unfocused heat, and this can cause collateral injury if not used carefully.

Bipolar RF ablation has the advantage of focused and discrete lesions that can be made in a fraction of the time of unipolar ablation. Moreover, by using a conductance algorithm, bipolar RF ablation is capable of creating reliable transmural lesions, both on the arrested and beating heart. Because of the focused nature of the energy, there is no chance for collateral injury. This energy source has the disadvantage that it can only ablate tissue that can be clamped and is difficult to use in proximity to valve tissue.

Microwave energy

Microwave ablation uses dielectric heating created by electromagnetic waves emitted from an antenna. The field that is created causes oscillation of molecular dipoles, generating heat and an area of ablated tissue. This technology produces efficient and uniform penetration without overheating and does not suffer from char formation [33, 34].

Device characteristics

Guidant Corporation (Indianapolis, IN) has developed the only US available microwave catheters, the Flex 4® and Flex 10® (Figure 24.5). The former has a flexible 4 cm long sheath, able to ablate in increments of 2 cm; the latter device is 20 cm long, also ablating in 2 cm increments. These probes consist of a flexible and malleable sheath containing a 2 cm microwave antenna that emits microwave radiation at 2450 MHz. The Flex 10® design allows for placement of the sheath around the heart and then positioning of the antenna within the sheath in 2 cm increments to create a continuous linear lesion up to 20 cm in length. Minimally invasive

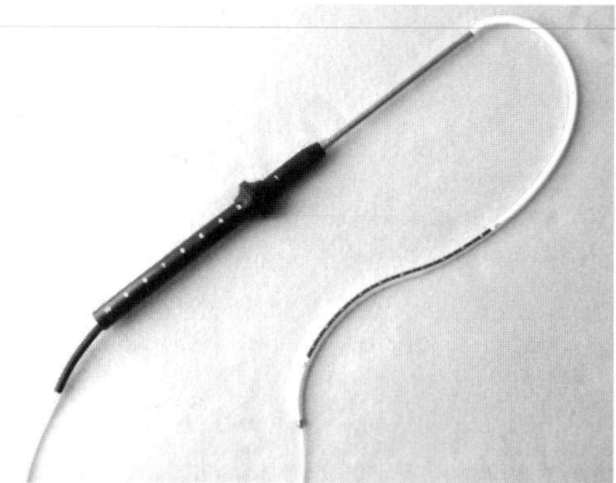

Figure 24.5 Guidant Flex 10® 20 cm flexible and malleable sheath containing a 2 cm microwave antenna.

techniques with the Flex 10® catheter have been described and involve accessing the heart through ports and a mini-thoracotomy. In this report, an encircling lesion around the pulmonary veins was created on the beating heart [35].

Mechanism and histology of tissue injury

Microwave encompasses electromagnetic waves between 30 and 3000 MHz; 915 MHz or 2450 MHz are used in ablation catheters. Microwave devices radiate an electromagnetic field into the surrounding tissue. Transmitted microwaves cause oscillation of molecular dipoles (e.g. water molecules) and electromagnetic energy is transferred into kinetic energy. The energy is independent of current flow from ablation catheter to tissue. As a result, catheter contact pressure, orientation, and tissue desiccation do not limit lesion formation. *In vitro* as well as *in vivo* studies of the bovine heart show that lesion size depends on the power, duration of delivery, and antenna length and width. The depth is dependent on power and duration. These results were obtained in a model similar to the arrested heart [33, 36].

Fifteen humans undergoing valve replacements with AF had microwave ablations created on the atrium prior to bypass with subsequent tissue sampling of the lesion in the atrial appendage. Histological studies showed that, similar to RF ablation, focal coagulation necrosis predominates acutely. Grossly, ablations had ill-defined borders, but cellular damage was distributed continuously throughout the myocardial wall. Consistent results included clear foci of coagulative necrosis and often irregular, or complete loss of, membranous borders. Ultrastructurally, ablated cells demonstrated architectural disarray, loss of contractile filaments, mitochondrial swelling, and focal interruption of plasma membrane [37].

Ability to create transmural lesions

Dose–response curves for microwave ablation have been developed on the arrested heart [33, 34]. In our laboratory, both the Flex 4® and Flex 10® created uniformly transmural lesions on the cardioplegic-arrested porcine atria after 90 s of ablation [34]. Thus, this energy source appears capable of creating endocardial transmural lesions on the arrested heart. However, there is controversy regarding its ability to create transmural lesions on the beating heart.

In a recent study of 16 dogs, the Flex 10® device was evaluated. The study's aim was to assess electrophysiologic isolation of ablation areas in relation to histologic proof of transmurality. After a single ablation, only half of the dogs were electrically isolated. After a second ablation, 13 of the 16 were shown to have isolating circumferential lesions. The histology showed full circumferential lesions after 1–3 weeks; however, they were not fully transmural [37]. In our laboratory, the Flex 10® has been incapable of creating transmural lesions on the beating heart in an acute porcine model.

Safety profile

Microwave technology ablates using heat and therefore is potentially susceptible to complications of collateral damage. There are reports of coronary artery stenosis after microwave ablation [38]. Concern for esophageal injury exists, although there are no published reports of such injury from this modality. Reports of over 600 patients from several clinical trials have not mentioned complications attributable to the microwave device, lending confidence to its safe use [39]. However, microwave ablation of cardiac tissue is still a relatively new modality and continued investigation of its safety is warranted.

Summary

Microwave ablation is an interesting technology that has several advantages over RF energy. It is less likely to create char formation, and is less sensitive to electrode positioning. It has the advantage of flexibility. It can reliably create endocardial lesions, but there is some question of whether it is capable of creating epicardial lesions on the beating heart.

It is still an unfocused heat energy that can cause collateral injury, and this has been documented in case reports. A disadvantage of this technology is that there is no way to judge transmurality of ablation during surgery.

Laser energy

Laser, or Light Amplified by Stimulated Emission of Radiation, consists of a power source, a laser medium (usually crystal or gas), and two mirrors at each end of the medium – one fully and one partially reflective. Lasers "boost" the energy state of the medium to a higher level, and then the device allows energy to be emitted when the medium drops back to its lower state. This mechanism allows controlled direction of energy output. Lasers produce narrow, deep lesions in a short amount of time, making this an attractive power source for ablation [40].

Device characteristics

Edwards Lifesciences (Irvine, CA) has developed the Optiwave 980™, an endocardial device with a malleable shaft and a 5 cm diffuser that allows for creation of linear ablation lines. Two forms of light are carried from the source via fiberoptics to the treatment site: visible red light to allow targeting of tissue, and invisible 980 nm wavelength laser energy which induces the destruction of tissue. The light is scattered within the tip and a diffuser disperses the infrared (IR) laser energy perpendicular to the shaft.

Mechanism and histology of tissue injury

The lesion created is a direct result of tissue heating, termed photocoagulation. Laser beam power decreases within tissue in an exponential decay manner, and absorption is tissue dependent. Because adipose tissue and cardiac muscle each have specific extinction coefficients (amount of scattering and absorption), the IR laser is able to penetrate myocardial tissue independent of overlying fat.

This technology produces no surface charring, and direct heating of the tissue from the laser is accompanied by conductive heating that allows penetration. The lesion size depends on the amount of energy delivered, the tissue heating, amount of scatter, transmission, reflection, and absorption. Damage to tissue includes intramyocardial hemorrhage, myocyte swelling, and contraction band necrosis [41].

Ability to create transmural lesions

The ability of laser to create transmural lesions has been investigated in a small number of preliminary studies. In an unpublished canine study by Williams *et al.* [42] from Columbia University, all of the ablation lines were found to be transmural ($n = 67$ tissue sections) and isolation was proven by inability to pace in all of the animals ($n = 16$). No damage to pulmonary veins, circumflex artery, or coronary sinus was found. Clinical trials with humans have been encouraging, but results are few.

Safety profile

Because laser has had very limited clinical use, its safety record is sparse. Ongoing trials will help elucidate its safety profile. Initial reports of difficulty being able to discern ablated tissue raise concerns regarding inadvertent injuries [42].

Summary

Laser ablation is a promising technology that may have some advantages over other energy sources. The energy is focused, unaffected by overlying fat, and may have enhanced penetration. A disadvantage of this technology is that the energy delivery is unconfined and thus could cause collateral damage. Another problem is that, at present, there is no way to judge transmurality of the ablation during procedures.

Conclusions

The development of new ablation technology has revolutionized the surgical treatment of AF. This new technology has taken an operation that was rarely performed and made it accessible to all cardiac surgeons. Whereas 5 years ago, few patients with AF who were having cardiac surgery had a concomitant ablation procedure, at the present time, most patients are undergoing AF surgery. These ablation technologies also have begun to allow for the development of less-invasive procedures, and hold the promise of enabling a port-access, beating-heart procedure with high efficacy in the future.

Each ablation technology has its own shortcomings and complications. In the future, it will be imperative to develop a more complete understanding of the effects of surgical ablation technology on atrial hemodynamics, function, and electrophysiology. The safety of ablation is dependent on an intimate knowledge of the technology being used. Thus, surgeons must develop accurate dose–response curves for all new devices in clinically relevant models on both the arrested and the beating heart. While most of the devices have been shown to be useful in the arrested heart, few have shown the capability of creating reliable transmural lesions on the beating heart. The effect of this technology on vital structures and on atrial function also needs to be better delineated.

While this new technology has led to progress, the field is still impaired by an inadequate understanding of the mechanisms of AF. Ideally in the future, surgeons will be able to design an operation based on the mechanism or substrate responsible for the arrhythmia in each patient and tailor that operation to the specific atrial geometry. In order to develop a truly minimally invasive operation, electrophysiological mapping may be necessary to confirm and guide therapy to allow for a more precise isolation or ablation of specific anatomic or electrophysiologic substrates. Finally, clinical and experimental research on the various different lesion sets that are being tried in the operating room will be essential for continuing progress.

The future presents AF surgeons with many opportunities and challenges. It is certain that the surgical treatment of AF will continue to undergo rapid evolution in the next decade, and much of this progress will be spurred by the use of new ablation technology.

Acknowledgment

This work was supported by NIH grants 2RO1HL032257 and 1F32HL78136.

References

1 Prasad SM, Maniar HS, Camillo CJ *et al.* The Cox Maze III procedure for atrial fibrillation: long-term efficacy in patients undergoing lone versus concomitant procedures. *Thorac Cardiovasc Surg* 2003; **126**: 1822–1828.

2 Raanani E, Albage A, David TE *et al.* The efficacy of the Cox/Maze procedure combined with mitral valve surgery: a matched control study. *Eur J Cardiothorac Surg* 2001; **19**(4): 438–442

3 Doty DB, Dilip KA, Millar RC. Mitral valve replacement with homograft and Maze III procedure. *Ann Thorac Surg* 2000; **69**(3): 739–742.

4 Schaff HV, Dearani JA, Daly RC *et al.* Cox–Maze procedure for atrial fibrillation: Mayo Clinic experience. *Semin Thorac Cardiovasc Surg* 2000; **12**(1): 30–37

5 Mitchell MA, McRury ID, Everett TH *et al.* Morphological and physiological characteristics of discontinuous linear atrial ablations during atrial pacing and atrial fibrillation. *J Cardiovasc Electrophysiol* 1999; **10**(3): 378–386.

6 Steinbach JP, Weissenberger J, Aguzzi A. Distinct phases of cryogenic tissue damage in the cerebral cortex of wild-type and *c-fos* deficient mice. *Neuropathol Appl Neurobiol* 1999; **25**: 468–480.

7 Holman WL, Ikeshita M, Douglas JM Jr *et al.* Ventricular cryosurgery: short-term effects on intramural electrophysiology. *Ann Thorac Surg* 1983; **35**: 386–393.

8 Wetstein L, Mark R, Kaplan A, Mitamura H *et al.* Nonarrhythmogenicity of therapeutic cryothermic lesions of the myocardium. *J Surg Res* 1985; **39**(6): 543–554.

9 Lustgarten DL, Keane D, Ruskin J. Cryothermal ablation: mechanism of tissue injury and current experience in the treatment of tachyarrhythmias. *Prog in Cardiovasc Dis* 1999; **41**: 481–98.

10 Manasse E, Colombo P, Roncalli M, Gallotti R. Myocardial acute and chronic histological modifications induced by cryoablation. *Eur J Cardiothorac Surg* 2000; **17**(3): 339–340.

11 Doll N, Kornherr P, Aupperle H *et al.* Epicardial treatment of atrial fibrillation using cryoablation in an acute off-pump sheep model. *Thorac Cardiovasc Surg* 2003; **51**(5): 267–273.

12 Doll N, Meyer R, Walther T *et al.* A new cryoprobe for intraoperative ablation of atrial fibrillation. *Ann Thorac Surg* 2004; **77**(4): 1460–1462.

13 Mikat EM, Hackel DB, Harrison L *et al.* Reaction of the myocardium and coronary arteries to cryosurgery. *Lab Invest* 1977; **37**(6): 632–641.

14 Holman WL, Ideshita M, Ungerleider RM *et al.* Cryosurgery for cardiac arrhythmias: acute and chronic effects on coronary arteries. *Am J Cardiol* 1983; **51**(1): 149–155.

15 Watanabe H, Hayashi J, Aizawa Y. Myocardial infarction after cryoablation surgery for Wolff–Parkinson–White syndrome. *Jpn J Thorac Cardiovasc Surg* 2002; **50**(5): 210–212.

16 Viola N, Williams MR, Oz MC, Ad N. The technology in use for the surgical ablation of atrial fibrillation. *Semin Thorac Cardiovasc Surg* 2002; **14**(3): 198–205.

17 Prasad SM, Maniar HS, Schuessler RB, Damiano RJ Jr. Chronic transmural atrial ablation by using bipolar radiofrequency energy on the beating heart. *J Thorac Cardiovasc Surg* 2002; **124**(4): 708–713.

18 Demazumder D, Mitrotznik MS, Schwartzman D. Biophysics of radiofrequency ablation using an irrigated electrode. *J Interv Card Electrophysiol* 2001; **5**(4): 377–389.

19 Ruchat P, Schlaepfer J, Delabays A *et al.* Left atrial radiofrequency compartmentalization for chronic atrial fibrillation during heart surgery. *Thorac Cardiovasc Surg* 2002; **50**(3): 155–159.

20 Khargi K, Deneke T, Haardt H *et al.* Saline-Irrigated, cooled-tip radiofrequency ablation is an effective technique to perform the maze procedure. *Ann Thorac Surg* 2001; **72**: 1090–1095.

21 Nakagawa H, Wittkampf FHM, Yamanashi WS *et al.* Inverse relationship between electrode size and lesion size during radiofrequency ablation with active electrode cooling. *Circulation* 1998; **98**(5): 458–465.

22 Prasad SM, Hersh S, Diodato MD *et al.* Physiological consequences of bipolar radiofrequency energy on the atria and pulmonary veins: a chronic animal study. *Ann Thorac Surg* 2003; **76**(3): 836–842.

23 Kress DC, Krum D, Chekanov V *et al.* Validation of a left atrial lesion pattern for intraoperative ablation of atrial fibrillation. *Ann Thorac Surg* 2002; **73**(4): 1160–1168.

24 Santiago T, Melo JQ, Gouveia RH, Martins AP. Intra-atrial temperatures in radiofrequency endocardial ablation: histologic evaluation of lesions. *Ann Thorac Surg* 2003; **75**(5): 1495–1501.

25 Thomas SP, Guy DJ, Boyd AC *et al.* Comparison of epicardial and endocardial linear ablation using handheld probes. *Ann Thorac Surg* 2003; **75**(2): 543–548.

26 Hoenicke EM, Strange RG Jr, Patel H *et al.* Initial experience with epicardial radiofrequency ablation catheter in an ovine model: moving towards an endoscopic Maze procedure. *Surg Forum* 2000; **51**: 79–82.

27 Santiago T, Melo J, Gouveia RH, Neves J *et al.* Epicardial radiofrequency applications: *in vitro* and *in vivo* studies on human atrial myocardium. *Eur J Cardiothorac Surg* 2003; **24**(4): 481–486.

28 Gaynor SL, Diodato MD, Prasad SM *et al.* A prospective, single-center clinical trial of a modified Cox–Maze procedure with bipolar radiofrequency ablation. *J Thorac Cardiovasc Surg* 2004; **128**: 535–542.

29 Kottkamp H, Hindricks G, Autschbach R *et al.* Specific linear left atrial lesions in atrial fibrillation: intraoperative radiofrequency ablation using minimally invasive surgical techniques. *J Am Coll Cardiol* 2002; **40**(3): 475–480.

30 Gillinov AM, Pettersson G, Rice TW. Esophageal injury during radiofrequency ablation for atrial fibrillation. *J Thorac Cardiovasc Surg* 2001; **122**(6): 1239–1240.

31 Laczkovics A, Khargi K, Deneke T. Esophageal perforation during left atrial radiofrequency ablation. *J Thorac Cardiovasc Surg* 2003; **126**(6): 2119–2120.

32 Damaria RG, Page P, Leung TK *et al.* Surgical radiofrequency ablation induces coronary endothelial dysfunction in porcine coronary arteries. *Eur J Cardiothorac Surg* 2003; **23**: 277–282.

33 Williams MR, Knaut M, Berube D *et al.* Application of microwave energy in cardiac tissue ablation: from *in vitro* analyses to clinical use. *Ann Thorac Surg* 2002; **74**: 1500–1505.

34 Gaynor SL, Byrd GD, Diodato MD *et al.* Microwave ablation for atrial fibrillation: dose–response curves in the cardioplegia-arrested and beating heart. (in press).

35 Saltman AE, Rosenthal LS, Francalancia NA, Lahey SJ. A completely endoscopic approach to microwave ablation for atrial fibrillation. *Heart Surg Forum* 2003; **6**(3): E38–E41.

36 Manasse E, Colombo PG, Barbone A *et al.* Clinical histopathology and ultrastructural analysis of myocardium following microwave energy ablation. *Eur J Cardiothorac Surg* 2003; **23**(4): 573–577.

37 Van Brakel TJ, Bolotin G, Salleng KJ *et al.* Evaluation of epicardial microwave ablation lesions: histology versus electrophysiology. *Ann Thorac Surg* 2004; **78**(4): 1397–1402.

38 Manasse E, Medici D, Ghiselli S *et al.* Left main coronary arterial lesion after microwave epicardial ablation. *Ann Thorac Surg* 2003; **76**(1): 276–277.

39 Williams MR, Argenziano M, Oz MC. Microwave ablation for surgical treatment of atrial fibrillation. *Semin Thorac Cardiovasc Surg* 2002; **14**(3): 232–237.

40 Thomas SP, Guy DJ, Rees A *et al.* Production of narrow but deep lesions suitable for ablation of atrial fibrillation using a saline-cooled narrow beam Nd:YAG laser catheter. *Lasers Surg Med* 2001; **28**(4): 375–380.

41 Reddy VY, Houghtaling C, Fallon C *et al.* Use of a diode laser balloon ablation catheter to generate circumferential pulmonary venous lesions in an open-thoracotomy caprine model. *PACE* 2004; **27**(1): 52–57.

42 Williams MR, Garrido M, Oz MC, Argenziano M. Alternative energy sources for surgical atrial ablation. *J Card Surg* 2004; **19**(3): 201–206.

25

CHAPTER 25

Epicardial access: present and future applications for interventional electrophysiologists

Robert A. Schweikert, MD *&* *Andrea Natale,* MD

Introduction

The Viennese physician Franz Schuh has been credited with performing the first successful percutaneous needle pericardiocentesis in 1840 [1]. Historically, percutaneous access to the pericardial space has been reserved primarily for therapeutic drainage of pericardial effusion, particularly as a life-saving measure in the instance of pericardial tamponade. However, prior to the use of fluoroscopic guidance and the addition of various methods of monitoring the patient, the procedure was associated with substantial morbidity and mortality. With refinements in the technique allowing greater safety with this procedure, additional applications of percutaneous pericardial access have been employed, even for patients without an abnormal collection of pericardial fluid. More recently, the percutaneous subxiphoid approach to the normal pericardial space in a catheterization or electrophysiology laboratory has been shown to be feasible and safe. Applications for this technique already include epicardial mapping and ablation of cardiac arrhythmias, as well as delivery of therapeutic drugs. Future applications will certainly evolve, such as the placement of epicardial pacing leads and perhaps other implantable cardiac devices.

Pericardial anatomy

The normal pericardium (Figure 25.1) is a double-layered flask-shaped sac composed of a fibrous outer layer and an inner serous membrane. The inner serous membrane covers the heart and proximal great vessels (visceral pericardium), which then reflects back upon itself to form the outer fibrous layer (parietal pericardium). The pericardial sac consists of the virtual space between these two layers and contains ~20–25 cc of physiologic fluid [3]. Pericardial reflections exist along the basal posterior of the heart at the location of the great vessels. Classically, two major serosal tunnels have been described: the transverse sinus and the oblique sinus [4], as shown in Figure 25.1. The transverse sinus is posterior to the aorta and main pulmonary artery and anterior to the atria and superior vena cava. The oblique sinus is posterior to the left atrium. More detailed reviews of the anatomy of the pericardium may be found elsewhere [5–7].

With the development of techniques to safely access the normal pericardial space for interventional cardiac and electrophysiological procedures, the pericardial anatomy has become quite relevant to the physicians performing such procedures. As Figure 25.1 illustrates, the pericardial space may permit access to most portions of the epicardial surface

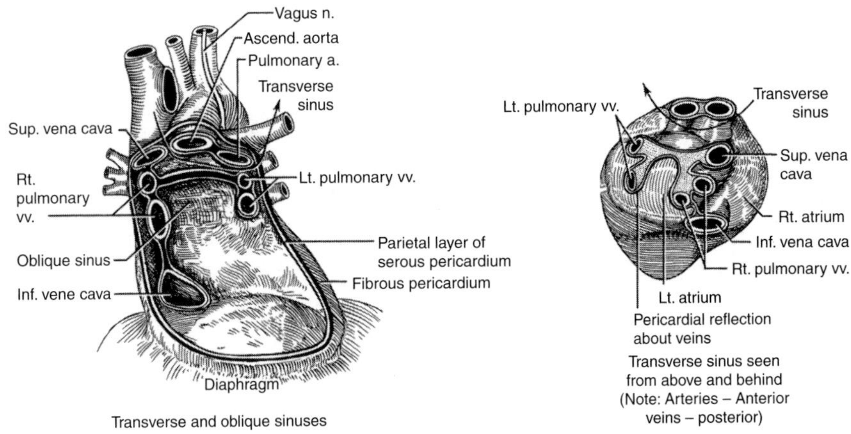

Figure 25.1 Illustrations of the pericardium demonstrating the pericardial reflections and the major sinuses, oblique and transverse. (Reprinted from [2], with permission from McGraw Hill Company.)

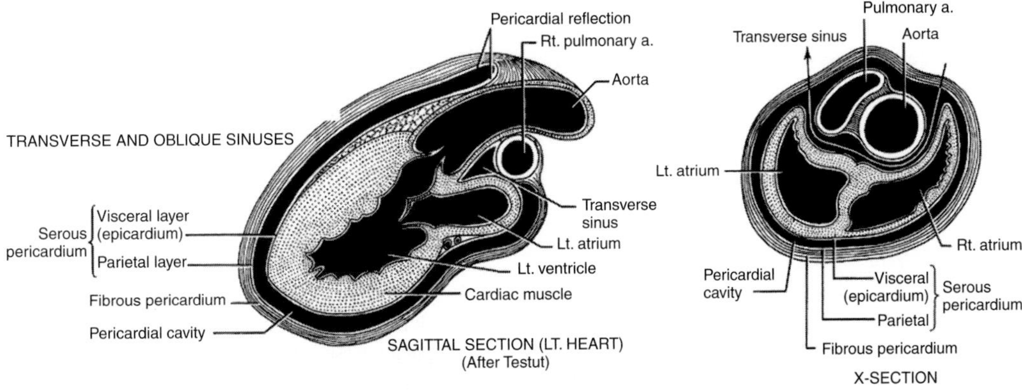

Figure 25.2 Illustrations of the pericardium in sagittal section and cross-section. (Reprinted from [2], with permission from McGraw Hill Company.)

of the heart, including the ventricles and atria. Figure 25.2 provides sagittal and cross-sectional views of the transverse and oblique sinuses that further illustrate the extent of the epicardial regions that may be accessible from a pericardial approach. D'Avila *et al.* [8] recently published an informative review regarding the pericardial anatomy relevant to the interventional electrophysiologist. Comprehensive reviews of the pericardium, including form, function, and disease states, have been published [3, 9].

Pericardial access

The history of accessing the pericardial space percutaneously is quite interesting. There are several publications that outline this history in more detail [9], but particularly comprehensive is the review by Kilpatrick and Chapman published in 1965 [1].

Pericardiocentesis performed blindly at the bedside via a percutaneous needle approach without the guidance of hemodynamic monitoring or echocardiography was associated with substantial morbidity and even mortality, with an incidence of life-threatening complications as high as 20%[1]. Marfan described the subcostal or subxiphoid approach to percutaneous pericardiocentesis in 1911 [9, 10]. More than 25 years ago this approach by a cardiologist in the cardiac catheterization laboratory was demonstrated to be feasible and safe with use of fluoroscopic guidance with hemodynamic and electrocardiographic monitoring [11]. Since the late 1970s, an echocardiographic-guided percutaneous approach has become the preferred technique for diagnostic and therapeutic pericardiocentesis due to increased efficacy and safety [12–14].

More recently, another technological advance has been with an instrument designed to achieve pericardial access percutaneously in the absence of pericardial effusion. This instrument, called the PerDUCER (Comedicus Inc., Columbia Hts., MN), utilizes a sheath inserted into the mediastinal space percutaneously at a subxiphoid location that allows the pericardium to be captured by suction, pericardiotomy performed with a needle under direct visualization, and a guidewire advanced into the pericardial space [15–18]. Figure 25.3 shows the PerDUCER device capturing the pericardium by suction (left panel) and a catheter inserted through the PerDUCER system into the pericardiotomy (right panel). Figure 25.4 shows the PerDUCER

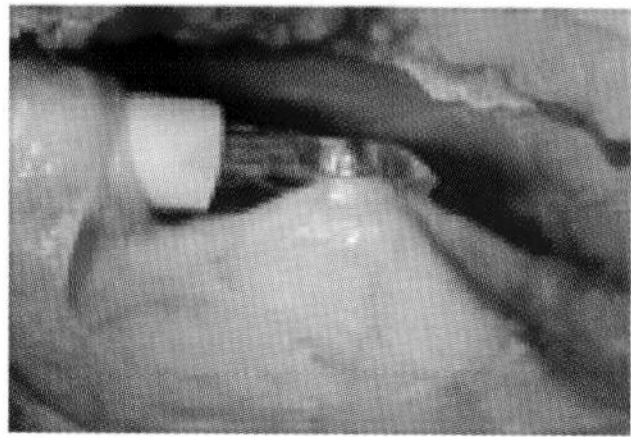

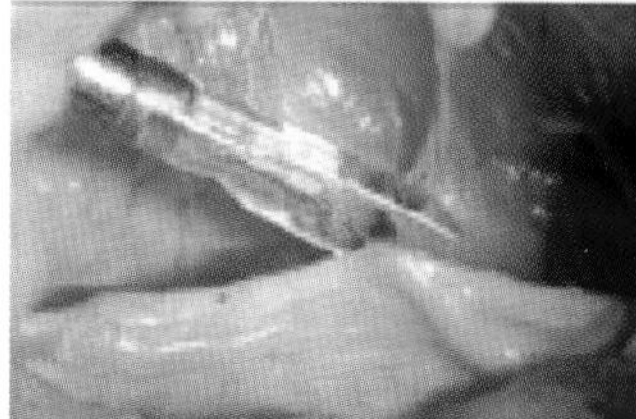

Figure 25.3 Photograph of the PerDUCER pericardial access device in an animal model. The left panel shows the device attached to the pericardium by suction. The right panel shows insertion of a catheter through the pericardium into the pericardial space via the PerDUCER system. (Reprinted with permission Comedicus Inc., Columbia Hts., MN.)

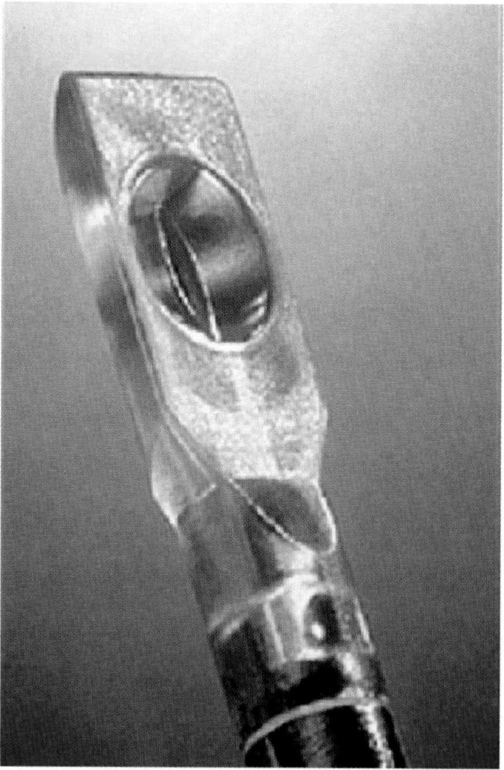

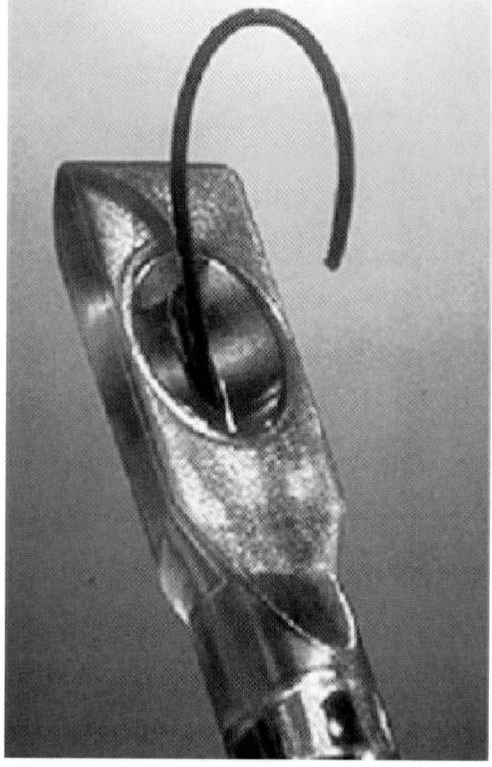

Figure 25.4 Photograph of the distal portion of the PerDUCER pericardial access device (left panel) and a catheter deployed through the device (right panel). (Reprinted with permission from Comedicus Inc., Columbia Hts, MN.)

device (left panel) and a catheter passed through it (right panel).

There are alternatives to the percutaneous approach to the pericardial space. One alternative approach to pericardial access involves a transvenous endocardial puncture from within a cardiac chamber, generally the right atrial appendage. This approach has been successfully employed in animals for drainage of pericardial effusions and delivery of cardiovascular medications [19–23], and a case report of emergent transcardiac puncture from the endocardium has been described for a patient with tamponade when percutaneous pericardiocentesis failed [24]. Additionally, the transbronchial method via the left lower lobe bronchus or distal trachea has been described as a diagnostic and therapeutic approach for posterior pericardial effusions that may not be accessible by other approaches [25].

Applications of pericardial access

Percutaneous pericardial access has traditionally been performed for the purpose of diagnostic and/or therapeutic removal of fluid from pericardial effusion. However, as the safety of percutaneous subxiphoid pericardiocentesis substantially improved, interest developed in accessing the normal pericardial space for therapeutic and interventional purposes. The percutaneous subxiphoid technique for instrumentation of the pericardial space has been applied to catheter ablation of arrhythmias in the electrophysiology laboratory for a variety of arrhythmias that have an epicardial substrate.

Endocardial catheter ablation via a percutaneous transvenous technique has become the preferred approach for the treatment of several types of arrhythmias, and has offered a considerable advantage over the more invasive surgical approach. However, the endocardial approach for catheter ablation has important limitations, including the inability to access epicardial portions of arrhythmia substrates. Technological improvements, such as cooled-tip or larger-tip ablation catheters and different energy sources for tissue ablation, have been useful but have not completely solved the problem.

Sosa *et al.* [26, 27] initially reported the use of the percutaneous approach in the electrophysiology laboratory for epicardial mapping and ablation of ventricular tachyarrhythmias associated with Chagasic heart disease. This group later reported their experience with this approach for ventricular tachyarrhythmias associated with ischemic heart disease [28]. The first report in the United States using this approach with electroanatomical mapping for a patient with ischemic heart disease and ventricular tachycardia was reported in 1999 [29].

Case reports documenting the use of the percutaneous pericardial approach for catheter ablation of other types of arrhythmia substrates followed, including accessory pathways [30, 31] and ventricular tachycardia associated with dilated nonischemic cardiomyopathy [32]. Our center was the first in the United States to report an experience with percutaneous epicardial mapping and ablation of a variety of different arrhythmias in a series of patients in which conventional endocardial ablation approaches had failed [33]. This series included patients with inappropriate sinus tachycardia, atrial tachycardia or fibrillation, supraventricular tachycardia associated with accessory pathways, and ventricular tachycardias associated with normal hearts, dilated nonischemic cardiomyopathy, and ischemic cardiomyopathy.

Further case reports from other centers have confirmed the feasibility, safety, and potential efficacy of this approach, as with inappropriate sinus tachycardia [34], accessory pathways [35, 36], ventricular tachyarrhythmias [37–40], and even pulmonary vein isolation for atrial fibrillation using percutaneous epicardial radiofrequency ablation lesions as an adjunct to endocardial lesions [41]. More recently, this same group reported preliminary results of a small series of patients with this approach, which was effective for only the left pulmonary veins and not the right pulmonary veins [42].

Percutaneous subxiphoid technique for pericardial access for catheter mapping and ablation of arrhythmias

At our institution, percutaneous pericardial puncture is performed in a manner similar to that previously described by Sosa *et al.* [26], which is a modification of the traditional pericardiocentesis technique described by Krikorian and Hancock [11].

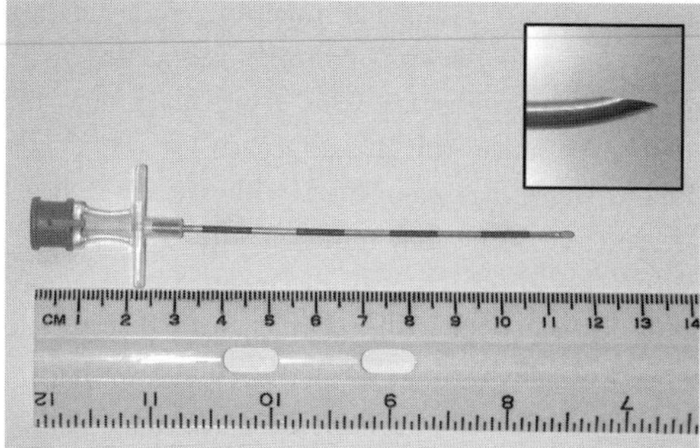

Figure 25.5 Photograph of the epidural needle (Arrow International, Reading, PA) used for percutaneous pericardial access. The removable obturator has been left in place. Inset shows close up side view of the needle tip.

The epigastric region is prepped and draped in a sterile fashion. The skin is anesthetized with a local anesthetic such as 1% procaine. Using a 15° left anterior oblique fluoroscopic projection, an 8.9 cm 17 gauge epidural needle (Arrow International, Reading, PA) is slowly advanced from the epigastric (subxiphoid) region toward the right ventricular apex. The needle has a blunt tip designed to approach a virtual space (shown in Figure 25.5 and described in more detail below). In some cases when the 8.9 cm needle does not reach the pericardium, a longer version of this needle (12.5 cm) is required. The vertebral column is used as a fluoroscopic landmark, as we generally aim the needle toward the cardiac silhouette with the needle tip along or to the left (patient's right) of the vertebral column on the fluoroscopic image in order to approach a region devoid of major epicardial vessels. When the needle is a few centimeters from the cardiac silhouette, intermittent injections of very small amounts of a contrast agent are used to determine the position of the needle tip. Care is taken to minimize the amount of contrast injected into the chest wall tissue and mediastinum. When the needle tip becomes in contact with the pericardium, "tenting" of the pericardium is generally observed with injection of contrast (Figure 25.6(a)). Puncture of the pericardium is often palpable and a sudden negative pressure may be observed with "sucking" of the contrast fluid into the needle. Entry into the pericardial space is then confirmed with injection of contrast, demonstrating a characteristic "layering" of contrast material within the pericardial space (Figure 25.6(b)).

A floppy tip guidewire is then advanced through the needle into the pericardial space with verification of position by fluoroscopy as the guidewire follows the contour of the cardiac silhouette (Figure 25.6(c)). A vascular sheath is then advanced over the wire into the pericardial space. We prefer to use an 8 French 45 cm Super Arrow-Flex wire reinforced vascular sheath (Arrow International, Reading, PA), as it is less likely to kink at the pericardial insertion site, which may prevent subsequent introduction of the mapping/ablation catheter. Aspiration of the sheath is then performed to remove as much as possible of the contrast material from the pericardial space. The ablation catheter is then immediately placed through the sheath and into the pericardial space. The catheter may be then manipulated throughout most of the pericardial space over the majority of the epicardial surface of the heart (Figure 25.6(d)).

Cleveland Clinic Foundation experience with percutaneous subxiphoid epicardial catheter mapping and ablation

We recently reported a series of 48 patients who underwent endocardial and percutaneous epicardial mapping and ablation in the EP laboratory for a variety of arrhythmias that could not be ablated by conventional endocardial methods [33]. The percutaneous epicardial approach appeared to be most useful for ventricular tachycardias and right atrial appendage to right ventricle accessory pathways. Our experience now includes 70 patients in whom we have attempted epicardial mapping and ablation: 66 patients via a subxiphoid percutaneous pericardial approach and 4 patients in whom this approach was unsuccessful due to difficult percutaneous access to the pericardial space. All four of these patients had prior cardiac surgery and the pericardial space was either obliterated or severely fibrosed due to adhesions. Two of these patients subsequently underwent successful epicardial mapping and ablation with a surgical approach. Table 25.1 presents the patient characteristics and type of target arrhythmia.

Of the 51 patients with ventricular tachycardia, 31 patients had no structural heart disease, 15 patients had ischemic cardiomyopathy, and 5 patients had

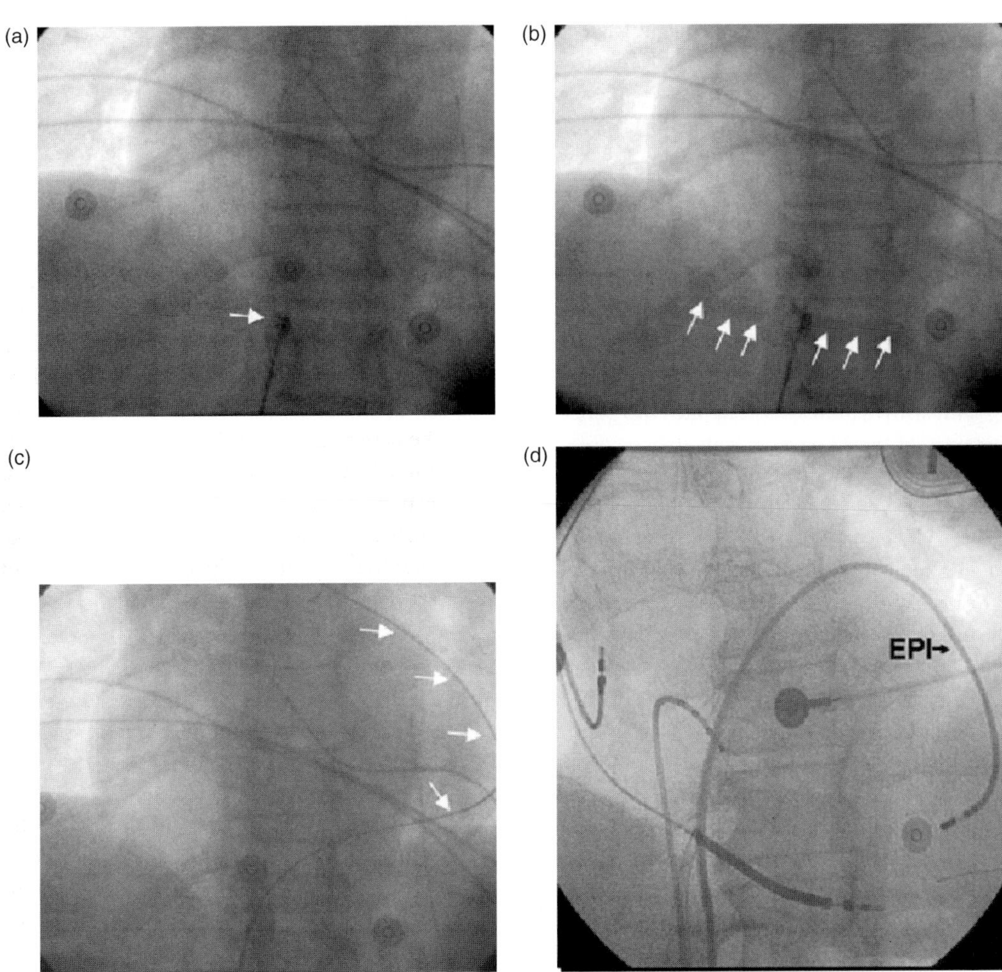

Figure 25.6 Fluoroscopic images (15° left anterior oblique projection) during various steps of percutaneous pericardial access from subxiphoid approach in a human patient. (a) Shows the needle tenting the pericardium (arrow) after a small injection of contrast. (b) Shows layering of contrast in the pericardial space (arrows) after needle entry. (c) Shows a guidewire (arrows) in the pericardial space with characteristic course along the lateral border of the cardiac silhouette. (d) Shows a catheter (EPI) in the pericardial space in a different patient. Also present are transvenous leads from a dual-chamber implantable cardioverter defibrillator (ICD), an EP catheter in the basal right ventricle, and a long intravascular sheath with tip in the IVC near the inferior right atrium.

Table 25.1 Patient characteristics.

Patients, *n*	70
Age (years), mean ± SD	46 ± 2
Previous ablations, mean (range)	1.5 ± 0.7 (0 − 3)
Type of arrhythmia substrate	
Ventricular tachycardia	51
Accessory pathways	11
Inappropriate sinus tachycardia	04
Atrial fibrillation	03
Atypical atrial flutter	01

dilated nonischemic cardiomyopathy. Of these 51 patients, 35 were found to have an epicardial arrhythmia substrate, generally with earliest sites of activation. Of these 35 patients, 22 (63%) were successfully ablated with epicardial radiofrequency ablation.

The most common reason for failure of percutaneous epicardial ablation of ventricular tachycardias was an inaccessible, protected or mid-myocardial target site. Our initial series included seven patients with coronary cusp variant of normal heart ventricular tachycardia that were mapped epicardially and from the coronary cusp, and as we previously reported the left atrial appendage and/or epicardial fat precluded delivery of effective ablation lesions epicardially in spite of epicardial sites being earlier [33, 43]. Other reasons for failure of percutaneous epicardial ablation of ventricular tachycardia included close vicinity to the phrenic nerve (two patients), inability to deliver adequate ablation lesions due to low power and/or high impedance values (three patients), and the presence of a mid-myocardial arrhythmia substrate site (two patients). Therefore, of the 22 patients with an accessible and early epicardial ventricular arrhythmia site, 18 (82%) were successfully ablated with percutaneous epicardial lesions.

Radiofrequency catheter ablation of posterior accessory pathways has been problematic from an epicardial approach, even when epicardial sites were earlier than endocardial sites. Delivery of radiofrequency energy at such sites was often ineffective, possibly due to interference from the posterior fat pad. However, nearly all of these accessory pathways could be ablated from a transvenous approach, often from within the coronary sinus or a tributary, or in some instances from a coronary sinus diverticulum [31]. Catheter ablation of the right atrial appendage to right ventricle accessory pathway may sometimes be unsuccessful from the endocardial approach, and in our experience may be readily ablated from a percutaneous pericardial approach [30, 33].

Overall, in our experience the reasons for failure of percutaneous epicardial ablation included inability to deliver adequate power, inability to deliver ablation lesions due to close vicinity to the phrenic nerve, and the presence of an inaccessible arrhythmia substrate. The latter included mid-myocardial sites, sites underneath epicardial fat or the left atrial appendage, sites beyond the pericardial recesses, and sites within areas of inaccessible pericardial spaces as with pericardial adhesions.

We have only encountered four patients in whom pericardial access could not be achieved with a percutaneous subxiphoid approach. All of these patients had previously undergone open-heart surgery and the pericardial space either could not be entered at all or catheter manipulation was severely restricted due to the presence of adhesions. Two of these patients underwent successful epicardial catheter mapping and ablation with a surgical approach. For all patients who underwent percutaneous pericardial access for epicardial mapping and ablation, we have not encountered severe complications.

Prediction of epicardial arrhythmia substrate

In light of the feasibility, efficacy, and safety of the percutaneous pericardial approach to catheter ablation at the epicardium demonstrated by the published experience of several centers, it is relevant to consider whether predictors of an epicardial substrate exist. Berruezo *et al.* [44] found that for ventricular tachycardia (predominantly ischemic cardiomyopathy) certain electrocardiographic characteristics were sensitive and specific for the prediction of an epicardial site of origin (Tables 25.2 and 25.3). These ECG parameters included the presence of a pseudo-delta wave, prolonged intrinsicoid deflection time, RS interval, and QRS complex duration. At our center, analysis of 107 normal heart ventricular tachycardias showed that

Table 25.2 Electrocardiographic recognition of epicardial ventricular tachycardia [44]

	Group A (Epi)	*Group B (Endo)*	*Group C (Neither)*
Pseudo-delta wave, ms	43 ± 9	16 ± 9	42 ± 9
ID time in V2, ms	97 ± 21	65 ± 15	98 ± 14
Shortest RS, ms	149 ± 39	91 ± 20	132 ± 30
QRS duration, ms	217 ± 24	174 ± 37	195 ± 27

Notes: Endo = endocardial, Epi = epicardial, ID = intrinsicoid deflection. $p < .05$ for Group A versus B and Group C versus B.

Table 25.3 Electrocardiographic recognition of epicardial ventricular tachycardia: predictive value [44]

	Sensitivity (%)	*Specificity (%)*
Pseudo-delta wave ≥ 34 ms	83	95
ID time in V2 ≥ 85 ms	87	90
RS ≥ 121 ms	76	85

Note: ID = intrinsicoid deflection.

Table 25.4 Prediction of epicardial origin of normal heart ventricular tachycardia [45]

	Endocardial VT	*Aortic Cusp VT*	*Epicardial VT*
Patients (*n*)	50	46	11
Male/Female	40/10	34/12	8/3
Ejection Fraction (%, ±SD)	52 ± 5	54 ± 5	53 ± 5
Mean QRS duration (ms, ±SD)	132 ± 14	142 ± 12*	145 ± 15*

Notes: VT = ventricular tachycardia, SD = standard deviation.
*$p < .05$ versus endocardial VT.

QRS duration was significantly longer for ventricular tachycardias arising from an epicardial substrate (Table 25.4) [45]. Further study is necessary as the prediction of the probability of an epicardial arrhythmia substrate may be important. Such information may help the interventional electrophysiologist to develop procedural strategies and counsel patients accordingly.

Unique challenges posed by percutaneous epicardial ablation

Percutaneous epicardial catheter ablation presents unique challenges that may not be encountered with the traditional endocardial approach. The pericardial space does not provide the convective cooling that occurs due to local blood flow with endocardial ablation, and this may therefore limit the amount of power delivered into the tissue and lesion depth achieved from an epicardial approach. Moreover, the epicardial surface of the heart may have extensive regions of fat that limit the delivery of effective ablation lesions. The presence of pericardial adhesions, as may occur with prior cardiac surgery or pericarditis, may significantly limit access to some or even all of the pericardial space.

Fortunately, many of these limitations may not be insurmountable, as new ablation technologies and alternative pericardial access techniques have been found to be useful for epicardial catheter ablation. New advances in this area should address the issues of effectiveness and safety.

Effectiveness of percutaneous epicardial ablation

Standard radiofrequency catheter ablation systems have important limitations within the pericardial space. The use of internal saline irrigation cooled-tip catheter ablation systems has been shown in animal models to provide more effective epicardial radiofrequency ablation lesions, particularly over regions of epicardial fat where standard radiofrequency catheter ablation systems have been known to fail [46]. A center in Germany reported effectiveness and safety with the use of an open irrigated-tip catheter ablation system within the pericardial space via subxiphoid percutaneous approach for ablation of ventricular tachycardia [39]. A preliminary report of a comparison of epicardial catheter ablation using open irrigated-tip versus standard catheter ablation systems demonstrated the irrigated system to produce deeper and larger ablation lesions from the epicardial space, and furthermore the standard radiofrequency lesions were less effective (smaller and nontransmural) from the epicardial approach compared with those delivered from the endocardial approach [47].

Cryothermy has been used for epicardial ablation during open-heart surgery. However, the effectiveness of epicardial cryothermy from a percutaneous pericardial approach is still being assessed. In animal models percutaneous epicardial cryothermy has been reported with mixed results. One study reported percutaneous cryothermy to be feasible and capable of delivering effective lesions, although attenuated over regions of epicardial fat [48]. However, another center reported their experience with a canine model, which showed less effective lesions with cryothermy, and transmural lesions only occurred from the posterior left atrium [49].

Other sources of energy for percutaneous epicardial ablation appear to be promising but there is very little data if any. For example, focused ultrasound may be effective and offer the advantage of being capable of delivering lesions through epicardial fat.

Regarding the potential limitation imposed by pericardial adhesions, a few experienced centers have reported successful use of the percutaneous pericardial approach for patients with difficult pericardial access due to previous cardiac surgery. In such patients, the presence of fibrous adhesions as a result of the cardiac surgical procedure may prevent the ability to access the pericardial space or freely manipulate a mapping/ablation catheter. One center reported their experience in which the pericardial puncture was targeted to the inferior left ventricle to avoid the expected anterior adhesions, and in all five patients the pericardial space was accessible with this approach and the inferolateral left ventricle could be mapped [50]. Another center reported the use of a subxiphoid approach for direct surgical exposure of the pericardial space to allow epicardial mapping and ablation for six patients in whom percutaneous needle pericardial approach was not feasible due to difficult access or prior cardiac surgery [51]. At our own center we have also successfully used this approach for two such patients (unpublished data).

Safety of percutaneous epicardial ablation

Although several centers have reported safety of the percutaneous pericardial approach for catheter mapping and ablation with very few serious complications, it is still prudent to consider the potential complications that are unique to epicardial ablation from the pericardial space. One potential concern is damage to epicardial vessels, either from the needle during the pericardial access or with delivery of ablation lesions. To our knowledge, puncture of an epicardial vessel during percutaneous pericardial access for epicardial catheter mapping and ablation has not been reported in the medical literature. The technique is quite important in this regard, as the pericardial puncture should be performed at a region devoid of major epicardial vessels as described above. In addition, most centers experienced in percutaneous pericardial access use an epidural type of blunt-tip needle, which is designed to approach a virtual space. Figure 25.5 is a photograph of the needle used at our center, with the obturator in place. The inset shows a closer view of the needle tip from the side. The use of such a needle makes puncture or laceration of the right ventricle or epicardial vessels less likely than with a conventional sharp-tip needle. The PerDUCER pericardial access system discussed above may be even less likely to result in epicardial vessel damage or ventricular perforation, as the pericardium is sucked away from the heart and pericardiotomy is performed in a more controlled manner.

The potential for damage to the epicardial coronary arteries during epicardial ablation lesion delivery remains a concern. D'Avila *et al.* [52] demonstrated in a canine model that injury to the epicardial arteries from delivery of radiofrequency energy is inversely proportional to the size of the vessel. Severe arterial damage and thrombosis occurred in vessels with a mean internal perimeter of 0.78 ± 0.49 mm compared with 1.79 ± 0.83 mm for arterial vessels without damage. Occlusion of the distal portion of the left circumflex coronary artery has been reported after delivery of epicardial radiofrequency ablation near the vessel [53]. The safety of cryothermy with a percutaneous pericardial approach has been studied in animal models. In the animal model (using goats and swine) for the use of percutaneous epicardial cryothermy discussed above, D'Avila *et al.* [48] reported no incidence of coronary artery thrombosis with cryoablation lesions delivered directly upon the epicardial coronary vessels. However, in the canine model reported by Lustgarten and colleagues, percutaneous epicardial cryoablation was associated with significant vascular damage when cryoablation lesions were applied directly over major epicardial coronary arteries. Importantly, cryoablation caused minimal damage to adjacent noncardiac structures, such as the lung [49]. Further study in a more extensive experience is required to more completely assess the efficacy of percutaneous epicardial cryoablation and determine whether cryoablation in this setting provides improved safety over radiofrequency ablation with regard to epicardial coronary vessels and adjacent noncardiac structures.

In our experience, we have not encountered damage to epicardial vessels from the pericardial access or from delivery of radiofrequency energy. In fact, for ventricular tachycardia the epicardial ablation sites tended to be near the course of the major epicardial vessels, often requiring delivery of ablation lesions adjacent to the vessels [33].

An additional concern is damage to adjacent noncardiac structures. Although this is not infrequently a concern with endocardial catheter ablation, the location of such structures is much closer when delivering ablation lesions to the epicardial surface of the heart from the pericardial space. Currently available catheter ablation systems deliver energy circumferentially from the catheter tip. Therefore, there is a greater likelihood of damage occurring to adjacent structures such as lung and, notably, the phrenic nerve.

The optimal percutaneous epicardial access and ablation system

Presently, the optimal system for percutaneous pericardial access and epicardial catheter mapping and ablation has not been determined. Percutaneous pericardial access has not been particularly difficult in our experience, except for those patients with pericardial adhesions, and complications have not occurred in a large series of patients. As for the optimal catheter ablation system, this remains to be determined. Such a system should offer the best combination of effectiveness, safety, and ease of use. Promising advances with radiofrequency ablation systems have occurred but more refinements are necessary. Cryothermy may indeed play an important role as well as this energy source is well established for epicardial use in open-heart surgery. Other energy sources for ablation may have a promising role for epicardial ablation, such as focused ultrasound. Further study is required in this area.

An exciting and interesting new technology is the catheter ablation system developed by Ablatrics (Chapel Hill, NC). This ablation system is designed to address a few of the important limitations posed by percutaneous epicardial ablation, particularly tissue contact, lesion depth, and lesion control. The system uses a novel 15 French catheter (Figures 25.7 and 25.8) that is flexible and uses a vacuum-induced suction mechanism at the ablation electrode to produce tissue contact. In addition, a perfusion lumen allows for saline irrigation (closed system due to the vacuum suction) to provide electrode–tissue interface cooling for delivery of a more effective ablation lesion. Also, the system has an insulated covering over a portion of the ablation

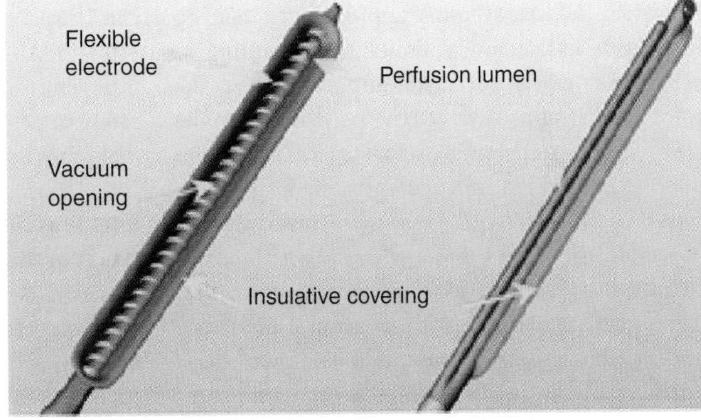

Figure 25.7 Illustration of two views of the distal portion of the Ablatrics ablation catheter, showing the flexible electrode, vacuum opening, perfusion lumen, and insulative covering. (Reprinted with permission from Ablatrics, Chapel Hill, NC.)

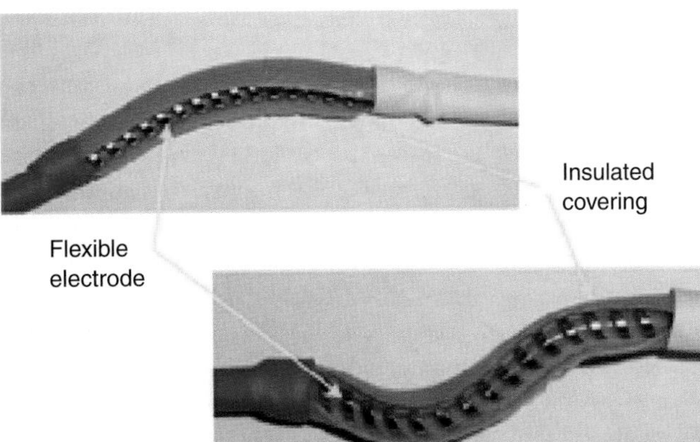

Figure 25.8 Photographs of the distal portion of the Ablatrics ablation catheter, showing the insulated covering and flexible electrode. (Reprinted with permission from Ablatrics, Chapel Hill, NC.)

electrode to allow directional delivery of ablation energy, perhaps minimizing the potential for damage to adjacent noncardiac structures. A preliminary report of the use of this system *in vitro* has been encouraging [54], and may prove quite useful for linear as well as more focal delivery of epicardial ablation lesions from a percutaneous pericardial approach.

Other applications of percutaneous pericardial access

Epicardial pacing leads

The clinical success of cardiac resynchronization therapy for patients with heart failure has led to increasing frequency of implantation of left ventricular pacing leads. The transvenous approach has been the preferred technique for placement of a left ventricular pacing lead into a tributary of the coronary sinus, generally a posterolateral or posterior left ventricular branch. However, the transvenous approach for placing such leads has technical limitations, resulting in ~5–10% rate of unsuccessful implantation via the transvenous approach. Such patients may be referred to a cardiac surgeon for surgical placement of an epicardial left ventricular pacing lead, which may be performed with a minimally invasive technique and in some centers with the assistance of robotic instrumentation. However, these surgical techniques are performed under general anesthesia and the thoracotomy requires left pneumothorax. Furthermore, in many instances a separate procedure is necessary for implantation of the remainder of the system, particularly for an implantable cardioverter defibrillator system, which is generally implanted in the EP laboratory.

There is therefore substantial interest in alternative techniques for the implantation of epicardial left ventricular pacing leads, particularly an approach that could be performed by electrophysiologists in the EP laboratory. The subxiphoid percutaneous pericardial approach may provide a feasible technique for placement of epicardial left ventricular pacing leads. Zenati *et al.* [55] recently described the use of subxiphoid videopericardioscopy for this purpose in animals. Further refinements in the pacing lead technology and pericardial access tools will need to occur to allow this approach to be feasible and practical for use in human patients.

Pericardial drug delivery

The use of the pericardial space as a drug reservoir for delivery of therapeutic substances to the heart may have application for the treatment of a variety of cardiac conditions. The delivery of amiodarone to the canine pericardial sac in an open chest model has been reported to produce myocardial electrophysiological effects and suppress electrically induced atrial fibrillation [56], although a similar study with ibutilide was ineffective in spite of demonstration of significant electrophysiological effects [57]. Delivery of therapeutic substances, such as angiogenic agents, growth factors, and gene therapy to the pericardial space via a percutaneous approach has been described in animals [58–61] and in humans with triamcinolone for autoreactive myocarditis [62]. Interestingly, several reports have described a transatrial approach to access the pericardial space for diagnostic or therapeutic purposes [19–23]. Although a feasible and potentially useful intervention, demonstration of the efficacy and safety of percutaneous drug delivery to the pericardial space in humans requires further study.

Echocardiography from the pericardial space

Intracardiac echocardiography has been used with increasing frequency for guidance of transvenous interventional electrophysiologic procedures, particularly catheter ablation. The development of a phased-array intracardiac echocardiography system has vastly improved the capabilities of intracardiac imaging. Intrapericardial echocardiography has been shown to be feasible in animals and was capable of imaging the right and left cardiac chambers and other cardiac structures, as well as intracardiac catheters [63]. Potential applications of intrapericardial echocardiography include the monitoring of position and tissue contact of intracardiac catheters, and monitoring of the catheter–tissue interface and lesion characteristics (e.g. size and depth of lesion) during delivery of ablation energy. For left ventricular endocardial catheter ablation, intrapericardial echocardiography could be superior to intracardiac echocardiography from the right cardiac chambers for such purposes. Further study is required to demonstrate the feasibility and safety of intrapericardial echocardiography in humans.

Use of percutaneous pericardial access for treatment of heart failure patients

Percutaneous access to the pericardial space presents the potential for exciting additional applications for the interventional electrophysiologist. One such application may be with a left ventricular support system that provides external passive ventricular restraint with a surgically implanted mesh. A system implanted at open-heart surgery is being investigated in a randomized clinical trial [64] and early reports have been favorable. For patients not requiring an open-heart surgical procedure otherwise, the morbidity and mortality of such an invasive approach may significantly offset the benefits of the passive ventricular restraint system. Another similar system, the Paracor Ventricular Support System (Paracor Medical, Inc., Sunnyvale, California) is designed for implantation via the pericardial space via mini-thoracotomy or a subxiphoid/subcostal incision (Figures 25.9 and 25.10). An exciting technological advance would be a similar system with a smaller profile that would allow implantation percutaneously via the subxiphoid or subcostal approach by interventional electrophysiologists. It is interesting to speculate whether such an epicardial mesh may also be used for other electrophysiological purposes, such as defibrillation, and perhaps multisite pacing, such as with cardiac resynchronization therapy.

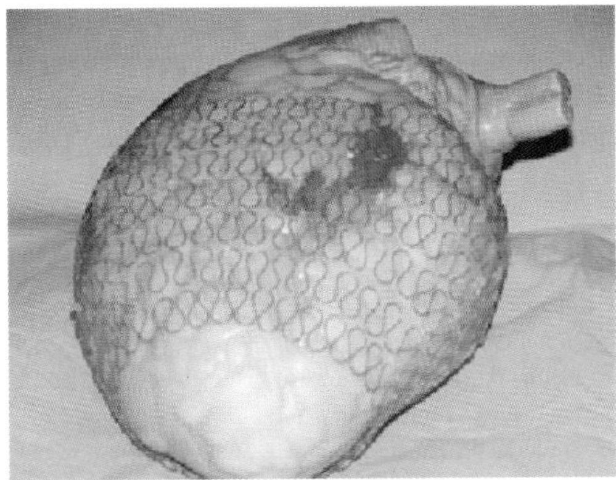

Figure 25.9 Photograph of the Paracor Ventricular Support System deployed around a heart model. (Reprinted with permission from Paracor Surgical, Inc., Sunnyvale, CA.)

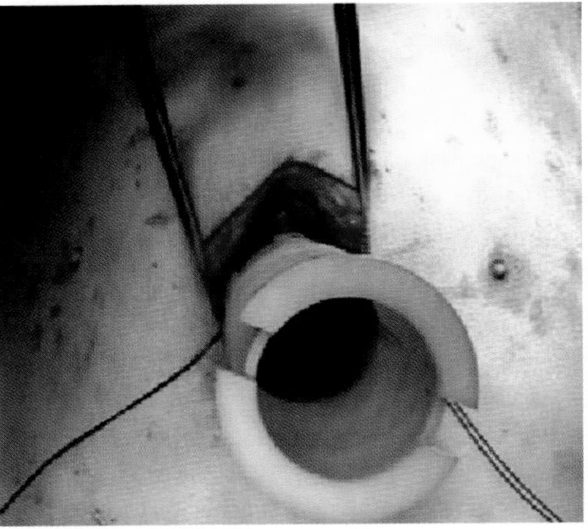

Figure 25.10 Photograph of a canine model with the introducer in place at the subxiphoid location for the Paracor Ventricular Support System. (Reprinted with permission from Paracor Surgical, Inc., Sunnyvale, CA.)

Summary

Percutaneous subxiphoid access to the normal pericardial space has been shown to be feasible and safe, and this approach has been safely and effectively utilized for epicardial mapping and ablation of a variety of arrhythmias with an epicardial substrate. The use of an epidural blunt-tip needle has been associated with a very low incidence of complications, and systems designed to facilitate percutaneous access to the normal pericardial space, such as the PerDUCER system, have been introduced. Further technological developments are necessary for improvement of efficacy and safety of catheter ablation from the pericardial space. This may include systems designed for such a purpose, perhaps with directional delivery of energy to focus upon cardiac tissue ablation and avoid damage to adjacent intrathoracic structures, as with the Ablatrics system. Alternative energy sources, including cryothermy and perhaps focused ultrasound, may also prove to be safer if not more effective. Additional applications for percutaneous pericardial access are an exciting area of interest, such as implantation of pacing leads, delivery of therapeutic agents, and placement of epicardial devices for treatment of heart failure patients. More extensive experience and further refinements to the technology will open new horizons for interventional electrophysiologists interested in the potential applications of percutaneous access to the pericardial space and the epicardial surface of the heart.

References

1 Kilpatrick ZM, Chapman CB. On pericardiocentesis. *Am J Cardiol* 1965; **16**(5): 722–728.
2 Pansky B. *Review of Gross Anatomy*, 5th edn. Macmillan Publishing Company, New York, 1984.
3 Spodick DH. *The Pericardium: A Comprehensive Textbook*. Marcel Dekker, New York, 1997.
4 *Nomina Anatomica*, 5th edn. Williams & Wilkins, Baltimore, MD, 1983.
5 Chaffanjon P, Brichon PY, Faure C, Favre JJ. Pericardial reflection around the venous aspect of the heart. *Surg Radiol Anat* 1997; **19**(1): 17–21.
6 Choe YH, Im JG, Park JH, Han MC, Kim CW. The anatomy of the pericardial space: a study in cadavers and patients. *AJR Am J Roentgenol* 1987; **149**(4): 693–697.
7 Vesely TM, Cahill DR. Cross-sectional anatomy of the pericardial sinuses, recesses, and adjacent structures. *Surg Radiol Anat* 1986; **8**(4): 221–227.
8 D'Avila A, Scanavacca M, Sosa E, Ruskin JN, Reddy VY. Pericardial anatomy for the interventional electrophysiologist. *J Cardiovasc Electrophysiol* 2003; **14**(4): 422–430.
9 Shabetai R. *The Pericardium*, 2nd edn. Kluwer Academic Publishers, Boston, MA, 2003.
10 Marfan A. Ponction du pericarde par l'epigastre. *Ann de Med et Chir Inf* 1911; **15**: 529–533.
11 Krikorian JG, Hancock EW. Pericardiocentesis. *Am J Med* 1978; **65**(5): 808–814.
12 Callahan JA, Seward JB, Tajik AJ. Cardiac tamponade: pericardiocentesis directed by two-dimensional echocardiography. *Mayo Clin Proc* 1985; **60**(5): 344–347.
13 Tsang TS, Freeman WK, Sinak LJ, Seward JB. Echocardiographically guided pericardiocentesis: evolution and state-of-the-art technique. *Mayo Clin Proc* 1998; **73**(7): 647–652.
14 Tsang TS, Enriquez-Sarano M, Freeman WK *et al.* Consecutive 1127 therapeutic echocardiographically guided pericardiocenteses: clinical profile, practice patterns, and outcomes spanning 21 years. *Mayo Clin Proc* 2002; **77**(5): 429–436.
15 Seferovic PM, Ristic AD, Maksimovic R *et al.* Initial clinical experience with PerDUCER device: promising new tool in the diagnosis and treatment of pericardial disease. *Clin Cardiol* 1999; **22**(1, Suppl. 1): I30–I35.
16 Macris MP, Igo SR. Minimally invasive access of the normal pericardium: initial clinical experience with a novel device. *Clin Cardiol* 1999; **22**(1, Suppl. 1): I36–I39.
17 Maisch B, Ristic AD, Rupp H, Spodick DH. Pericardial access using the PerDUCER and flexible percutaneous pericardioscopy. *Am J Cardiol* 2001; **88**(11): 1323–1326.
18 Hou D, March KL. A novel percutaneous technique for accessing the normal pericardium: a single-center successful experience of 53 porcine procedures. *J Invasive Cardiol* 2003; **15**(1): 13–17.
19 Moreno R, Waxman S, Rowe K, Verrier RL. Intrapericardial beta-adrenergic blockade with esmolol exerts a potent antitachycardic effect without depressing contractility. *J Cardiovasc Pharmacol* 2000; **36**(6): 722–727.
20 Pulerwitz TC, Waxman S, Rowe KA, Quist WC, Lipinska I, Verrier RL. Transatrial access to the normal pericardial space for local cardiac therapy: preclinical safety testing with aspirin and pulmonary artery hypertension. *J Interv Cardiol* 2001; **14**(5): 493–498.
21 Verrier RL, Waxman S, Lovett EG, Moreno R. Transatrial access to the normal pericardial space: a novel approach for diagnostic sampling, pericardiocentesis, and therapeutic interventions. *Circulation* 1998; **98**(21): 2331–2333.
22 Waxman S, Moreno R, Rowe KA, Verrier RL. Persistent primary coronary dilation induced by transatrial delivery of nitroglycerin into the pericardial space: a novel approach for local cardiac drug delivery. *J Am Coll Cardiol* 1999; **33**(7): 2073–2077.
23 Waxman S, Pulerwitz TC, Rowe KA, Quist WC, Verrier RL. Preclinical safety testing of percutaneous transatrial access to the normal pericardial space for local cardiac drug delivery and diagnostic sampling. *Catheter Cardiovasc Interv* 2000; **49**(4): 472–477.
24 Hsu LF, Scavee C, Jais P, Hocini M, Haissaguerre M. Transcardiac pericardiocentesis: an emergency lifesaving technique for cardiac tamponade. *J Cardiovasc Electrophysiol* 2003; **14**(9): 1001–1003.
25 Ceron L, Manzato M, Mazzaro F, Bellavere F. A new diagnostic and therapeutic approach to pericardial effusion: transbronchial needle aspiration. *Chest* 2003; **123**(5): 1753–1758.
26 Sosa E, Scanavacca M, D'Avila A, Pilleggi F. A new technique to perform epicardial mapping in the electrophysiology laboratory. *J Cardiovasc Electrophysiol* 1996; **7**(6): 531–536.
27 Sosa E, Scanavacca M, D'Avila A *et al.* Endocardial and epicardial ablation guided by nonsurgical transthoracic epicardial mapping to treat recurrent ventricular tachycardia. *J Cardiovasc Electrophysiol* 1998; **9**(3): 229–239.
28 Sosa E, Scanavacca M, D'Avila A, Oliveira F, Ramires JA. Nonsurgical transthoracic epicardial catheter ablation to treat recurrent ventricular tachycardia occurring late after myocardial infarction. *J Am Coll Cardiol* 2000; **35**(6): 1442–1449.
29 Tomassoni G, Stanton M, Richey M, Leonelli FM, Beheiry S, Natale A. Epicardial mapping and radiofrequency catheter

ablation of ischemic ventricular tachycardia using a three-dimensional nonfluoroscopic mapping system. *J Cardiovasc Electrophysiol* 1999; **10**(12): 1643–1648.

30 Lam C, Schweikert R, Kanagaratnam L, Natale A. Radiofrequency ablation of a right atrial appendage-ventricular accessory pathway by transcutaneous epicardial instrumentation. *J Cardiovasc Electrophysiol* 2000; **11**(10): 1170–1173.

31 Saad EB, Marrouche NF, Cole CR, Natale A. Simultaneous epicardial and endocardial mapping of a left-sided posteroseptal accessory pathway associated with a large coronary sinus diverticulum: successful ablation by transection of the diverticulum's neck. *PACE* 2002; **25**(10): 1524–1526.

32 Swarup V, Morton JB, Arruda M, Wilber DJ. Ablation of epicardial macroreentrant ventricular tachycardia associated with idiopathic nonischemic dilated cardiomyopathy by a percutaneous transthoracic approach. *J Cardiovasc Electrophysiol* 2002; **13**(11): 1164–1168.

33 Schweikert RA, Saliba WI, Tomassoni G *et al.* Percutaneous pericardial instrumentation for endo-epicardial mapping of previously failed ablations. *Circulation* 2003; **108**(11): 1329–1335.

34 Koplan BA, Parkash R, Couper G, Stevenson WG. Combined epicardial – endocardial approach to ablation of inappropriate sinus tachycardia. *J Cardiovasc Electrophysiol* 2004; **15**(2): 237–40.

35 de Paola AA, Leite LR, Mesas CE. Nonsurgical transthoracic epicardial ablation for the treatment of a resistant posteroseptal accessory pathway. *PACE* 2004; **27**(2): 259–261.

36 Valderragano M, Cesario DA, Ji S *et al.* Percutaneous epicardial mapping during ablation of difficult accessory pathways as an alternative to cardiac surgery. *Heart Rhythm* 2004; **1**(3): 311–316.

37 Brugada J, Berruezo A, Cuesta A *et al.* Nonsurgical transthoracic epicardial radiofrequency ablation: an alternative in incessant ventricular tachycardia. *J Am Coll Cardiol* 2003; **41**(11): 2036–2043.

38 Soejima K, Stevenson WG, Sapp JL, Selwyn AP, Couper G, Epstein LM. Endocardial and epicardial radiofrequency ablation of ventricular tachycardia associated with dilated cardiomyopathy: the importance of low-voltage scars. *J Am Coll Cardiol* 2004; **43**(10): 1834–1842.

39 Ouyang F, Bansch D, Schaumann A *et al.* Catheter ablation of subepicardial ventricular tachycardia using electroanatomic mapping. *Herz* 2003; **28**(7): 591–597.

40 Ouyang F, Antz M, Deger FT *et al.* An underrecognized subepicardial reentrant ventricular tachycardia attributable to left ventricular aneurysm in patients with normal coronary arteriograms. *Circulation* 2003; **107**(21): 2702–2709.

41 Reddy VY, Neuzil P, Ruskin JN. Extra-ostial pulmonary venous isolation: use of epicardial ablation to eliminate a point of conduction breakthrough. *J Cardiovasc Electrophysiol* 2003; **14**(6): 663–666.

42 Reddy V, Neuzil P, D'Avila A, Kralovec S, Ruskin J. Extra-ostial pulmonary vein isolation: efficacy of epicardial ablation to eliminate points of conduction breakthrough across endocardial lesion sets. *Heart Rhythm* 2004; **1**(1): S203.

43 Kanagaratnam L, Tomassoni G, Schweikert R *et al.* Ventricular tachycardias arising from the aortic sinus of valsalva: an under-recognized variant of left outflow tract ventricular tachycardia. *J Am Coll Cardiol* 2001; **37**(5): 1408–1414.

44 Berruezo A, Mont L, Nava S, Chueca E, Bartholomay E, Brugada J. Electrocardiographic recognition of the epicardial origin of ventricular tachycardias. *Circulation* 2004; **109**(15): 1842–1847.

45 Alchekakie O, Marrouche N, Schweikert R *et al.* Measurement of the QRS width predicts epicardial origin of normal heart ventricular tachycardia. *J Am Coll Cardiol* 2003; **41**(6, Suppl. A): 123A.

46 D'Avila A, Houghtaling C, Gutierrez P *et al.* Catheter ablation of ventricular epicardial tissue: a comparison of standard and cooled-tip radiofrequency energy. *Circulation* 2004; **109**(19): 2363–2369.

47 Madrid AH, Peng J, Nannini S *et al.* Experimental evaluation of epicardial ablation. Comparison of irrigated tip versus standard catheter ablation. *Heart Rhythm* 2004; **1**(1): S173.

48 D'Avila A, Holmvang G, Houghtaling MS *et al.* Focal and linear endocardial and epicardial catheter-based cryoablation of normal and infarcted ventricular tissue. *Heart Rhythm* 2004; **1**(1): S173.

49 Lustgarten D, Bell S, Hardin N, Calame J, Spector P. Safety and efficacy of epicardial cryoablation. *Heart Rhythm* 2004; **1**(1): S143.

50 Sosa E, Scanavacca M, D'Avila A, Antonio J, Ramires F. Nonsurgical transthoracic epicardial approach in patients with ventricular tachycardia and previous cardiac surgery. *J Interv Card Electrophysiol* 2004; **10**(3): 281–288.

51 Soejima K, Couper G, Cooper JM, Sapp JL, Epstein LM, Stevenson WG. Subxiphoid surgical approach for epicardial catheter-based mapping and ablation in patients with prior cardiac surgery or difficult pericardial access. *Circulation* 2004; **110**(10): 1197–1201.

52 D'Avila A, Gutierrez P, Scanavacca M *et al.* Effects of radiofrequency pulses delivered in the vicinity of the coronary arteries: implications for nonsurgical transthoracic epicardial catheter ablation to treat ventricular tachycardia. *PACE* 2002; **25**(10): 1488–1495.

53 Scanavacca M, D'Avila A, Sosa E. Epicardial mapping and ablation to treat sustained ventricular tachycardia. In: Liem LB & Downar E, eds. *Progress in Catheter*

Ablation. Kluwer Academic Publishers, Boston, MA, 2001: 377–387.

54 Zou JG, McGreevy BS, Hummel JP, Whayne JG, Haines DE. Linear ablation with a novel low profile suction ablation electrode. *PACE* 2003; **26**(4, Part II): 954.

55 Zenati MA, Bonanomi G, Chin AK, Schwartzman D. Left heart pacing lead implantation using subxiphoid videopericardioscopy. *J Cardiovasc Electrophysiol* 2003; **14**(9): 949–953.

56 Ayers GM, Rho TH, Ben-David J, Besch HR, Jr., Zipes DP. Amiodarone instilled into the canine pericardial sac migrates transmurally to produce electrophysiologic effects and suppress atrial fibrillation. *J Cardiovasc Electrophysiol* 1996; **7**(8): 713–721.

57 Vereckei A, Gorski JC, Ujhelyi M, Mehra R, Zipes DP. Intrapericardial ibutilide administration fails to terminate pacing-induced sustained atrial fibrillation in dogs. *Cardiovasc Drugs Ther* 2004; **18**(4): 269–277.

58 Laham RJ, Rezaee M, Post M, Xu X, Sellke FW. Intrapericardial administration of basic fibroblast growth factor: myocardial and tissue distribution and comparison with intracoronary and intravenous administration. *Catheter Cardiovasc Interv* 2003; **58**(3): 375–381.

59 Laham RJ, Simons M, Hung D. Subxyphoid access of the normal pericardium: a novel drug delivery technique. *Catheter Cardiovasc Interv* 1999; **47**(1): 109–111.

60 Laham RJ, Hung D, Simons M. Therapeutic myocardial angiogenesis using percutaneous intrapericardial drug delivery. *Clin Cardiol* 1999; **22**(1, Suppl. 1): I6–I9.

61 Tio RA, Grandjean JG, Suurmeijer AJ, van Gilst WH, van Veldhuisen DJ, van Boven AJ. Thoracoscopic monitoring for pericardial application of local drug or gene therapy. *Int J Cardiol* 2002; **82**(2): 117–121.

62 Maisch B, Ristic AD, Seferovic PM, Spodick DH. Intrapericardial treatment of autoreactive myocarditis with triamcinolon. Successful administration in patients with minimal pericardial effusion. *Herz* 2000; **25**(8): 781–786.

63 Rodrigues AC, d'Avila A, Houghtaling C, Ruskin JN, Picard M, Reddy VY. Intrapericardial echocardiography: a novel catheter-based approach to cardiac imaging. *J Am Soc Echocardiogr* 2004; **17**(3): 269–274.

64 Mann DL, Acker MA, Jessup M, Sabbah HN, Starling RC, Kubo SH. Rationale, design, and methods for a pivotal randomized clinical trial for the assessment of a cardiac support device in patients with New York health association class III–IV heart failure. *J Card Fail* 2004; **10**(3): 185–192.

26

CHAPTER 26

Advances in catheter control devices

Girish Narayan, MD, *Paul J. Wang*, MD, & *Amin Al-Ahmad*, MD

Catheter-based ablation procedures are approaching increasingly complex tasks such as pulmonary vein isolation and ventricular tachycardia ablation. In these procedures, catheters must be manipulated to distinct positions, often separated by several millimeters. In addition, catheters are used for the creation of linear lesions over a relatively long distance, which can be complex and challenging. The anatomic locations involved in these procedures can also involve areas of the heart that are not readily accessible via simple advancement through venous or arterial conduits. These types of procedures have highlighted the need for technologies that offer fine control of the catheter tip to facilitate accurate positioning. For example, the tips of catheters must be navigated through tortuous paths in three dimensions. In addition, once in place, the catheters must be held in close contact with the myocardium using a sufficient amount of force in order to achieve transmural lesions. Furthermore, the only access to catheters is from several feet away from the tip. Current technologies provide only limited solutions to these issues.

Current technologies

The mainstay of current electrophysiology catheter manipulation technologies is the pull-wire catheter. These catheters offer a single or double curve that is affected by a pull wire. The radius and plane of curvature is fixed. While catheters of different curvature radii can be selected, it is often cumbersome and expensive to use multiple catheters for the task. Preformed shaped sheaths offer some advantages, especially in providing a local source of stability for the catheter tip in areas that are accessed with multiple bends. However, in some cases where there is considerable anatomic variation, sheaths may not provide a robust solution. In addition, sheaths, while providing increased stability, also restrict movement greatly. Another factor decreasing the ability of the operator to achieve precise positioning of the catheter tip is the lack of 1 : 1 torque transmission to the distal end of the catheter. All of these factors greatly limit the ability of the operator to precisely position and orient the catheter in three-dimensional space. New catheter design ideas, such as catheters that have multiple lumens for pull wires that can then cause the catheter to assume different curves or catheters with a stabilizing element on the distal tip, may have a role in the future [1, 2]. Also catheter designs with multiple flexible curves, that is, catheters that have the ability to change shape may be valuable as well [3, 4].

Newer technologies

Magnetic guidance

Recently, newer technologies have allowed finer manipulation and positioning of catheter tips. Magnetic manipulation systems have been proposed in the literature as early as 1951 where an external magnet was used to deflect the articulated tip of an intravascular catheter [5]. Recent advances and refinement of this strategy has lead to magnetic manipulation and navigation systems that were introduced for primarily neurosurgical and interventional cardiology applications [6]. Recently, a system has become available for electrophysiology application. The NIOBE® system (Steriotaxis, Inc. St Louis, MO) uses external magnetic manipulation of the catheter [7]. The system uses two permanent magnets of 0.15 Tesla field strength positioned on either side of the patient (Figure 26.1). The position and orientation of the magnets are computer controlled, allowing the creation of a unique magnetic vector. The catheters are equipped with a small permanent magnet that aligns itself with this custom magnetic vector. The operator uses the user interface to prescribe the desired orientation of the catheter. The angular resolution of the system is $<1°$. The computer- controlled manipulation of the external magnets typically require from 5 to 20 s. By manipulating the external magnetic vector, the catheter tip can be deflected to a desired orientation. In addition, the catheter can also be advanced along a desired path using a remote drive unit that allows axial advancement or withdrawal of the catheter using a motorized system positioned at the femoral venous entry site. The system can also have several preset instructions that move the magnetic vector in different directions in a set order that allow the catheter to advance to certain anatomic structures that vary only slightly in location between different individuals.

Faddis *et al.* [8] describe the use of an early version of this magnetic navigation system to direct the catheter to preselected sites within the right atrial (RA) and right ventricular (RV) in 20 patients. In addition, they performed sustained ventricular tachycardia mapping in 13 patients, including 4 with accessory pathways. The magnetic navigation system was successfully used to perform radiofrequency (RF) ablation in 7 patients. No procedural complications were noted. They note that the data offers preliminary validation of the safety and feasibility of this system. Their study, however, was not designed to assess whether this system offered any significant benefit over conventional manual manipulation strategies. In fact, they claim that in the majority of the cases, manual manipulation would have worked as well.

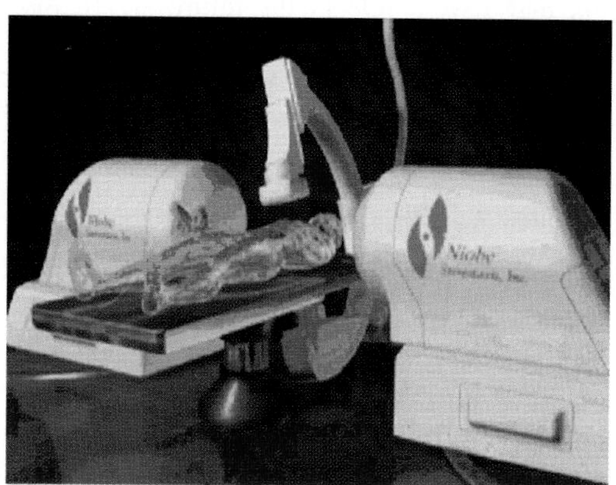

Figure 26.1 The Niobe System. (Reprinted with permission from Steriotaxis Inc.)

Recently, Ernst *et al.* [9] have described their experience with the NIOBE system in performing AVNRT ablation in 42 patients. Notably, they report that after the insertion of the catheters, the entire EP study and ablation procedure were performed from the control room. Slow pathway modification or ablation was performed in all patients using RF ablation with an average fluoroscopy time of 8.9 min and 7 RF applications. They note that there were no recurrences after the ablation procedure [9].

The main advantages that were described in the procedure include the complete elimination of fluoroscopic exposure for the operator. In addition, the system did not cause any complications. Again, the study did not compare traditional catheter manipulation strategies with the novel system. Further studies with more complex ablation procedures would allow a greater degree of differentiation between traditional and magnetic manipulation strategies. Nonetheless, the strategy seems to offer a promising modality of "remote-control" catheter-based ablation in the case of AVNRT.

The system, however, presents areas that require further examination. For example, it requires a large financial commitment with substantial required infrastructural modifications. Furthermore, the technology requires the use of two large magnets in each electrophysiology laboratory, raising issues of space and accommodation.

As this technology develops in the future, integration with more advanced imaging systems and advanced mapping systems may allow full utilization of the fine catheter control and maneuverability of this catheter control system.

Prior authors have suggested using a strategy of guidewire steering within an MR imaging environment. This technique works by passing varying direct currents though three different orthogonally oriented coils within the MR scanner. The catheter tip then experiences a deflecting force as the magnetic vector induced by the coils is different than the magnetic vector of the MR scanner. This causes the tip of the catheter to be deflected to the point where the two vectors are aligned. By changing the current in each of the coils, a unique magnetic vector can be generated facilitating a specific deflection of the catheter tip [10]. The construction of the tip of the catheter does become quite complex, however, especially if ablation capability also needs to be included. The flexibility of such a system is apparent given that separate, large moving magnets are not required. In addition, real-time MR imaging techniques can be employed to permit image guidance during catheter ablation procedures [11]. However, the magnetic environment of conventional MR scanners is at least 10 times larger than that proposed in the magnetic guidance system discussed above. This presents significant technical hurdles in terms of compatibility of RF ablation catheters, guidewires, and other equipment (i.e. displays, etc.) within the immediate vicinity of the scanner.

Emerging technologies

Robotic control systems

Other technologies are also being developed to provide fine catheter control and positioning. Recent advancement in robotics have enabled a multitude of surgical procedures, including many minimally invasive cardiac procedures, to be performed by remotely controlled robotic manipulators. The advantages of such a platform theoretically include oversight of surgical hand motion (i.e. reduction of tremor, limitation of translation, etc.), operative intervention via extremely small portals, and decreased overall patient recovery time [12]. This strategy is currently being explored for catheter-based procedures.

Initial studies have demonstrated the utility of using this strategy for catheter manipulation tasks within an *ex vivo* specimen [13]. The system employs a robotically controlled guide catheter through which any conventional catheter can be inserted. The guide catheter is controlled via a computer system that is directed by the operators. In recent experiments, the ability of the system to maneuver the tip of conventional catheters to desired locations was compared against traditional means. The two strategies were compared on time and precision based on eight different targets (high RA, RA free-wall, RA septum, RA appendage, RV septum, LA appendage, mitral valve annulus, and pulmonary vein ostium). The new strategy significantly reduced the time needed for navigation (6.1 s versus 22 s for the conventional strategy). Overall the system promises to offer a compact strategy for three-dimensional positioning of a catheter tip within the heart. In addition, the remote manipulation strategy promises to decrease fluoroscopy time and operator fatigue (Figure 26.2).

Further work has focused on *in vivo* settings. The same catheter control system was placed via a femoral vein into the heart in six healthy swine. The ability to navigate to five prespecified right-sided locations (high right atrium, superior vena cava, RA septum, atrial septal fossa, tricuspid valve annulus) was evaluated using fluoroscopic and intracardiac echo visualization. The system was also evaluated for navigation to four prespecified left-sided locations (LA appendage, mitral valve, pulmonary veins, left ventricle) via a transseptal puncture. The control technology successfully navigated to 28 of 30 (93%) right-sided locations and 20 of 24 (83%) left-sided locations in under 5 min of initiation. Navigation of a robotically controlled remote catheter control system in the beating heart to clinical relevant targets appears feasible and safe. Further study in humans is currently underway and aims to evaluate the utility of this technology for complex ablations. As this technology develops, integration with electroanatomical mapping systems as well as advanced imaging systems may increase the utility of remote robotic catheter control system.

Experimental technologies

Electroactive polymers

The recent advent of polymers with an electroactive reaction with substantial displacements has opened the possibilities of creating highly flexible,

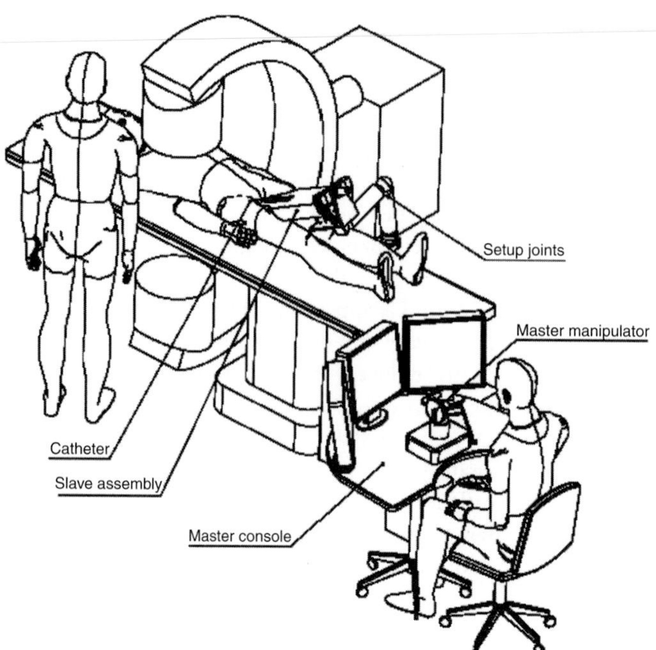

Figure 26.2 Early prototype system of robotic catheter control system. (Reprinted with permission from Hansen Medical.)

low density, strong structures that can be used for a variety of purposes including catheter manipulation. These electroactive polymers offer considerable promise for precision manipulation tasks. These polymers adopt varying configurations (i.e. either a relaxed or contracted state) depending on the administration of voltage. By combining polymers, one can create a structure that can adopt a variety of curvatures. Various configurations can be combined to allow precise control of a catheter tip [14].

However, while the latest generation polymers demonstrate substantial displacements and actuation strains, these still fall short in terms of meeting the requirements for robust clinical application. The current limitations of electroactive polymers include the low catheter deflection force achievable with currently available polymers. In addition, current control systems are nonlinear in their response, making feedback control, especially while maintaining multiple curves, an inherently difficult problem. Nonetheless, these technologies offer promise for offering a convenient, highly flexible and modular approach for precise catheter control that can be easily integrated in existing catheterization labs without the requirement for large infrastructure modification. Improvements in these areas will likely provide an important, flexible, and compact alternative catheter manipulation technology.

References

1 Gibson C, Seang H. Steerable catheter Patent 6783510, in United States Patent and Trademark Office. 1999, C. R. Bard, Inc., USA.

2 Gambale RA, Forcucci SJ, Shah CB, Weiser MF, Forde S. Catheter positioning systems Patent 06629987, in United States Patent and Trademark Office. 2003, C. R. Bard, Inc., USA.

3 Chen P. de la Rama A. Ablation catheter with multiple flexable curves Patent 5782828, in United States Patent and Trademark Office. 1996, Irvine Biomedical, Inc., USA.

4 Maitland DJ, Lee AP, Schumann DL, Matthews DL, Decker DE, Jungreis CA. Shape memory polymer actuator and catheter Patent 6740094, in United States Patent and Trademark Office. 2001, The Regents of the University of California, USA.

5 Tillander H. Magnetic guidance of a catheter with articulated steel tip. *Acta Radiol* 1951; **35**: 62–64.

6 Grady MS, Howard MA 3rd, Dacey RG Jr. Experimental study of the magnetic stereotaxis system for catheter manipulation within the brain. *J Neurosurg* 2000; **93**(2): 282–288.

7 Faddis MN, Blume W, Finney J. Novel, magnetically guided catheter for endocardial mapping and radiofrequency catheter ablation. *Circulation* 2002; **106**(23): 2980–2985.

8 Faddis MN, Chen J, Osborn J, Talcott M, Cain ME, Lindsay BD. Magnetic guidance system for cardiac electrophysiology: a prospective trial of safety and efficacy in humans. *J Am Coll Cardiol* 2003; **42**(11): 1952–1958.

9 Ernst S, Ouyang F, Linder C, *et al.* Initial experience with remote catheter ablation using a novel magnetic navigation system: magnetic remote catheter ablation. *Circulation* 2004; **109**(12): 1472–1475.

10 Roberts TP, Hassenzahl WV, Hetts SW, Arenson RL. Remote control of catheter tip deflection: an opportunity for interventional MRI. *Magn Reson Med* 2002; **48**(6): 1091–1095.

11 Kerr AB, Pauly JM, Hu BS *et al.* Real-time interactive MRI on a conventional scanner. [Erratum appears in *Magn Reson Med* 1998; **40**(6): 952–955.] *Magn Reson Med* 1997; **38**(3): 355–367.

12 Lanfranco AR, Castellanos AE, Desai JP, Meyers WC. Robotic surgery: a current perspective. *Ann Surg* 2004; **239**(1): 14–21.

13 Al-Ahmad A, Grossman JD, Wang PJ. Early experience with a computer driven robotically assisted sterable catheter system. *Heart Rhythm* 2004, Poster Sessions, Moscone 134–135.

14 Bar-Cohen Y. Transition of EAP material from novelty to practical applications – are we there yet? Proceedings of EAPAD, SPIE's 8th Annual International Symposium on Smart Structures and Materials, 5–8 March, 2001, Newport, CA. Paper No. 4329–02.

27

CHAPTER 27

Advances in energy sources in catheter ablation

David E. Haines, MD

Introduction

Catheter ablation has evolved into one of the most successful modes of antiarrhythmic therapy. In each case, the goal of ablation is to irreversibly modify or destroy a specific anatomical substrate that is required for arrhythmia propagation. In order to achieve that goal, the mechanism of the arrhythmia must be understood so that the optimal ablation target is known. Then the ablation catheter must approximate the target of ablation. Finally, the ablative lesion must incorporate the targeted substrate. The technology of catheter ablation has progressed greatly on all fronts. In the early days of catheter ablation, 4 mm tip catheters and a radiofrequency energy source were employed. The resultant lesions were relatively small. This apparent limitation had a beneficial effect on the development of the field because it forced operators to map the arrhythmia origin with a high degree of accuracy, and drove industry to create better catheter delivery systems. The small lesions limited collateral damage and therefore were a factor in the low complication rate of the procedure and its high acceptance among patients and physicians. As the indications for catheter ablation have expanded beyond superficial targets, such as accessory pathways and slow atrioventricular (AV) nodal pathways, the need for deeper and larger lesion formation has increased. With larger lesions, there is the anticipated increased risk of increased collateral damage with increased complication rate. Therefore, the challenge with new ablation technologies is to create large but precise lesions, to optimize the efficiency, safety, and success of the ablation procedure.

Many new technologies have been proposed to achieve these goals. The most common mechanism of myocardial ablation is with hyperthermic sources. The entire span of the electromagnetic spectrum has been tested regarding its ability to heat the myocardium (Figure 27.1). Mechanical energy in the form of ultrasound is a promising hyperthermic approach. Conversely, removal of heat with cryothermic ablation may offer unique advantages over the hyperthermic techniques. The following review will discuss the theoretical and practical advantages and disadvantages of each new technology. Until the technologies are tested in the clinical setting, however, their unique place in the management of patients with symptomatic arrhythmias will not be defined.

Mechanisms of myocardial injury

The goal of catheter ablation is to irreversibly damage or destroy myocardium. Ideally, this should be easily titrated and produce a discrete lesion boundary. The initial approach to catheter ablation employed high voltage D.C. shocks. The mechanism of injury to the cell was a combination of electrical injury and barotrauma. This mode of ablation was difficult to control and resulted in a wide range of depth of injury with a high prevalence of arrhythmia recurrence. It was soon replaced by radiofrequency catheter ablation.

Radiofrequency catheter ablation accomplishes myocardial injury by tissue heating. The radiofrequency electrical current creates a narrow rim of direct resistive heating in the tissue closest to the electrode. The heat generated by resistive heating

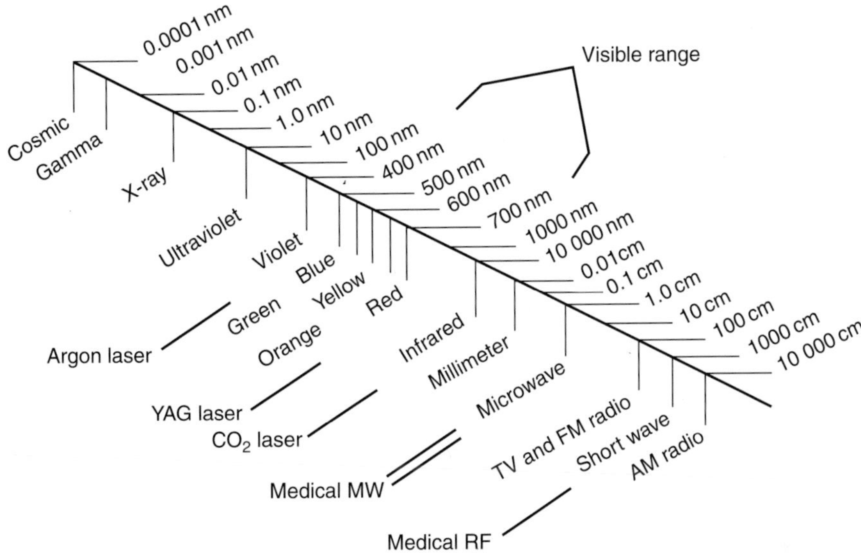

Figure 27.1 A schematic of the electromagnetic wave spectrum is shown, along with the common forms of electromagnetic energies used in catheter ablation.

then conducts thermally to deeper tissue layers. The radial temperature gradient reaches its peak 0–4 mm from the endocardial surface then falls off steadily with increasing distance from the heat source, eventually returning to the basal temperature [1]. No matter what the energy source, hyperthermic ablation modalities, such as microwave, laser, and ultrasound, follow similar principles. Different energy forms will result in different depths of volume heating. The temperature of tissues surrounding the ablation source is dependent upon the source temperature, size of the heat source (i.e. the radius of volume-heated tissue) [2], distance from the source, and duration of heating. The temperature boundary (isotherm) for irreversible myocardial injury from hyperthermic ablation has been reported as ~50–52°C [3]. Thus, one can predict the size and geometry of ablative lesions by mapping the final tissue temperature profile at the end of the ablation. Tissue temperatures and lesion size increase in direct proportion to the source temperature and radius of the heat source. The temperature falls in an inverse proportion to the distance from the heat source [1]. The lesion size increases over time in a monoexponential fashion. A small radius ablation source has a short half time of lesion growth (8–10 s), but as volume heating increases, the rate of lesion growth slows. In general, however, a steady-state radial tissue temperature gradient and stable lesion size is approached at 1 min with conventional radiofrequency catheter ablation and within 2 min for larger lesion technologies [4, 5].

A number of pathophysiological effects occur in myocardium in response to hyperthermia. Most notably, the cells begin to depolarize in the moderate hyperthermic range of 45–50°C. They show evidence of abnormal automaticity and reversible loss of excitability. Above 50°C, the cells depolarize further, become unexcitable, and show evidence of cell contracture and death (Figure 27.2) [6]. In tissue preparations, the effect of hyperthermia on conduction velocity parallels the findings of depolarization seen in the cellular recordings [7]. It has been hypothesized that cellular injury and death observed with hyperthermia is mediated by calcium overload. With increasing temperature, an increase in cytosolic calcium can be measured. At temperatures below 50°C, the magnitude of increased cytosolic free calcium is modest unless the buffering mechanisms of the cell preventing calcium overload are blocked. At temperatures above 50°C, the cells are overwhelmed and injury occurs. When myocytes are exposed to hyperthermic conditions in the presence of calcium channel blockers, depolarization and calcium overload are

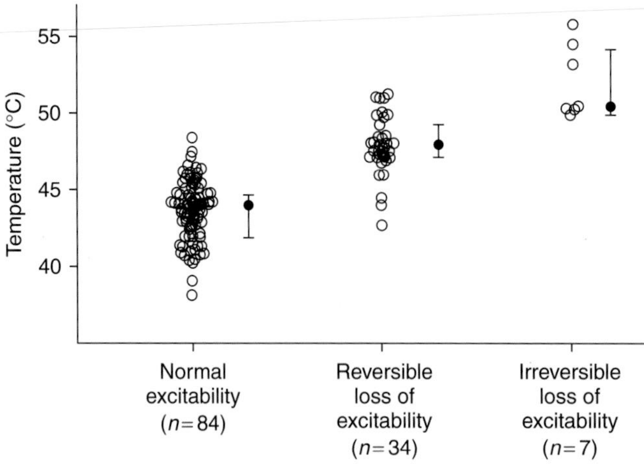

Figure 27.2 Response of an isolated guinea pig papillary muscle to field stimulation during hyperthermic exposure at varying temperatures. Normal excitability was seen in the low hyperthermic range, reversible effects in the intermediate range, and irreversible loss of excitability (consistent with cell death) at temperatures above 50°C. (Reprinted from *Circulation* [6], with permission.)

not prevented. Therefore, these phenomena do not appear to be channel specific. It is hypothesized that hyperthermia causes nonspecific poration of the sarcolemmal membrane, allowing unregulated passage of ions that result in further depolarization, calcium overload, cell contracture, and death [6, 8]. Observations of morphological changes in the cell after hyperthermic exposure are consistent with this hypothesis. The ultrastructural changes described include disruption of the plasma membrane, gap junctions, and microvasculature [9, 10].

Aside from hyperthermia, the only other mechanisms of tissue injury employed in catheter ablation are freezing with cryothermic ablation, and a combination of electrical and mechanical (barotrauma) injury with direct current shock ablation. Shock ablation is very difficult to control, and was associated with significant complications such as perforation. For that reason, the procedure is no longer performed and is of historical interest only. Cryothermic catheter ablation is unique compared with the hyperthermic techniques since tissue injury depends on the formation of an ice ball. As the temperature is lowered, a crystal ice lattice forms within the cell, disrupting the cytoskeleton and other critical subcellular components. The critical temperature for irreversible injury is −40°C. A faster rate of cooling will increase the magnitude of intracellular destruction. An extracellular ice matrix forms as well, and disrupts the sarcolemmal membrane. A secondary phase of cellular injury occurs during the thawing process [11]. The thermodynamics of cryothermic ablation are analogous to hyperthermic ablation as lesion formation is both time and temperature dependent. A colder source temperature results in a deeper penetration of the freezing temperature (Figure 27.3). Convective heating from the circulating blood pool opposes the cooling effect of the ablation catheter. The ice ball and lesion size continue to grow over time at a slower rate than that seen with hyperthermic ablation technologies. Therefore, the recommended duration of cryoablation is 4 min [12].

Cooled-tip radiofrequency ablation

Conventional radiofrequency catheter ablation is limited by the fact that temperatures exceeding 100°C result in boiling of blood with formation of coagulated blood proteins known as coagulum. This coagulum is electrically insulating, and with its rapid accumulation and adherence to the electrode tip, a sudden rise in electrical impedance and fall off in delivered power will be observed. If, however, the electrode tip is actively cooled by saline perfusion in either a closed or open system, more radiofrequency power can be delivered without exceeding a 100°C electrode–tissue interface temperature. As a result, the depth of volume heating can be significantly increased. This results in a larger virtual heat source and a significantly deeper and wider lesion (Figure 27.3) [13]. Active-electrode-tip cooling is useful when there is good energy coupling of the ablation catheter to the tissue. If the majority of energy is being dissipated with passive electrode cooling by the circulating blood pool, then additional active-tip cooling may decrease ablation efficiency to the point where tissue heating is limited and

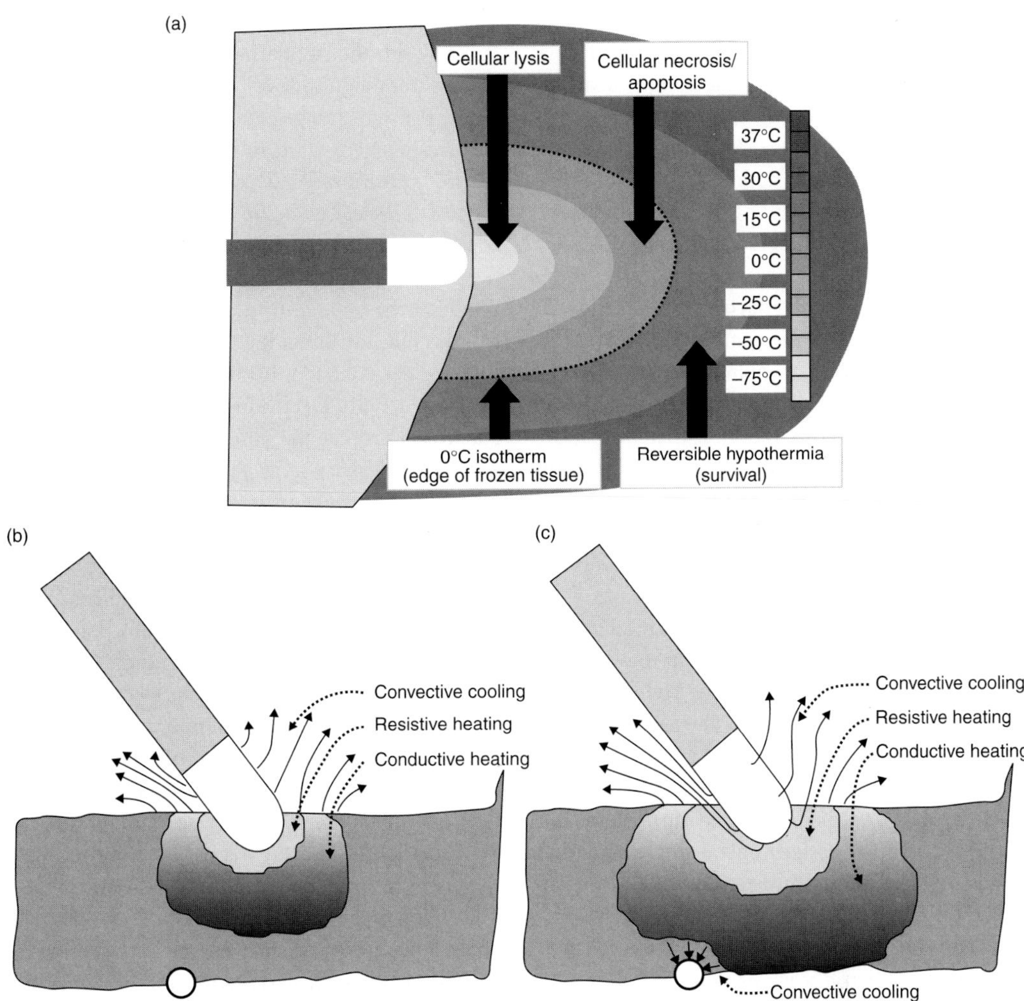

Figure 27.3 Schematic representation of cryothermic catheter ablation demonstrating the different biological effects seen at different isotherms. Schematic demonstrating the thermodynamics of radiofrequency catheter ablation with a standard catheter (top panel) versus a high-power ablation with a perfused-tip catheter. The tip perfusion results in greater convective cooling at the electrode–tissue interface. This in turn allows deeper volume heating without exceeding a surface temperature of 100°C.

lesion size is inadequate. The goal, therefore, is to work to achieve excellent electrode– tissue contact in order to assure that a high proportion of the radiofrequency energy is dissipated as heat within the myocardium. Because the peak tissue temperature may occur below the endocardial surface, intramyocardial temperatures can exceed 100°C resulting in sudden steam pops and possible crater formation or perforation. Caution must therefore be exercised to limit power and surface temperature to avoid excessive tissue heating.

The introduction of active radiofrequency ablation catheter cooling had a significant positive effect on achieving ablation efficacy with difficult arrhythmia substrates such as atrial flutter and ventricular tachycardia. Studies have demonstrated the superiority of cooled-tip catheters over conventional catheters in atrial flutter ablation. A retrospective nonrandomized trial compared ablation with standard 4 mm tip radiofrequency ablation catheters versus cooled radiofrequency ablation catheters. The authors found that patients treated with the cooled-tip technology required shorter fluoroscopy and procedure times, had a higher acute success rate (93% versus 80%), and a lower late recurrence rate (10% versus 26%) than those treated with noncooled radiofrequency ablation [14]. A prospective randomized trial employed an irrigated-tip catheter and achieved 100% block of the TV-IVC isthmus whereas success rate with a conventional 4 mm tip catheter was 85% before crossover. In addition, procedure time was reduced with tip cooling [15]. No increased procedural risk was observed with the cooled-tip technologies. Similar observations have been reported with ventricular tachycardia ablation. A trial of 66 patients with ventricular tachycardia due to prior myocardial infarction examined the efficacy of cooled-tip radiofrequency ablation versus standard radiofrequency catheter ablation. When ablation was performed at a critical isthmus (defined by entrainment mapping) with mid-diastolic potentials, the cooled-tip ablation terminated tachycardia in 89% of cases compared with 54% with conventional ablation ($p = .003$) [16].

To date, prospective randomized clinical studies have not compared closed cooled-tip to open irrigated-tip radiofrequency ablation. The theoretical advantages of the closed-tip system are that infusion of volume and risk of introduction of air into left-sided ablations are eliminated. The possible advantages of the open irrigated-tip systems are that it is a simpler design (only a single perfusion line is required in the catheter body), and the tip irrigation may reduce the risk of coagulum accumulation on the electrode tip. However, it is unknown whether efficacy or safety is better with one or another design.

Large-tip and multiple electrode radiofrequency ablation

It has been demonstrated that lesion size is proportional to the radius of the electrode during radiofrequency catheter ablation [2] because a larger contact surface area of the electrode to the tissue allows for greater power to be delivered. Power density (the main determinant of tissue heating) is distributed around the active electrode surface. The total power delivered for any given power density, therefore, is proportional to the electrode surface area. Therefore, larger electrode size allows higher power delivery, more volume of direct tissue heating and larger lesions. A secondary phenomenon is passive electrode cooling. As described above, tip cooling also allows for higher power delivery. A greater electrode surface area in contact with the circulating blood pool may result in a greater magnitude of convective cooling by the blood. A disadvantage of large electrode tips is that electrical current tends to cluster at points of geometric transition. As a result, current density is highest at the electrode tip and proximal edge. The edge effect results in non-uniform heating along the electrode length (Figure 27.4) [17]. The other disadvantage of large-tip electrodes is that in order to take full advantage of the increased electrode surface area, contact must be maintained along the electrode length. Electrode-tip orientation is difficult to control in the clinical setting, and hence much of the extra energy passed into the large electrode tip may just be dissipated into the circulating blood pool. Use of intracardiac echocardiography may be useful to optimize tip orientation [18].

In order to minimize edge effect and maximize ablation length, multiple electrode ablation arrays have been tested with varying efficacy. All linear electrodes depend upon excellent electrode–tissue contact, and various means for optimizing that contact have been tested [19]. If radiofrequency energy is delivered in a bipolar fashion between contiguous electrodes, then the current passes through the tissue superficially. If energy is passed from multiple electrodes in a unipolar fashion to a dispersive electrode, then gaps in ablation between electrodes may occur. Since radiofrequency energy is an alternating current, an intermediate shift in phases of the current between contiguous electrodes can result in a blend of bipolar and unipolar energy delivery. Phased radiofrequency ablation has been proposed

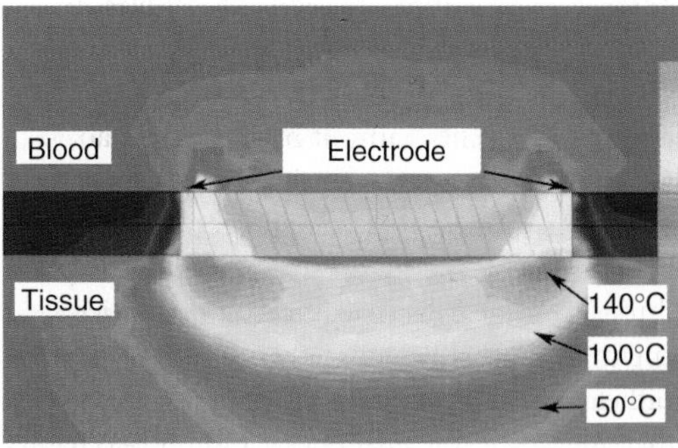

Figure 27.4 Finite element analysis of radiofrequency catheter ablation with a long electrode applied tangentially to the tissue. Because there is increased heating at points of sudden geometric transition (the edge effect), nonuniform heating is observed along the length of the catheter.

as one method of creating long, large, and deep radiofrequency ablation lesions. Other investigators have developed multiple electrode catheters in a variety of orientations to target specific sites such as pulmonary vein ostia. One such catheter employs multiple electrodes in a mesh that deploys in a circumferential fashion engaging a cuff of atrium at the base of the pulmonary vein. A single energy delivery to the electrode array can effectively create an encircling lesion around the vein [20].

Large-tip electrodes coupled with high output radiofrequency generators have proven to be effective in a wide number of clinical settings. One trial tested ablation of atrial flutter with an 8 mm tip catheter compared with a conventional 4 mm tip catheter. The group treated with the large tip had a 92% initial success rate before crossover versus a 67% success rate for the conventional electrode tip. TV-IVC isthmus block was reached significantly faster (24 ± 15 versus 31 ± 12, $p < .05$) [21]. Other groups have confirmed this observation, showing higher acute procedure success rates with 8 mm tip catheters (100%) versus the standard 4 mm tip variety (93%) [22]. However, the larger tip size results in less consistent tissue contact and therefore may increase technical difficulty of the procedure in some cases [23].

Microwave ablation

Like radiofrequency ablation, microwave ablation is a hyperthermic ablation technology that employs a form of electromagnetic energy for tissue heating. However, the mechanism of heating differs in that microwave energy oscillates at much higher frequencies and causes motion of dipoles in the medium (water) converting electrical energy to kinetic energy (heat). Therefore, microwave catheter ablation is another form of hyperthermic ablation, and the same biological principles of myocardial injury observed with radiofrequency ablation apply [3]. In contrast to radiofrequency energy that passes through tissue like any electrical current, microwave energy is radiated into tissue from an antenna catheter. Because microwave energy is radiated, the theoretical depth of energy penetration into the tissue should be greater [24, 25]. This depth of penetration depends upon lossiness of the tissue (the tendency to dissipate microwave energy as heat) and the microwave frequency selected. Of the two frequencies approved for medical applications, 915 MHz should yield a greater penetration depth than 2450 MHz, although a greater dissipation of energy along the transmission line with higher frequencies may negate this advantage [3]. The near-field patterns of microwave energy deposition in tissue are complex and complex antenna designs, such as helical coils and wave guides, have been a challenge to apply to the ablation setting. However, *in vitro* testing with selected coil designs has shown promise [26]. *In vivo* studies of ventricular ablation with microwave energy resulted in lesions averaging 8.8 mm in depth with a 44% prevalence of transmural lesion formation [27].

Transvenous intracardiac microwave catheter ablation has not been tested in the clinical setting. Microwave energy has been used successfully in the intraoperative setting for the treatment of atrial fibrillation. A modified maze lesion set was created with a hand-held microwave probe in 90 patients after open thoracotomy. Lesions were successfully created with with a mean microwave ablation time of 13 ± 5 min. Sinus rhythm was restored in 74% of patients at 6 months ($n = 35$) and in 67% of patients at 1 year ($n = 27$) [28, 29]. Another surgical trial randomized patients undergoing open-heart surgical procedures to intraoperative linear atrial ablation with a hand-held microwave probe coupled with atrial size reduction ($n = 24$) or to medical therapy with amiodarone or sotalol ($n = 19$). At 12 months, 80% of the ablation group was in sinus rhythm compared with only 33% of the medically treated cohort [30].

Laser ablation

Laser energy has shown great promise but limited practical application in the field of catheter ablation. Laser light energy heats tissue with optical heating. The depth of volume heating (skin depth) is determined by the frequency of the laser irradiation. High-frequency laser light such as excimer laser (wavelength 157–351 nm) has a very superficial skin depth and ablates with superficial vaporization of tissue in close apposition to the laser source. Low-frequency laser light such as 1.06 μm neodymium-YAG has a greater depth of volume heating, and with an adequate duration of energy delivery can result in very large lesions. More recently, inexpensive solid state diode laser generators radiating at 805 nm have become available, and may allow for more widespread testing and adoption of this technology. High-amplitude laser irradiation can be easily transmitted through flexible fiber optics and is therefore well suited for delivery tools with small diameters. However, it is dissipated by blood and therefore requires close contact of the fiberoptic to the tissue. Another disadvantage of laser catheter ablation is that it is highly directional. This results in a narrow beam of heating at the endocardial surface. The light scatters as it passes through tissue and produces a broader lesion at deeper layers. The classic flask-shaped lesion observed with laser catheter ablation is not effective in many arrhythmic substrates since the subendocardium is most often the myocardial layer that is the source of the arrhythmia. In order to address this limitation, diffusers have been attached to the terminus of ablation catheters to spread the laser beam and distribute the photonic energy over a larger endocardial surface area.

One laser ablation catheter design successfully employed a longitudinal diffuser to create long linear lesions *in vivo* [31]. Another design used an extendable fiber-optic diffuser element that was designed to puncture into the myocardium. Intramural diode laser irradiation was able to create reliable intramural lesions [32]. Laser irradiation has been explored for circumferential ablation of pulmonary veins in canine preparations. An occlusive fluid-filled balloon can be placed in the pulmonary vein ostium, and laser irradiation accomplished by circumferential diffuser or by ring fiber tips. Vein isolation was achieved in one study with 30–50 W of Nd : YAG irradiation for 60–90 s. However, successful isolation with this design is dependent upon close contact of the balloon wall to the vein wall [33, 34]. A new laser balloon ablation catheter design employs a similar mode of circumferential laser irradiation from a diode laser source, but reflects the light forward to achieve a ring of laser irradiation around the base of the vein. Initial testing of this device in 19 open chest goats yielded successful electrical pulmonary vein isolation in 19 of 27 (70%) veins ablated. However, use of real-time reflectance spectroscopy monitoring to assess blanching of the endocardium and optimize the balloon placement and orientation increased acute success rate to 5 of 5 (100%) (Figure 27.5) [35].

Clinical data regarding laser photocoagulation for the treatment of arrhythmias is very scarce. As a proof of concept, laser irradiation has been employed intraoperatively for ablation of ventricular tachycardia. One series reported successful ablation of 38 tachycardias in 20 patients with coronary artery disease using a 15 W argon laser and limited subendocardial resection [36]. Another study employed Nd-YAG laser for epicardial ablation of ventricular tachycardia without ventriculotomy in patients with prior infarction. Most scar locations were on the inferior wall, which is difficult to approach with surgical resection without disruption of the submitral apparatus. Tachycardias were terminated in all patients and 86% remained free of ventricular tachycardia during long-term follow-up [37]. Catheter ablation with laser energy sources has been limited to one small study that tested a unique end-fire laser catheter that employs a strut structure at its terminus to allow the laser beam to spread. A pilot series of 10 patients with AV nodal reentrant tachycardia

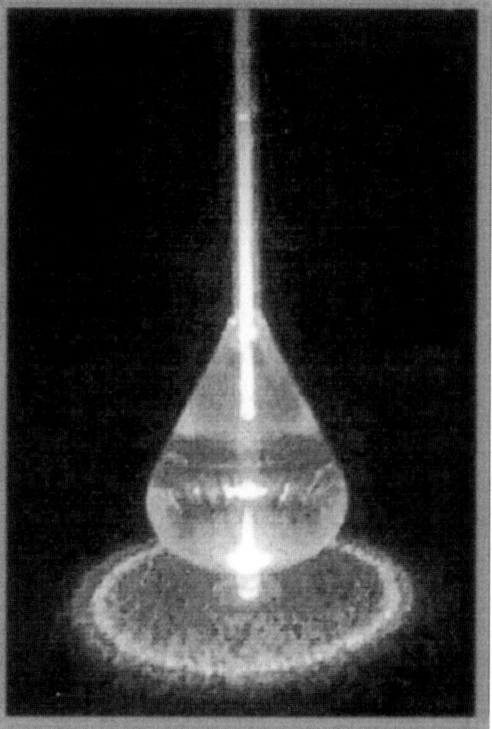

Figure 27.5 Laser balloon catheter prototype designed for circumferential ablation of the pulmonary vein orifice. The laser irradiation is directed laterally, then reflected forward in a circular pattern. (Reprinted from *PACE* [35], with permission.)

reported successful arrhythmia ablation with a mean of 2.2 laser pulses per patient. No complications or late arrhythmia recurrences were observed [38].

Other electromagnetic energy sources for ablation

Innovative technologies have been tested for catheter ablation. Utilizing electromagnetic energy at a frequency between conventional radiofrequency and microwave, Satake *et al.* tested ablation with a 13.56 MHz current passed from a coil electrode into a balloon electrode that was 5–10 mm greater in diameter than the vein ostium. Power was adjusted to maintain temperature within the balloon between 60°C and 75°C. Successful superior pulmonary vein isolation was achieved in 39 of 40 veins. During a mean clinical follow-up of 8 months, 17 of 20 patients were free from arrhythmia recurrence [39]. On the other extreme of the electromagnetic wave spectrum, pulmonary vein ablation has been attempted experimentally with beta irradiation. An encapsulated P-32 beta radiation source was inserted into the central lumen of a balloon catheter placed in the pulmonary veins of experimental animals. A radiation dose of 40, 50, or 60 Gy was administered to the vein wall. Higher dose lesions resulted in a 75% rate of lesion formation, but technical difficulties in balloon centering and consistent dose delivery translated into a low rate of circumferential vein isolation [40].

Ultrasound ablation

Within an ultrasound transducer, alternating current induces high-frequency oscillation of a piezoelectric crystal thereby converting electromagnetic energy into mechanical energy. The ultrasound waves, in turn, transmit the mechanical energy through the medium. Of the energy passes, some is reflected and some is absorbed by the tissue medium. The mechanical energy that is absorbed is converted to kinetic energy in the tissue underlying in tissue heating. Unlike diagnostic ultrasound, the power is delivered continuously at high amplitude in order to achieve tissue heating. A significant theoretical advantage of ultrasound heating is that there is a 10 : 1 tissue to blood energy absorption ratio. Ultrasound energy can be transmitted through the blood pool with minimal attenuation before being dissipated in the tissue. Thus, close catheter–tissue contact is not required for tissue heating. The depth of energy dissipation is dependent upon the frequency of the ultrasound. Lower-frequency energy will have deep penetration whereas higher-frequency energy will yield more superficial heating. The mechanism of tissue injury is thermal, similar to the other hyperthermic technologies. Like other hyperthermic approaches, tissue heating with ultrasound ablation is opposed by tissue cooling from convection by the circulating blood flow. Because deep tissue heating can be achieved with ultrasound energy, an anomalous phenomenon can arise where the mid-myocardium is ablated, but the endocardium is spared.

Catheter ablation with ultrasound energy has been tested with two specialized tools for the treatment of atrial fibrillation. An ultrasound balloon catheter was developed that employed a cylindrical piezoelectric crystal with a central resonating chamber that delivers therapeutic ultrasound circumferentially. When the balloon is filled with saline and occludes a pulmonary vein, the energy passes through the saline with little energy dissipation and a rim of pulmonary vein tissue contacting the balloon wall is heated. In a pilot clinical study, treatment of atrial fibrillation by pulmonary vein ablation was attempted with the ultrasound balloon catheter in 15 patients. The operators had difficulty with catheter placement in the right inferior pulmonary vein, so only three veins were ablated in 14 patients. Despite the face that this design was intended to ablate the entire vein with a single energy delivery, between 3 and 39 energy deliveries (mean 14.7 ± 12.6) were administered per patient. Short-term follow-up showed a procedure success rate of 66% [41]. Comparable outcomes were achieved with a similar balloon ultrasound ablation catheter in another pilot study of nine patients with paroxysmal atrial fibrillation [42]. Failure analysis suggested that failure of the balloon to completely occlude the vein resulted in regions of convective cooling and inadequate vein wall heating. Variability of venous anatomy, with early branching, and irregular ostia, contributed to these technical failures. A novel type of ultrasound energy delivery for pulmonary vein isolation has been developed that employs a balloon-within-balloon design with an inner saline-filled balloon and an outer gas-filled balloon. Ultrasound energy is delivered circumferentially and is reflected off of the saline–gas interface resulting in a forward

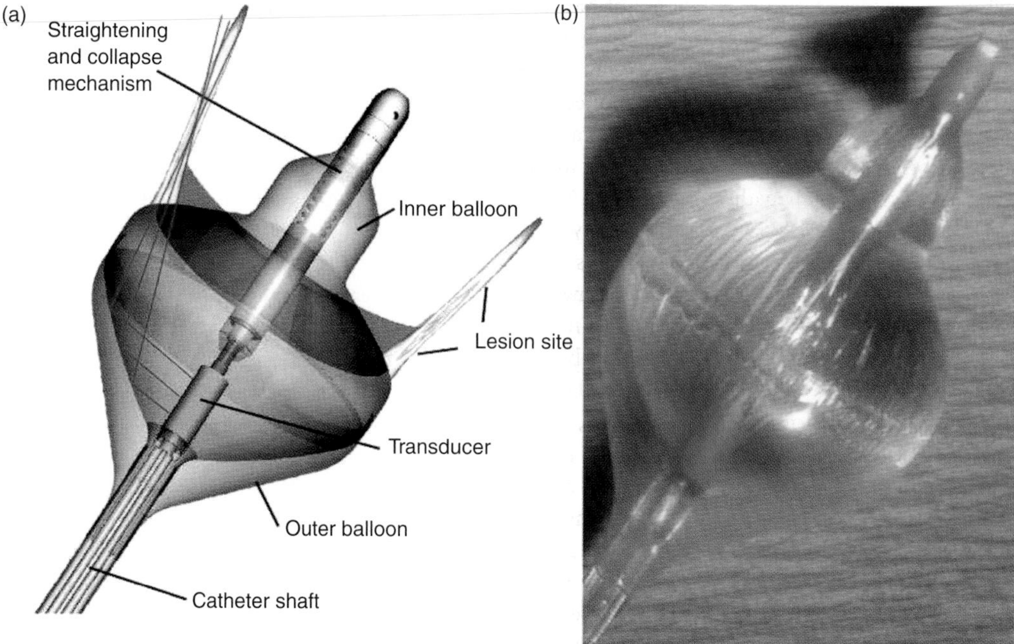

Figure 27.6 (a) Schematic representation and (b) photograph of prototype of a high-intensity focused ultrasound ablation catheter for circumferential ablation of the pulmonary vein ostia. The ultrasound energy is directed in a circumferential fashion. The double balloon design allows the energy to be transmitted with minimal loss through saline in the inner balloon, but then reflects the energy forward at the transition to the outer balloon, which is air filled. The curvature of the fluid–gas interface is hyperbolic, resulting in a focused ultrasound beam at a prescribed depth. (Reprinted from *J Interv Card Electrophysiol* [43], with permission.)

focused ultrasound beam in a ring pattern (Figure 27.6). Like all balloon technologies, successful encirclement of the vein was dependent upon optimal balloon seating and orientation [43].

Cryothermic ablation

Cryothermy has been an important adjunctive ablative technology since the origin of surgical ablation of arrhythmic substrates. As myocardium is frozen, an intracellular ice crystal matrix forms and disrupts the microtubule cytoskeleton. The extracellular ice matrix disrupts the sarcolemmal membrane. Cell injury occurs during both freezing and thawing phases. The time course of tissue injury in response to cryothermic ablation is slow with approach of the steady-state lesion size after 5 min or more [12]. Conventional ablation has been tested with 4, 6, or 8 mm tip cryothermic ablation catheters. The catheter tips are cooled to −70°C or below by gaseous expansion of liquid nitrous oxide. In comparison to radiofrequency catheter ablation *in vivo*, the cryo-lesions tended to be smaller in volume and surface area. However, catheter ablation with cryothermy did result in a significant reduction in the incidence of thrombus (30% versus 76%, $p = .0005$) and thrombus volume 1 week postablation [44]. Linear ablation in the cavo-tricuspid isthmus was able to effect isthmus conduction block in a canine study. Pathology at 6 weeks demonstrated continuous and transmural lesions [45].

Cryothermic ablation allows the operator to test the safety and efficacy of ablation at specific ablation sites with cryomapping. The catheter is first slowly cooled to −30°C at which point electrophysiological effects are fully reversible. If the desired ablation effect is observed, therapeutic cyrothermy can be applied with rapid catheter cooling to −70°C. Conversely, if an adverse effect such as heart block is observed, the catheter can be rewarmed with reliable resolution of conduction block. With tip freezing, the catheter adheres to the tissue. This is advantageous because the catheter will not be displaced during ablation, but has the disadvantage of preventing active mapping with a roving catheter during ongoing ablation. Slow AV nodal pathway ablation was attempted in 18 patients with AV nodal reentrant tachycardia. Success was achieved in 94% [46]. A similar study reported successful slow pathway ablation in 31 of 32 patients [47]. Gaita *et al.* tested the safety and efficacy of cryothermic ablation in 20 patients with para-Hisian or midseptal accessory pathways. Ablation was successful in all patients with a mean of 1.2 cryo-applications per patient. No heart block was observed. However, accessory pathway conduction recurred in four patients (20%), and repeat ablation was required [48]. Friedman *et al.* reported the overall efficacy of cryothermic ablation in 164 patients with AV nodal reentrant tachycardia, AV reciprocating tachycardia or atrial fibrillation requiring AV junctional ablation. They observed that if the ablation target was successful identified by cryomapping, acute ablation success was 94%, but if mapping was unsuccessful, success rate dropped to 67% [49]. An advantage of cryothermic ablation over hyperthermic methods is that it is relatively painless. When cryothermic catheter ablation was compared with radiofrequency catheter ablation for the treatment of atrial flutter in a small series of 14 patients, only 1 of 7 patients perceived pain with cryothermy compared with 7 of 7 receiving radiofrequency therapy [50].

One of the promising applications of cryothermic ablation is pulmonary vein isolation for the treatment of atrial fibrillation. Pulmonary vein isolation with radiofrequency energy may be complicated by pulmonary vein stenosis. In addition, point-by-point circumferential ablation around the pulmonary vein with conventional radiofrequency ablation catheters is laborious and time consuming. New cryoablation tools are being tested to encircle the pulmonary vein with a single or limited number of ablative lesions. One cryoablation catheter design is a linear ablation catheter that ablates the base of the pulmonary vein with an expanding loop [51]. Another promising design employs a balloon catheter that expands at the orifice of the vein. Refrigerant is introduced into the balloon, and the entire expanded balloon acts as the cryoablation source. This effectively created circumferential conduction block in all ablated veins in all experimental animals. The finding of hemoptysis in all animals postablation showed evidence of collateral damage of the lung parenchyma. This was confirmed at pathological examination. The veins were effectively isolated by both electrophysiological and anatomical criteria [52]. Balloon cryoablation of pulmonary veins is an emerging technology that may improve efficacy and decrease procedure time with pulmonary vein isolation procedures. As with all balloon-based ablation technologies, the limiting factor of this approach will likely be successful balloon seating at the pulmonary vein–left atrial junction. Any persisting blood flow around the balloon will certainly diminish the efficacy of circumferential tissue freezing.

Conclusion

Catheter ablation has been a successful modality for the curative treatment of arrhythmias for the past two decades. The goal of catheter ablation is to create controlled destruction of an adequate volume of tissue to capture the arrhythmogenic substrate. For most arrhythmias, conventional radiofrequency ablation is very safe and highly effective. Catheter ablation with all technologies balances the risk of the procedure with the anticipated benefits. Excellent targeting, enhanced by new three-dimensional, allows the operator to achieve procedural success in most cases with a small, discrete lesion. Some ablation cases are limited by difficult targeting, unstable catheter positioning or large/deep arrhythmogenic anatomical substrates. Unfortunately, all technologies that result in large lesions are limited by controllability and may increase procedure risk. The balance must be achieved between large lesions with an increased risk of significant collateral damage and small lesions with diminished efficacy. New ablation technologies including new energy sources or new catheter designs may be useful for ablation of difficult targets including pulmonary veins or substrates for ventricular tachycardia.

References

1 Haines DE, Watson DD. Tissue heating during radiofrequency catheter ablation: a thermodynamic model and observations in isolated perfused and superfused canine right ventricular free wall. *PACE* 1989; **12**(6): 962–976.

2 Haines DE, Watson DD, Verow AF. Electrode radius predicts lesion radius during radiofrequency energy heating. Validation of a proposed thermodynamic model. *Circ Rese* 1990; **67**(1): 124–912.

3 Whayne JG, Nath S, Haines DE. Microwave catheter ablation of myocardium in vitro. Assessment of the characteristics of tissue heating and injury. *Circulation* 1994; **89**(5): 2390–2395.

4 Haines DE. Determinants of lesion size during radiofrequency catheter ablation: the role of electrode tissue contact pressure and duration of energy delivery. *J Cardiovasc Electrophysiol* 1991; **2**: 509–515.

5 Wittkampf FH, Simmers TA, Hauer RN, Robles De Medina EO. Myocardial temperature response during radiofrequency catheter ablation. *PACE* 1995; **18**(2): 307–317.

6 Nath S, Lynch C III, Whayne JG, Haines DE. Cellular electrophysiological effects of hyperthermia on isolated guinea pig papillary muscle. Implications for catheter ablation. *Circulation* 1993; **88**(4 Pt 1): 1826–1831.

7 Simmers TA, de Bakker JM, Wittkampf FH, Hauer RN. Effects of heating on impulse propagation in superfused canine myocardium. *J Am Coll Cardiol* 1995; **25**(6): 1457–1464.

8 Everett TH, Nath S, Lynch C III, Beach JM, Whayne JG, Haines DE. Role of calcium in acute hyperthermic myocardial injury. *J Cardiovasc Electrophysiol* 2001; **12**(5): 563–569.

9 Nath S, Redick JA, Whayne JG, Haines DE. Ultrastructural observations in the myocardium beyond the region of acute coagulation necrosis following radiofrequency catheter ablation. *J Cardiovasc Electrophysiol* 1994; **5**(10): 838–845.

10 Nath S, Whayne JG, Kaul S, Goodman NC, Jayaweera AR, Haines DE. Effects of radiofrequency catheter ablation on regional myocardial blood flow. Possible mechanism for late electrophysiological outcome. *Circulation* 1994; **89**(6): 2667–2672.

11 Skanes AC, Klein GJ, Krahn AD, Yee R. Advances in energy delivery. *Coron Artery Dis* 2003; **14**(1): 15–23.

12 Matsudaira K, Nakagawa H, Yamanashi WS *et al.* Effect of application time on catheter cryoablation lesion size. *Circulation* 2004; **102**: II–526.

13 Nakagawa H, Yamanashi WS, Pitha JV *et al.* Comparison of *in vivo* tissue temperature profile and lesion geometry for radiofrequency ablation with a saline-irrigated electrode versus temperature control in a canine thigh muscle preparation. *Circulation* 1995; **91**(8): 2264–2273.

14 Spitzer SG, Karolyi L, Rammler C, Otto T. Primary closed cooled tip ablation of typical atrial flutter in comparison to conventional radiofrequency ablation. *Europace* 2002; **4**(3): 265–271.

15 Jais P, Haissaguerre M, Shah DC *et al.* Successful irrigated-tip catheter ablation of atrial flutter resistant to conventional radiofrequency ablation. *Circulation* 1998; **98**(9): 835–838.

16 Soejima K, Delacretaz E, Suzuki M *et al.* Saline-cooled versus standard radiofrequency catheter ablation for infarct-related ventricular tachycardias. *Circulation* 2001; **103**(14): 1858–1862.

17 McRury ID, Mitchell MA, Panescu D, Haines DE. Nonuniform heating during radiofrequency ablation with long electrodes: monitoring the edge effect. *Circulation* 1997; **96**: 4057–4064.

18 Chan RC, Johnson SB, Seward JB, Packer DL. The effect of ablation electrode length and catheter tip to endocardial orientation on radiofrequency lesion size in the canine right atrium. *PACE* 2002; **25**(1): 4–13.

19 Avitall B, Urbonas A, Millard S, Urboniene D, Helms R. Ablation of atrial fibrillation in the rapid pacing canine model using a multi-electrode loop catheter. *J Am Coll Cardiol* 2001; **37**(6): 1733–1740.

20 Arruda M, Wilber DJ, Nakagawa H *et al.* A multicenter pre-clinical safety study using a single mesh catheter for mapping and radiofrequency delivery: a simplified approach to pulmonary vein isolation. *Heart Rhythm* 2004; **1**(1): s171.

21 Tsai CF, Tai CT, Yu WC *et al.* Is 8-mm more effective than 4-mm tip electrode catheter for ablation of typical atrial flutter? *Circulation* 1999; **100**(7): 768–771.

22 Kasai A, Anselme F, Teo WS, Cribier A, Saoudi N. Comparison of effectiveness of an 8-mm versus a 4-mm tip electrode catheter for radiofrequency ablation of typical atrial flutter. *Am J Cardiol* 2000; **86**(9): 1029–1032, A10.

23 Rodriguez LM, Nabar A, Timmermans C, Wellens HJ. Comparison of results of an 8-mm split-tip versus a 4-mm tip ablation catheter to perform radiofrequency ablation of type I atrial flutter. *Am J Cardiol* 2000; **85**(1): 109–112, A9.

24 Keane D, Ruskin J, Norris N, Chapelon PA, Berube D. *In vitro* and *in vivo* evaluation of the thermal patterns and lesions of catheter ablation with a microwave monopole antenna. *J Interv Card Electrophysiol* 2004; **10**(2): 111–119.

25 Erdogan A, Grumbrecht S, Neumann T, Neuzner J, Pitschner HF. Microwave, irrigated, pulsed, or conventional radiofrequency energy source: which energy source for which catheter ablation? *PACE* 2003; **26**(1 Pt 2): 504–506.

26 VanderBrink BA, Gu Z, Rodriguez V *et al.* Microwave ablation using a spiral antenna design in a porcine thigh muscle preparation: *in vivo* assessment of temperature profile and lesion geometry. *J Cardiovasc Electrophysiol* 2000; **11**(2): 193–198.

27 VanderBrink BA, Gilbride C, Aronovitz MJ *et al.* Safety and efficacy of a steerable temperature monitoring microwave catheter system for ventricular myocardial ablation. *J Cardiovasc Electrophysiol* 2000; **11**(3): 305–310.

28 Knaut M, Tugtekin SM, Spitzer S, Gulielmos V. Combined atrial fibrillation and mitral valve surgery using microwave technology. *Semin Thorac Cardiovasc Surg* 2002; **14**(3): 226–231.

29 Knaut M, Spitzer SG, Karolyi L *et al.* Intraoperative microwave ablation for curative treatment of atrial fibrillation in open heart surgery – the MICRO-STAF and MICRO-PASS pilot trial. MICROwave application in surgical treatment of atrial fibrillation. MICROwave application for the treatment of atrial fibrillation in bypass-surgery. *Thorac Cardiovasc Surg* 1999; **47**(Suppl 3): 379–384.

30 Schuetz A, Schulze CJ, Sarvanakis KK *et al.* Surgical treatment of permanent atrial fibrillation using microwave energy ablation: a prospective randomized clinical trial. *Eur J Cardiothorac Surg* 2003; **24**(4): 475–480; discussion 480.

31 Fried NM, Lardo AC, Berger RD, Calkins H, Halperin HR. Linear lesions in myocardium created by Nd : YAG laser using diffusing optical fibers: *in vitro* and *in vivo* results. *Lasers Surg Medi* 2000; **27**(4): 295–304.

32 Ware DL, Boor P, Yang C, Gowda A, Grady JJ, Motamedi M. Slow intramural heating with diffused laser light: a unique method for deep myocardial coagulation. *Circulation* 1999; **99**(12): 1630–1636.

33 Fried NM, Tsitlik A, Rent KC *et al.* Laser ablation of the pulmonary veins by using a fiberoptic balloon catheter: implications for treatment of paroxysmal atrial fibrillation. *Lasers Surg Med* 2001; **28**(3): 197–203.

34 Lemery R, Veinot JP, Tang AS *et al.* Fiberoptic balloon catheter ablation of pulmonary vein ostia in pigs using photonic energy delivery with diode laser. *PACE* 2002; **25**(1): 32–36.

35 Reddy VY, Houghtaling C, Fallon J *et al.* Use of a diode laser balloon ablation catheter to generate circumferential pulmonary venous lesions in an open-thoracotomy caprine model. *PACE* 2004; **27**(1): 52–57.

36 Saksena S, Gielchinsky I, Tullo NG. Argon laser ablation of malignant ventricular tachycardia associated with coronary artery disease. *Am J Cardiol* 1989; **64**(19): 1298–1304.

37 Pfeiffer D, Moosdorf R, Svenson RH *et al.* Epicardial neodymium. YAG laser photocoagulation of ventricular tachycardia without ventriculotomy in patients after myocardial infarction. *Circulation* 1996; **94**(12): 3221–3225.

38 Weber HP, Kaltenbrunner W, Heinze A, Steinbach K. Laser catheter coagulation of atrial myocardium for ablation of atrioventricular nodal reentrant tachycardia. First clinical experience. *Eur Heart J* 1997; **18**(3): 487–495.

39 Satake S, Tanaka K, Saito S *et al.* Usefulness of a new radiofrequency thermal balloon catheter for pulmonary vein isolation: a new device for treatment of atrial fibrillation. *J Cardiovasc Electrophysiol* 2003; **14**(6): 609–615.

40 Mangrum JM, Sih H, Molloy J *et al.* Beta radiation for pulmonary vein isolation. *Circulation* 2002; **106**: II-631.

41 Natale A, Pisano E, Shewchik J *et al.* First human experience with pulmonary vein isolation using a through-the-balloon circumferential ultrasound ablation system for recurrent atrial fibrillation. *Circulation* 2000; **102**(16): 1879–1882.

42 Wang JA, Sun Y, He H. Ultrasound ablation of pulmonary veins for treatment of paroxysmal atrial fibrillation. *J Zhejiang Univ (Sci)* 2003; **4**(6): 745–748.

43 Meininger GR, Calkins H, Lickfett L *et al.* Initial experience with a novel focused ultrasound ablation system for ring ablation outside the pulmonary vein. *J Interv Card Electrophysiol* 2003; **8**(2): 141–148.

44 Khairy P, Chauvet P, Lehmann J *et al.* Lower incidence of thrombus formation with cryoenergy versus radiofrequency catheter ablation. *Circulation* 2003; **107**(15): 2045–2050.

45 Timmermans C, Rodriguez LM, Van Suylen RJ *et al.* Catheter-based cryoablation produces permanent bidirectional cavotricuspid isthmus conduction block in dogs. *J Interv Card Electrophysiol* 2002; **7**(2): 149–155.

46 Skanes AC, Dubuc M, Klein GJ *et al.* Cryothermal ablation of the slow pathway for the elimination of atrioventricular nodal reentrant tachycardia. *Circulation* 2000; **102**(23): 2856–2860.

47 Riccardi R, Gaita F, Caponi D *et al.* Percutaneous catheter cryothermal ablation of atrioventricular nodal reentrant tachycardia: efficacy and safety of a new ablation technique. *Italian Heart J: Off J Italian Fed Cardiol* 2003; **4**(1): 35–43.

48 Gaita F, Haissaguerre M, Giustetto C *et al.* Safety and efficacy of cryoablation of accessory pathways adjacent to the normal conduction system. *J Cardiovasc Electrophysiol* 2003; **14**(8): 825–829.

49 Friedman PA, Dubuc M, Green MS *et al.* Catheter cryoablation of supraventricular tachycardia: results of the multicenter prospective "frosty" trial. *Heart Rhythm* 2004; **1**: 129–138.

50 Timmermans C, Ayers GM, Crijns HJ, Rodriguez LM. Randomized study comparing radiofrequency ablation with cryoablation for the treatment of atrial flutter with emphasis on pain perception. *Circulation* 2003; **107**(9): 1250–1252.

51 Wong T, Markides V, Peters NS, Wright AR, Davies DW. Percutaneous isolation of multiple pulmonary veins using an expandable circular cryoablation catheter. *PACE* 2004; **27**(4): 551–554.

52 Avitall B, Urboniene D, Rozmus G, Lafontaine D, Helms R, Urbonas A. New cryotechnology for electrical isolation of the pulmonary veins. *J Cardiovasc Electrophysiol* 2003; **14**(3): 281–286.

53 Meininger GR, Calkins H, Lickfett L *et al.* Initial experience with a novel focused ultrasound ablation system for ring ablation outside the pulmonary vein. *J Interv Card Electrophysiol* 2003; **8**(2): 141–148.

28

CHAPTER 28

New ablation paradigms: Anatomic ablation of complex arrhythmia substrates

David J. Callans, MD

Introduction

The initial strategies for selection of ablation targets focused entirely on electrophysiologic mapping: analysis of electrogram timing and response to pacing maneuvers. Catheter mapping was guided exclusively by fluoroscopy and the operator's "mind's eye." The governing principle was that ablation at a single site critical to arrhythmia maintenance would result in success. This strategy remains useful for most simple arrhythmia syndromes. However, viewing ablation targets in a more anatomic perspective has significantly improved ablation of complex arrhythmia substrates. The first example of this paradigm switch was atrial flutter. Mapping and ablation of a single site within the "zone of slow conduction" was supplanted by linear ablation of the anatomy necessary for arrhythmia maintenance, the cavotricuspid isthmus, resulting in a simpler, more effective procedure [1, 2].

Targeting the anatomic substrate responsible for arrhythmia syndromes has allowed ablation of clinical arrhythmias that were essentially impossible with conventional electrophysiologic mapping. Electrophysiologic mapping facilitated ablation of well-tolerated ventricular tachycardia (VT) in patients with structural heart disease; substrate-based ablation of the infarct anatomy extended the efficacy of ablation to patients with poorly tolerated uniform VT. Further concentration on the anatomy dictating the location of specific arrhythmia triggers (pulmonary vein (PV) triggers for atrial fibrillation (AF), Purkinje triggers for polymorphic VT), allowed ablation of nonuniform arrhythmias, where electrophysiologic mapping is not possible. More complete understanding of the relationship of electrophysiologic and anatomic substrate may well help to extend these initial advances. Often advances in this understanding have been fostered by new imaging techniques that link cardiac anatomy to the electrophysiologic data acquired by catheter mapping. Three-dimensional mapping systems (e.g. CARTO, Biosense Webster; NAVEX and EnSite, Endocardial Solutions) that allow reconstruction of anatomic "casts" of the chamber being mapped, the use of preprocedural cardiac MRI or CT images can be integrated into these systems, and intracardiac echocardiography (ICE) all have developing applications for increasing our capacity for anatomic ablation.

The purpose of this chapter is to explore recent developments in new anatomic ablation paradigms for the ablation of complex arrhythmia substrates. These new paradigms add anatomic constructs to augment, rather than replace, electrophysiologic mapping principles. Examples of advances in cardiac mapping systems and cardiac imaging that facilitate this paradigm switch will also be discussed.

Substrate ablation for VT

The development of electrophysiologic catheter mapping techniques for ablation of VT in healed infarction in the early 1990s produced modestly successful ablation procedures in a well-defined subset of patients [3–6]. These techniques involved detailed mapping during VT, searching for sites with mid-diastolic potentials that could be proven to be within protected isthmuses with entrainment mapping. Electrophysiologic mapping techniques require that the clinical VT is reproducibly inducible, sufficiently well tolerated to permit prolonged mapping and stable (i.e. does not change morphology or accelerate) during pacing techniques. Some estimated that these preconditions limited the patients eligible for ablation to ~10% of patients with VT [3]. However, even in this subset of patients with clinically well-tolerated VT referred for catheter ablation, inability to induce or tolerate the clinical VT morphology prevented successful ablation in 41% during the initial procedure using an intention to treat analysis [7].

Experience from surgical ablation of VT in healed infarction demonstrated the obligate relationship of the VT circuit and the anatomic substrate of the infarct border zone. Subendocardial resection resulted in freedom from arrhythmia recurrence in >90% of patients that survived surgery [8]. There were significant obstacles encountered in replicating surgical ablation with catheter techniques. First, as direct visualization of the infarct was not possible (as it was from the surgeon's viewpoint), imaging techniques to represent the infarct anatomy were developed. Endocardial voltage mapping using electroanatomic mapping during sinus rhythm was validated as an accurate representation of the infarct substrate by statistical analysis of normal right ventricular (RV) and left ventricular (LV) bipolar electrograms [9], direct observation in a porcine model of VT [10], and comparison with nuclear perfusion imaging (Figure 28.1). Confluent sites with bipolar electrogram amplitude of ≤0.5 mV represent dense scar; areas with electrograms between 0.5 and 1.5 mV represent the infarct border zone. Second, subendocardial resection removed 5–8 cm^2 of infarct substrate; the amount of substrate modification possible with current catheter ablation technology is orders of magnitude less. Linear lesions constructed of individual point RF lesions represented the closest approximation possible in the EP laboratory. The "anchors" of these linear lesion sets was the anatomy of the infarct and the presumed exit site of the VT circuit, as approximated by pace mapping to match the 12 ECG morphology of the targeted VTs (Figure 28.1). Single point ablation guided by analysis of individual electrograms during sinus rhythm or pace mapping has proven insufficient to guide VT ablation; ablation of regions of the border zone mapped during sinus rhythm can successfully interrupt individual VT circuits. This is the final difference between surgical- and catheter-based substrate ablation. Removal of the subendocardial scar conceptually resulted in destruction of essentially all present and future circuits (although additional VT foci were located at sites adjacent to the infarct and treated with cryoablation). Linear lesions are directed to the exit site of

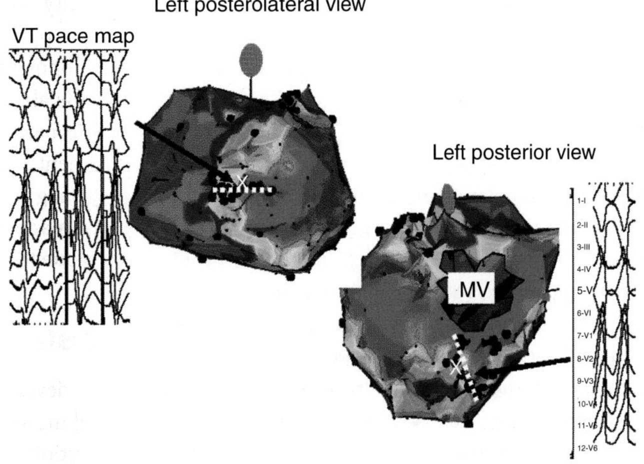

Figure 28.1 Substrate mapping for ablation of unstable VT. Electroanatomic voltage mapping in a patient with an inferior infarction and VT. Endocardial mapping is performed in sinus rhythm to construct a voltage map of the infarct (color code: purple ≥ 1.7 mV, red ≤ 0.5 mV). Pace mapping is performed to approximate exit sites in the infarct border zone; the sites for pace mapping are selected by analysis of 12 lead ECGs VT morphologies. Linear lesions are delivered from the dense scar out to normal myocardium through the exit site for each specific VT morphology.

Table 28.1 Steps for substrate ablation of unmappable VT using electroanatomic mapping.

Create endocardial voltage map in sinus rhythm (>100 points/chamber).
Programmed stimulation to capture 12 lead ECG of all clinically pertinent VT morphologies (if not available from spontaneous events).
Pace map at border zone of substrate to determine VT exit site = site of best pace map match.
Linear ablation from dense scar out to normal tissue passing through each identified exit site.

each specific VT morphology. Table 28.1 lists the procedural steps for substrate-based VT ablation.

The initial experience with this technique included 16 patients with drug-refractory, unmappable VT. Nine patients had healed infarction, seven had predominantly RV cardiomyopathy with endocardial scarring (see below). Prior to ablation, patients had experienced 6–55 episodes of VT/month, resulting in frequent implantable cardioverter defibrillator (ICD) shocks. Delivery of a median of 55 radiofrequency (RF) lesions to construct 4 linear lesions (each linear lesion through the exit site of a specific VT morphology) resulted in successful arrhythmia control in all but one patient over 8 month mean follow-up [9]. More extensive follow-up in a larger and more diverse patient population (53 patients with healed infarction, RV cardiomyopathy, and idiopathic LV cardiomyopathy) demonstrated freedom from any arrhythmia recurrence in 60% and infrequent VT recurrence in 25% [11]. Other investigators have modified the anatomic approach, extending linear lesions between "islands" of unexcitable segments within the infarct [12] or interrupting relatively high-voltage "channels" of preferential conduction [13]. Preliminary data suggests that similar functional channels of preferential conduction through the infarct may be identified during sinus rhythm or pacing within the infarct using noncontact mapping. Presumably this approach may be helpful in predicting areas critical for maintenance of VT circuits prior to initiation of VT. All of these strategies explore the relationship of various sites within the construct of the infarct anatomy, rather than the electrophysiologic characteristics of single sites. All depend greatly on three-dimensional mapping systems, to allow visualization of the infarct substrate as well as the interrelationship of individual RF applications to construct linear lesions.

Another paradigm shift that this new technique allowed was extension of substrate ablation techniques to patients with unmappable VT in clinical settings less well understood than healed infarction. Electrophysiologic mapping has been successful in patients with arrhythmogenic RV cardiomyopathy/dysplasia [14]. Nonetheless, VT is often unmappable because of the multiplicity of morphologies that interchange during pacing techniques. In 18 patients with RV cardiomyopathy and recurrent VT, electrophysiologic mapping and focal ablation was possible in only 3 patients. Endocardial mapping during sinus rhythm identified scars extending from the tricuspid and/or pulmonic valves; VT sites of origin were identified within these sites using limited activation mapping or pace mapping. Linear lesions extending through each VT circuit to the anatomic barrier of the valve plane prevented recurrent VT in 16/18 patients (mean 27 month follow-up) [15]. The pathophysiology of uniform VT in the setting of nonischemic cardiomyopathy is incompletely understood. However, qualitatively similar though quantitatively less endocardial scar, typically surrounding the mitral annulus, can be identified by electroanatomic mapping and serves as the foundation for anatomic ablation of VT in this setting [16]. More of the substrate may be identified with epicardial mapping in patients with dilated cardiomyopathy and VT, and anatomic ablation may be more successful using this approach [17].

Semianatomic approach to ablation of polymorphic VT

Electrophysiologic mapping techniques cannot be applied to localization of nonuniform arrhythmias such as polymorphic VT. Haissaguerre *et al.* demonstrated that premature ventricular beats from relatively predictable anatomic locations may serve as the initiating events in patients with idiopathic ventricular fibrillation (VF). In a series of 27 patients, many of whom demonstrated "electrical storm" of frequent premature ventricular contractions (PVCs) and runs of VF clustered within several days, distinct initiating beats could be identified in 24. These originated from the RV outflow

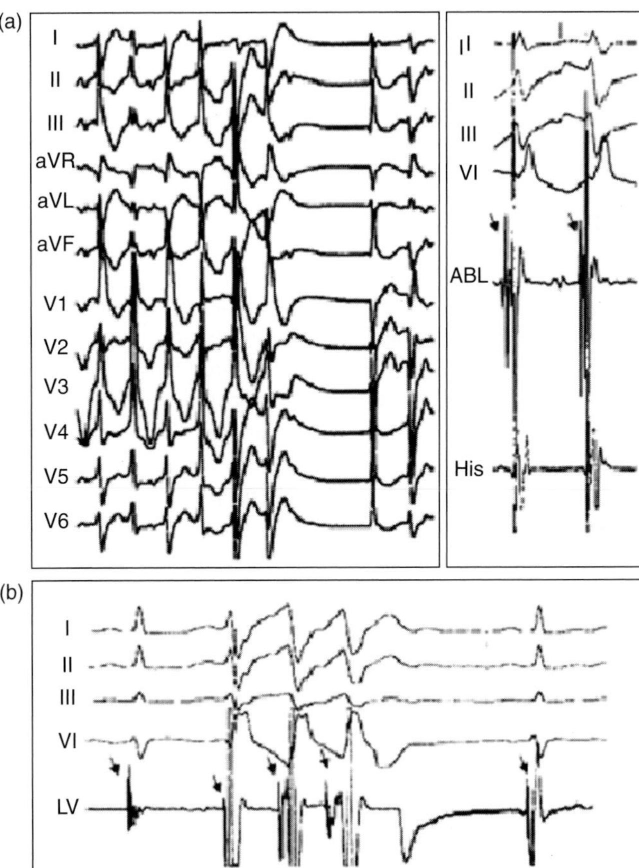

Figure 28.2 Top tracing: Holter monitor strip recording an episode of idiopathic VF. Note that the episode is "triggered" by a uniform initiating beat (different in morphology than the isolated premature beat earlier in the tracing). Bottom tracing: surface and intracardiac recordings during a run of premature beats originating from the Purkinje system in the same patient. Each QRS complex is slightly different in morphology, and is preceded by a Purkinje potential (arrow) with subtle changes in the Purkinje–ventricular interval. (Reprinted from *Circulation* [18], with permission.)

tract ($n = 4$), or the peripheral Purkinje system (right ventricle in seven, left ventricle in nine, and both ventricles in four patients). When initiating beats that arose from the Purkinje system, individual beats often had variable morphologies and Purkinje–ventricular intervals (Figure 28.2). The three patients without premature beats during electrophysiologic study were considered to have Purkinje beats based on ECG characteristics during spontaneous episodes. Ablation at these sites resulted in freedom from recurrent VF in 24 of 27 patients. Three patients had late recurrence of identical PVC triggers that had previously been ablated leading to recurrent VF; all three were managed with antiarrhythmic drugs. Although traditional electrophysiologic mapping is helpful in determining ablation targets in this experience, the realization that triggering beats arise from predictable anatomic sources (particularly the Purkinje system) greatly facilitated this experience, particularly given the changing morphology of the initiating beats.

This experience has been extended to patients with Brugada syndrome and long QT syndrome [19]. In seven patients, RV outflow tract or Purkinje system ventricular beats triggered polymorphic VT in these disease processes as well. Even more variability in Purkinje–ventricular interval (30–110 ms during premature beats) was observed in this series. Ablation was targeted to the site of earliest activation during premature beats, but particularly in patients with Purkinje-system triggers, an anatomic area of the Purkinje-system rather than a single site of origin was ablated. Ablation prevented recurrent polymorphic VT in all patients, although one patient had persistent premature beats. These investigators have reported similar Purkinje-system triggers in selected patients with structural heart disease with polymorphic ventricular arrhythmias. It is possible that Purkinje-system triggers are important in the genesis of nonuniform ventricular arrhythmias in all clinical settings; certainly this hypothesis requires further investigation.

Anatomic ablation of AF

Historical arguments regarding the nature of AF aside, AF is the ultimate chaotic arrhythmia and a purely electrophysiologic approach cannot support successful ablation. The initial surgical ablation for AF, the Maze procedure, was entirely anatomic. The incisions of the Maze procedure divided the atrium into sufficiently small spaces that the meandering wavelets could not successfully propagate. With a few notable exceptions, attempts at recapitulation of the surgical experience with catheter ablation were unsuccessful [20]. More recently two distinct anatomic approaches to AF ablation have been developed: PV isolation (which is partially guided by anatomy, partially electrophysiologic recordings) and left atrial substrate ablation.

Although several investigators reported isolated cases of ablation of a focal site firing rapidly that resulted in cure of AF, it was the seminal observations of the Bordeaux group that recognized the importance of PV triggers in patients without structural heart disease and frequent AF episodes [21]. Initially, ablation of these triggers, even with the "hint" of their anatomic location, required painstaking electrophysiologic mapping for point ablation of specific sites; this mapping was difficult because the frequency of the triggers was variable, and initiation of AF was frequent, interrupting mapping. In addition, even after successful ablation recurrence (development of a new trigger site) and PV stenosis frequently complicated the clinical course. Because triggering atrial premature beats originated primarily from atrialized segments several centimeters from the PV ostium, the Bordeaux group made the approach more anatomic by ablating the electrical connections of the PV to the atrium rather than single site ablation of the triggers [22]. Many new techniques have assisted visualization of the complex PV anatomy to assist in this largely anatomic ablation: venography, multipolar electrode circular mapping catheters, nonfluoroscopic navigation systems with or without preprocedural computed tomography or MR imaging integration, and ICE (Figure 28.3). Accurate visualization of the anatomy of the PV ostium has markedly reduced the incidence of PV stenosis after ablation. Although harder to directly evaluate, better understanding of PV–atrial anatomy has lead to better ablation success, as the pulmonary venous atrium can be more completely isolated. In a series of patients with recurrent AF after PV isolation, Gerstenfeld *et al.* [23] observed that triggers arose from segments proximal within ablated PVs in 11%; greater experience in intracardiac echo imaging guidance has significantly reduced this phenomenon. A more frequent limitation in PV isolation is recurrent conduction following ablation. In another series, 77% of patients with recurrent AF had APD triggers that arose from previously ablated but reconnected PVs [24]. More powerful ablation catheters, such as 8 mm tip or cooled-tip catheters may decrease the incidence of PV electrical reconnection [25].

Left atrial substrate ablation represents an even more completely anatomic approach to ablation

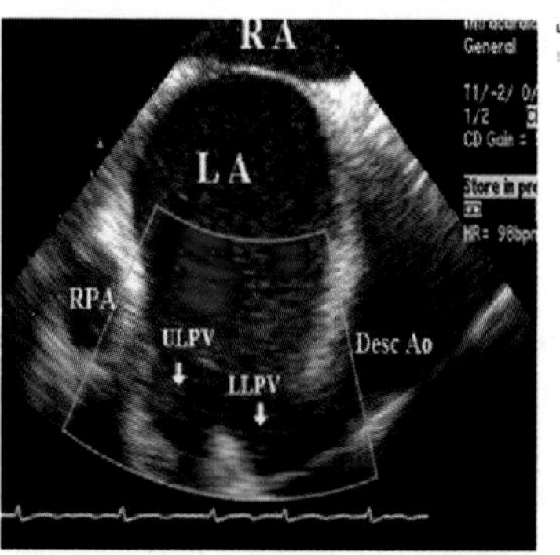

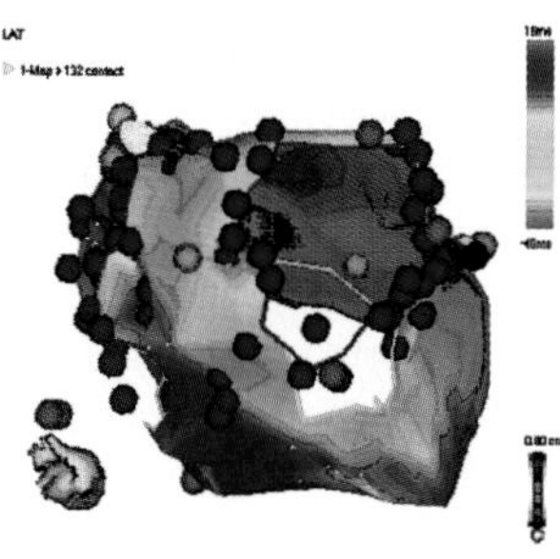

Figure 28.3 "Multimedia imaging" for PV isolation. In addition to multipolar electrogram recordings from the PVs, the ablation strategy for AF incorporates ICE imaging and three-dimensional mapping. The ICE image (left) demonstrates the view of the left PVs from an ultrasound catheter positioned in the right atrium at the level of the fossa ovalis. Typically, the left superior and inferior PVs leave the atrium from a common antrum. Electroanatomic mapping (right) shows the lesions delivered for segmental isolation of the left common PV.

Table 28.2 Possible mechanisms for the effect of left atrial substrate ablation.

Reduction in functional atrial size.
PV isolation or change in the ability of PV triggers to conduct to the atrium.
Elimination of anchor points for rotors or mother waves in the posterior venous atrium
Ablation of the ligament of Marshall
Autonomic denervation

of AF. This technique relies on circumferential ablation of the PVs without electrophysiologic mapping guidance or verification of PV isolation. Substrate ablation is typically guided by three-dimensional mapping systems to catalog the lesion set with relation to the location of the PV ostia. Initially this technique was developed in response to the incidence of PV stenosis encountered with ablation closer to the PV ostia. However, the initial studies presented by Pappone *et al.* [26, 27] seemed to indicate that procedural success correlated with the area of left atrial tissue encircled in the ablation lesion set rather than the presence or absence of PV – atrial electrical connection. This lead to the hypothesis that modification of the left atrial substrate was responsible for successful treatment of AF, perhaps independent of the effect on PV triggers. Influenced by this concept, subsequent investigators have added additional linear lesions, based on anatomic principles alone [28, 29]. The mechanism of substrate ablation is not clear, but several possibilities have been proposed (Table 28.2). One of the most promising is the hypothesis that substrate ablation changes the focal AF syndrome not by effects on atrial or PV electrophysiology, but by altering the cardiac intrinsic autonomic nervous system, which has ganglia located in epicardial fat pads near the PVs (Figure 28.4). This hypothesis is supported by experiments performed in animal models. High-frequency subthreshold electrical stimulation of the atrium over areas of autonomic ganglia induce AF in normal dogs [30]; this effect can be abolished by lidocaine injection into the fat pads that house autonomic ganglia. A clinical study suggested that patients who experience slowing of the ventricular response during AF when RF energy is applied to areas around the PV (presumably on the basis of damage to underlying autonomic ganglia) are more likely to have freedom from

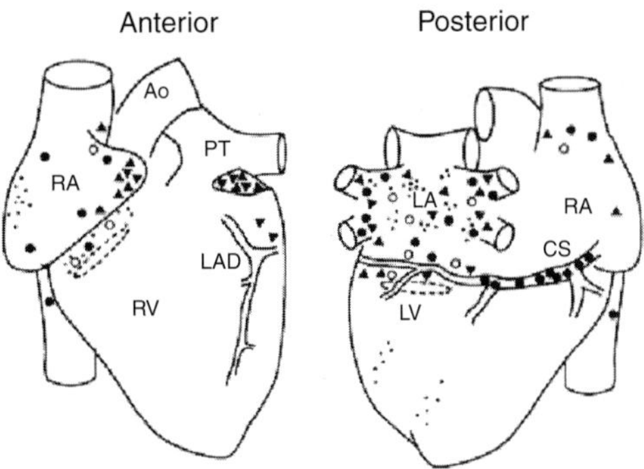

Figure 28.4 Schematic diagrams showing the relative distribution of nerve terminals in the human heart. Endocardial terminals arise from either myelinated (•, ○) or nonmyelinated (*) nerve fibers; coronary sinus (•) and epicardial nerve terminals (▲) were identified only as arising from myelinated nerves. (Reprinted from K Marron, J Wharton, MN Sheppard, *et al.* Distribution, morphology, and neurochemistry of endocardial and epicardial nerve terminal arborizations in the human heart. *Circulation* 1995; **92**: 2343–2351, with permission.)

symptomatic AF following ablation than those in whom this phenomenon is not observed [31]. This hypothesis may also explain why results with different lesion sets result in essentially identical results, both for surgical and catheter ablation.

Summary

Consideration of the underlying anatomic substrate represents a paradigm shift in interventional electrophysiology that has allowed successful ablation of increasingly more complex arrhythmias. Anatomic ablation has grown in lock step with new cardiac mapping and imaging technologies, both to allow visualization of functional cardiac anatomy and to organize the delivery of complex lesion sets. Anatomic ablation techniques are used to augment rather than supplant electrophysiologic mapping techniques. Even in completely anatomic ablation procedures, such as left atrial substrate ablation for AF, constant appreciation of the underlying electrophysiology is necessary for procedural success.

The anatomic substrate for arrhythmias typically exists long before development of clinical arrhythmia syndromes. The anatomic substrate for sustained VT is present immediately after infarction; the initial presentation with VT may occur as long as 20 years after this index infarction. Anatomic substrates for other arrhythmias, such as PMVT/VF and AF are not as well understood. However, the greatest future hope for an anatomic paradigm for catheter ablation is that it will eventually allow recognition of specific anatomic conditions that predictably lead to clinical arrhythmias. This would allow substrate modification, using ablation or other methods, to prevent arrhythmias in susceptible patients even before they happen. The impact of this paradigm on the treatment strategy for ventricular arrhythmias in particular would be profound.

References

1 Poty H, Saoudi N, Abdel Aziz A, Nair M, Letac B. Radiofrequency catheter ablation of type 1 atrial flutter. Prediction of late success by electrophysiological criteria. *Circulation* 1995; **92**(6): 1389–1392.

2 Schwartzman D, Callans DJ, Gottlieb CD, Dillon SM, Movsowitz C, Marchlinski FE. Conduction block in the inferior vena caval-tricuspid valve isthmus: association with outcome of radiofrequency ablation of type I atrial flutter. *J Am Coll Cardiol* 1996; **28**(6): 1519–1531.

3 Morady F, Harvey M, Kalbfleisch S, el-Atassi R, Calkins H, Langberg JJ. Radiofrequency catheter ablation of ventricular tachycardia in patients with coronary artery disease. *Circulation* 1993; **87**(2): 363–372.

4 Stevenson W, Khan H, Sager P *et al.* Identification of reentry circuit sites during catheter mapping and radiofrequency ablation of ventricular tachycardia late after myocardial infarction. *Circulation* 1993; **88**(4): 1647–1670.

5 Kim YH, Sosa-Suarez G, Trouton TG *et al.* Treatment of ventricular tachycardia by transcatheter radiofrequency ablation in patients with ischemic heart disease. *Circulation* 1994; **89**(3): 1094–1102.

6 El-Shalakany A, Hadjis T, Papageorgiou P, Monahan K, Epstein L, Josephson ME. Entrainment/ mapping criteria for the prediction of termination of ventricular tachycardia by single radiofrequency lesion in patients With coronary artery disease. *Circulation* 1999; **99**(17): 2283–2289.

7 Callans DJ, Zado E, Sarter BH, Schwartzman, D, Gottlieb CD, Marchlinski FE. Efficacy of radiofrequency catheter ablation for ventricular tachycardia in healed myocardial infarction. *Am J Cardiol* 1998; **82**(4): 429–432.

8 Miller J, Kienzle M, Harken A *et al.* Subendocardial resection for ventricular tachycardia: predictors of surgical success. *Circulation* 1984; **70**(4): 624–631.

9 Marchlinski FE, Callans DJ, Gottlieb CD Zado E. Linear ablation lesions for control of unmappable ventricular tachycardia in patients with ischemic and nonischemic cardiomyopathy. *Circulation* 2000; **101**(11): 1288–1296.

10 Callans DJ, Ren J-F, Michele J Dillon SM. Electroanatomic left ventricular mapping in the porcine model of healed anterior myocardial infarction : correlation with intracardiac echocardiography and pathological analysis. *Circulation* 1999; **100**(16): 1744–1750.

11 Alonso C, Lin D, Poku J Beshai J, Rajawat Y, Marchlinski FE. The role of transcatheter ablation in the prevention of sudden death. In: Santini M, ed. *Sudden Death – Non Pharmacological Treatment.* Adrianna Editrice, Rome, 2002.

12 Soejima K, Stevenson WG, Maisel WH Sapp JL, Epstein LM. Electrically unexcitable scar mapping based on pacing threshold for identification of the reentry circuit isthmus: feasibility for guiding ventricular tachycardia ablation. *Circulation* 2002; **106**(13): 1678–1683.

13 Arenal A, del Castillo S, Gonzalez-Torrecilla E *et al.* Tachycardia related channel in the scar tissue in patients with sustained monomorphic ventricular tachycardias. Influence of the voltage scar definition. *Circulation* 2004; **110**: 2568–2574.

14 Fontaine G, Tonet J, Gallais Y *et al.* Ventricular tachycardia catheter ablation in arrhythmogenic right ventricular dysplasia. A 16 year experience. *Curr Cardiol Rep* 2000; **2**: 498–506.

15 Marchlinski FE, Zado E, Callans DJ *et al.* Ablation outcome in patients with right ventricular cardiomyopathy and ventricular tachycardia. *Heart Rhythm* 2004; **1**: S234, abstract.

16 Hsia HH, Callans DJ, Marchlinski FE. Characterization of endocardial electrophysiological substrate in patients with nonischemic cardiomyopathy and monomorphic ventricular tachycardia. *Circulation* 2003; **108**(6): 704–710.

17 Soejima K, Stevenson WG, Sapp JL Selwyn Ap, Couper G, Epstein LM. Endocardial and epicardial radiofrequency ablation of ventricular tachycardia associated with dilated cardiomyopathy: the importance of low-voltage scars. *J Am Coll Cardiol* 2004; **43**(10): 1834–1842.

18 Haissaguerre M, Shoda M, Jais P. Mapping and ablation of idiopathic ventricular fibrillation. *Circulation* 2002; **106**(8): 962–967.

19 Haissaguerre M, Extramiana F, Hocini M *et al.* Mapping and ablation of ventricular fibrillation associated with long-QT and Brugada syndromes. *Circulation* 2003; **108**(8): 925–928.

20 Ernst S, Ouyang F, Lober F, Antz M, Kuch KH. Catheter-induced linear lesions in the left atrium in patients with atrial fibrillation: an electroanatomic study. *J Am Coll Cardiol* 2003; **42**(7): 1271–1282.

21 Haissaguerre M, Jais P, Shah DC *et al.* Spontaneous initiation of atrial fibrillation by ectopic beats originating in the pulmonary veins. *N Engl J Med* 1998; **339**(10): 659–666.

22 Haissaguerre M, Shah DC, Jais P *et al.* Elecrophysiological breakthroughs from the left atrium to the pulmonary veins. *Circulation* 2000; **102**(20): 2463–2465.

23 Gerstenfeld EP, Callans DJ, Dixit S, Zado E, Marchlinski FE. Incidence and location of focal atrial fibrillation triggers in patients undergoing repeat pulmonary vein isolation: implications for ablation strategies. *J Cardiovasc Electrophysiol* 2003; **14**(7): 685–690.

24 Callans DJ, Gerstenfeld EP, Dixit S, Zado E, Vanderhoff M, Ren J-F, Marchlinski FE. Efficacy of repeat pulmonary vein isolation procedures in patients with recurrent atrial fibrillation. *J Cardiovasc Electrophysiol* 2004; **15**: 1050–1055.

25 Marrouche NF, Dresing T, Cole C *et al.* Circular mapping and ablation of the pulmonary vein for treatment of atrial fibrillation: impact of different catheter technologies. *J Am Coll Cardiol* 2002; **40**(3): 464–474.

26 Pappone C, Rosanio S, Oreto G *et al.* Circumferential radiofrequency ablation of pulmonary vein ostia: a new anatomic approach for curing atrial fibrillation. *Circulation* 2000; **102**(21): 2619–2628.

27 Pappone C, Oreto G, Rosanio S *et al.* Atrial electroanatomic remodeling after circumferential radiofrequency pulmonary vein ablation: efficacy of an anatomic approach in a large cohort of patients with atrial fibrillation. *Circulation* 2001; **104**(21): 2539–2544.

28 Oral H, Scharf C, Chugh A *et al.* Catheter ablation for paroxysmal atrial fibrillation: segmental pulmonary vein ostial ablation versus left atrial ablation. *Circulation* 2003; **108**(19): 2355–2360.

29 Haissaguerre M, Sanders P, Hocini M *et al.* Changes in atrial fibrillation cycle length and inducibility during catheter ablation and their relation to outcome. *Circulation* 2004; **109**(24): 3007–3013.

30 Schauerte P, Scherlag BJ, Patterson E *et al.* Focal atrial fibrillation: experimental evidence for a pathophysiologic role of the autonomic nervous system. *J Cardiovasc Electrophysiol* 2001; **12**(5): 592–599.

31 Pappone C, Santinelli V, Manguso F *et al.* Pulmonary vein denervation enhances long-term benefit after circumferential ablation for paroxysmal atrial fibrillation. *Circulation* 2004; **109**(3): 327–334.

Index

Note: Page references in *italics* refer to figures and tables.